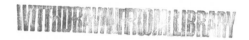

Change *of* Heart

Change of Heart
The Bypass Experience

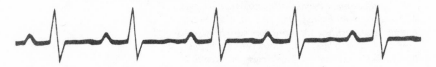

NANCY YANES HOFFMAN

HARCOURT BRACE JOVANOVICH, PUBLISHERS

San Diego   New York   London

Copyright © 1985 by Nancy Yanes Hoffman
All rights reserved. No part of this publication may be reproduced
or transmitted in any form or by any means, electronic or
mechanical, including photocopy, recording, or any information
storage and retrieval system, without permission in writing from
the publisher.

Requests for permission to make copies of any part of the work
should be mailed to: Permissions, Harcourt Brace Jovanovich,
Publishers, Orlando, Florida 32887

Library of Congress Cataloging in Publication Data
Hoffman, Nancy Yanes.
  Change of heart.

  Bibliography: p.
  1. Aortocoronary bypass—Psychological aspects.
2. Aortocoronary bypass—Patients—United States—
Family relationships.   3. Aortocoronary bypass—Social
aspects—United States.   4. Aortocoronary bypass—
Patients—United States—Interviews.   5. Health
surveys—United States.   I. Title.
RD598.H584   1985   617'.412   85-8759
ISBN 0-15-116641-2

Designed by Francesca M. Smith
Printed in the United States of America

First edition

A B C D E

This book is dedicated to my best teachers:

To my husband, Dr. Marvin Hoffman, who taught me how to love medicine and care about patients.

To my mother, Edith Yanes, my Maine rock, who taught me to be as stalwart as she.

To my father, William Yanes (1895–1950), who taught me that words and books do last, and whose heart gave out before the era of Bypass.

Contents

A Few Words About . . .   ix
A Note of Thanks   xi
I Point of Departure   1
II The Travelers, Ages at Bypass, Occupations   9
    1. *Chris Kozanis, 47, business executive*   11
    2. *Stowe Phillips, 30, gem dealer*   31
    3. *Tom Fouretier, 50, IRS supervisor*   52
    4. *Jed Anderson, 54, 58, 59, business executive*   72
    5. *Carole Cosby, 42, part-time sales clerk*   97
    6. *Jordan Bredely, Ph.D., 37, headmaster, boy's preparatory school*   112
    7. *Sven Thorgesen, 35, 35, television weatherman*   128
    8. *Thomas Windsor, 60, businessman*   143
    9. *Abraham Stearin, M.D., 53, psychiatrist*   160
    10. *Ben Rand, M.D., 46, internist*   198
    11. *Jason Master, M.D., 49, 55, chief of gynecology*   222
    12. *Kurt Ranter, M.D., 62, family physician*   235
    13. *Pierre Borget, M.D., 51, internist*   251
    14. *Sister Cecilia O'Brien, 55, nun*   279

15. *Willard Dreiser, 58, shoestore owner-operator*   292
16. *Orville Dreiser, 58, shoestore owner-operator*   301
17. *Phil and Bernice Milard, 50/49, engineer/housewife*   313
18. *John Boggs, 55, retired army colonel, retired*
        hospital administrator   332
19. *Kevin McDonough, 36, time-study supervisor*   340
20. *Bill Doell, 54, advertising executive*   354
21. *Moira Kitt, 50, editor*   367
III Transfer Point   389
From the Admitting Office to the Cashier's Office   391
Conference Call   403
Comfort Station: Easy Ways to Relieve Common
    Complaints   412
Concentration and Relaxation Techniques   417
Sex: The Three-Letter Word Doctors Are Reluctant to Use   420
Activity Sheet   425
A Talk About Heart Disease and Its Prevention   426
IV Envoi: Looking Back, Looking Ahead   439
Glossary of Medical Terms   447
Pharmaceutical Addenda   459
Bibliography   461

A Few Words About . . .

The use of "Bypass"

The procedure known as coronary artery bypass surgery (CABS) is the medical focus of this book. For convenience and brevity, it is frequently called Bypass, and the patients who have elected such surgery are called Bypassers.

The use of pronouns

Writing about these Bypassers, I've been troubled by how to use proper pronouns. Of the more than 2,000 Board-certified cardiovascular surgeons in this country, fewer than ten are women; of the one million Bypassers, some 79 percent are male. In speaking of both physicians and patients, therefore, except when writing of female Bypassers, I have tended to use the masculine pronoun.

The use of disguises

To protect confidentiality, the names of hospitals, physicians, and Bypassers have been disguised, as have their hometowns, states, and other identifying marks. All hospitals connected to medical schools have been called University Hospital. Other hospitals and all physicians are given fictitious names. In rare instances where the actual names are used, these are denoted by an asterisk and an explanatory footnote.

A Note of Thanks

This book is a collective enterprise. I set out with tape recorder and typewriter to rally the memories of Bypass veterans so that their voices would speak to prospective Bypassers—and to the rest of us. Barring a five-thousand-page volume, most of the hundreds of Bypassers who have talked and written to me could not be included. Yet each is important. Each cared that this book be written, and for that purpose gave unstintingly of himself or herself. Each examined his or her life before and after Bypass for old and new meanings. Each participated in the making of these pages.

To every Bypasser who spoke into my tape recorder, who answered my interminable questionnaires, who offered suggestions along the way, even opened his or her home to me, *Thank you.* Whether you are explicitly or implicitly here, you have enriched this book. Surely, you have enriched my life.

I am indebted to many others.

To the non-Bypassers on my team: my student, mentee, friend, Lisa Crecco, without whose help this book might have taken ten more years to complete; and my friend Abraham Rothberg, selfless and severe, the best of Socratic gadflies.

To Dr. Meyer Friedman, who taught me about Type-A, became my friend, even lent me his office. To Dr. George Engel, who honed my interviewing skills, gave me a job when I was eighteen, even remembers what I looked like then. To Col. Rostik Zajtchuk (USAMC), who lit my way through Walter Reed Army Hospital. To Col. Julius Bedynek (USAMC), who taught me about the Army's Over-40 Program and sent me to Dr. Friedman. To Judy Dorsett, who fed and housed me. To Mort Brodsky, who gave me a Rochester office. To Dr. Elijah Saunders, who introduced me to a group of black Bypassers. To Dr. Richard Hornick, who led me to the Army's program. To Peter Freund, a Bypass-refuser, who urged me to take a year's unpaid leave to finish this book.

To Miriam Mitchell, Linda Mocejunas, and Cathy Erdman, who typed their way through miles of transcription tape and pounds of paper and who promised faithfully they'd stop smoking "when this darn book gets done."

To my first friends at Harcourt Brace Jovanovich—Joan Judge for her unflagging good cheer, many skills, and generous help, and Julian Muller, a serendipitous blind date, who taught me that an editor can guide a writer and her work (when she'll listen).

And, of course, to Dr. John Ochsner, whose idea this book was, who started me on this road, who urged me to write about Bypass so that Bypassers could help one another.

I

Point of
Departure

This book is about getting your heart fixed, about the fears and uncertainties before, the alarms and triumphs afterwards. In these pages, Bypass veterans talk about how they came to coronary artery bypass surgery, how Bypass dealt with them during surgery and its aftermath, how they and their families dealt with it. In some measure, this is two books. Starting out to write about how Bypassers coped, I discovered through them some broader and deeper perceptions about the way we live now, where we think we're going, what prices we pay, wittingly and unwittingly, to get there.

The heart of the matter is that the fault is not in our genes but in ourselves, for many of us see Bypass as a metaphor for the way we live our lives. If we listen to the voices of the men and women in this book, we can hear something of the modern temper and its character—impatient, perfectionistic, competitive, anxious, stressful, rushing, irritable, insecure.

What we have inherited from our forebears, we can do little about. How we work with our heredity and our culture is something else again: whether we fail to alter our "Type-A" personalities, eat excesses of saturated fats, smoke two packs of cigarettes a day, yield frequently to anger or consuming ambition, is a quite different issue. In some measure, this book demonstrates how our hereditary predispositions shape our lives. But far more important, it shows how we can change our mode of living to influence that heredity and so prolong and better our lives.

This book is based on the effects of Bypass on one thousand patients—eight hundred questionnaire-respondents and two hundred interviewees. Inquiries were conducted as early as four weeks and as long as fifteen years after heart surgery. The nearly two dozen accounts printed here combine the essence of all those experiences and memories. These Bypassers not only describe the factors primarily responsible for coronary artery disease, factors that can lead to Bypass, but they also delineate the physical, emotional, social, and economic consequences of Bypass surgeries. The Bypass veterans here discuss whether they should have had Bypass, what it accomplished, whether they would, if advised, return to the Bypass table. They speak of how they got through the mill, what helped and what hindered them, what they wish they had done for themselves or had been done for them by others.

Not an argument for or against Bypass, this book's basic premise is that veterans of Bypass can help prospective Bypassers contend with a critical event in their lives, that individual lives tell us more about what we need to know than does the recital of statistics. In confronting crucial choices, most of us lack the essential data that apply specifically to ourselves.

Each interviewee represents particular problems and responses that, taken together, reveal a whole range of medical, psychological, social, and economic dilemmas. Henry Kissinger, Alexander Haig, Jerry Lewis, Rock Hudson, and Barbara Bel Geddes, all Bypassers, do not appear here. One Bypasser enjoined me: "Don't focus on celebrities. Write about us, the unknown Bypassers, going through heart surgery, picking ourselves up, brushing ourselves off, getting going again." I have followed that injunction.

The voices you hear are those of your neighbors and mine, men and women from their thirties to their sixties, although other interviewees are from their twenties to their eighties. These people come from various walks of life—an engineer, storekeepers, an editor, business executives, doctors (whose viewpoint is particularly illuminating because they see Bypass from both sides of the desk), the clergy and nonbelievers, working people and retired people. In my full survey, some occupations are, regrettably, not particularly well represented—farmers and professors, for instance—and I could not find as many blacks to interview as I'd have liked, or any American Indians or Orientals. Thus, though this book does represent a cross section, it does not pretend to be comprehensive in an economic, social, racial, or ethnic sense. Moreover, no one is a statistic to himself; each story is individually as well as collectively significant: each Bypasser is unique.

Yet statistics do matter. There are a million Bypassers in the United States. For the fifteen-year period since 1968, when Dr. René Favaloro reported the first Bypass of the modern Bypass era, the National Heart, Lung and Blood Institutes (NHLBI) estimates that at least one million Americans—about 800,000 men and 200,000 women—had coronary artery bypass surgery. In 1984, approximately 200,000 Bypasses were performed, a huge leap from 54,000 in 1975. On February 17, 1983, Dr. Denton Cooley and his Texas colleagues performed their fifty-thousandth Bypass operation. By 1987, an expected half-million Bypass procedures will be done each year in the United States alone, and a million heart patients will be deciding whether or not to have Bypass. Today, more Bypasses are performed than any other major operation.

Where did the Bypassers in this survey come from? Almost everywhere. They answered my calls for Bypassers in corporate newsletters of the first and second Fortune 500s, replied to notices in military newspapers and veterans' organizations. These in turn sent me other Bypassers—relatives, friends, co-workers and business acquaintances, fellow patients who had been in the hospital with them, people who belonged to support groups with them after they got out of the hospital.

In medical terms, these Bypassers do resemble one another: every Bypasser here was characterized by at least three of the Framingham Study's or the American Heart Association's risk factors. Most were afflicted by more. According to these surveys, the following characteristics place an individual at higher coronary risk than the general population:
• Male sex—before sixty, one in five men and one in seventeen women will have a heart attack.
• Age—as one grows older, the risk of heart disease increases.

- Family history—heart disease may run in families. The tendency to high blood cholesterol and diabetes may also be inherited.
- Smoking—the more cigarettes smoked per day, the greater the risk of heart disease.
- Hypertension—even mildly elevated blood pressure may, if untreated, aggravate the possibility of a heart attack.
- Elevated cholesterol[1] and triglycerides—we are what we eat, and we eat the wrong foods.
- Obesity.
- Type-A behavior.[2]
- Diabetes.
- Low income and educational level.
- A sedentary way of life.

Like most studies, statistical or anecdotal, this one is awry. Mostly, these Bypassers are "satisfied customers." If need be, they would have or have had a second Bypass. This holds true even for female Bypassers, who fare less well than men. For reasons as yet unclear, despite a variety of educated guesses, females at every age and stage are twice as likely as their male counterparts to get into trouble during and after Bypass.

About one-third of all patients undergo post-Bypass depression. Some didn't tell me their tales, perhaps because the melancholy was too deep, perhaps because their malaise had lifted and, as one man wrote, "To talk about it would be to relive the most painful experience of my life. I couldn't stand it." Others spoke to me long after the operation, when, blessedly, dejection had vanished. Yet even a decade later, some Bypassers remembered the depression as a terrible, debilitating, unforeseen aftermath. Those who had been forewarned grappled more swiftly and successfully with depression, although frequently even they couldn't recall how they had pulled themselves out of it. In imparting their experiences, this book informs and aids the prospective patient and his or her family about the various vexing questions of post-Bypass depression.

[1] Every discipline has its own language. Medicine is no exception. Technical terms and drugs are explained in the Glossary and Pharmaceutical Addenda.
[2] This book's indebtedness to Friedman's pioneer work on Type-A behavior and its modification is obvious. The reader is urged to read *Type-A Behavior and Your Heart*, by Meyer Friedman and Ray Rosenman.

What is Bypass?[3] Why should anybody go through the pain and expense of having one? Coronary artery bypass surgery constructs open channels around blocked arteries to restore the flow of life-giving oxygen-carrying blood necessary to fuel the heart's essential pumping. To forge new roadways around partial constrictions or complete obstructions, segments of saphenous leg vein and/or internal mammary artery are attached, thereby creating a Bypass. Surgeons sew one end to a small hole cut in the aorta, the main trunk line from the heart, and the other end to an opening made in the coronary arteries beyond the roadblock. Bypass is just what its name suggests: a detour. No more, no less.

Bypass does not cure heart disease. It is one way that physicians and patients fight heart disease, our number-one killer. The two fundamental objectives of coronary artery bypass surgery are (1) to help someone with coronary artery blockage reduce or eliminate symptoms significantly interfering with that individual's way of life, symptoms resistant to nonsurgical treatment, and (2) to improve the heart patient's chances of living longer. For those with certain kinds of heart disease, Bypass can prolong life.

Bypass can thus buy time for the patient to change his or her ways, to stop smoking, to avoid eating so much fat and salt, to begin regular exercising, to stop hating and start enjoying life— before it's too late.[4] Whatever the arguments about Bypass—its costs, its overuse, and what Dr. Thomas Preston calls its marketing—studies demonstrate that such surgery usually accomplishes its immediate goals and improves the possibilities for healthier living.

In reading these accounts, the reader will note how often, deliberately or inadvertently, we choose various high-stress "environments" for ourselves. Sometimes such environments seem almost to choose us. We live with marital stife, family strains, divorce, addictions to food, drink, tobacco, and drugs, lusts for money, power, and sex. Competition drives us. Fears of loss—of jobs, of youth, of love, of companionship, of children—haunt us. Why are so many of us so chafed by stress? How much of our disappointed great expectations are self-generated and self-perpetuated? How

---

[3] More details about Bypass can be found in Part III.
[4] A Talk About Heart Disease and Its Prevention, in Part III, discusses ways of preventing or ameliorating heart disease.

much does modern society impose on us? How much is engendered by our inability to savor what we have while we still have it? There are no simple answers. Most studies thus far, however broad-based, result in conclusions that frequently are debatable.

Yet we do know that the tensions of the way we live now can and do damage us severely, can eventually result in serious and sometimes life-threatening impairment. Heart disease is a prime example of this. If we do not yet have a perfect understanding of all its many causes, we do recognize clearly many of its contributing factors. And that leads us to a critical question: Do we have the requisite discipline, the motivation, to change the direction and content of our lives, to bring ourselves the physical health and psychological serenity we yearn for?

This book is committed to the belief that such changes of heart are possible, that the Bypassers' experiences so stirringly revealed to us can point us in the right direction and can even to some degree, like good companions, take us part of the way on our journey. For as with Chaucer's pilgrims on the road to Canterbury, they tell us things we ought to know. By listening to their tales, by understanding what they actually have lived through, we may find both counsel and comfort.

II

The
Travelers

1. Chris Kozanis
Business executive
Age at Bypass: 47

The executive offices of Chris Kozanis's Chicago corporation have been moved from their teak-and-glass enclave high above Michigan Avenue to the fourth floor of an old building on North Dearborn Street. At the receptionist's desk a red-haired Irish girl, barely looking up as I enter, purrs a brogued lament into the telephone. Hearing me say my name through his open office door, Christopher Kozanis, the chief executive officer (CEO), strides out, booms a loud cheerful greeting, shakes my hand hard, and guides me into his office, where he shuts the door and settles me in a chair opposite him across a broad desk.

"Let me warn you," he says, smiling warmly, "I have a copy of your questionnaire and my replies in front of me, so I can check you out." Taking off his blue glen-plaid suit jacket, he puts on horn-rimmed glasses to reread the form. In his blue shirt, its short sleeves showing his muscular hairy arms, a thick lock of black hair falling over his olive-skinned forehead, he looks more the son of a Salonikan fisherman than the president of a heavy-equipment company.

Did you have any inkling this was going to happen to you?

"The interview or the heart attack?"

The need for Bypass.

"Never! I was sure nothing could touch me. I was indestructible. As CEO here, I'm always working for time. There aren't enough hours in a day, so how could I figure that there might be too few hours to live my life?"

Are you pressured by self-imposed deadlines?

"People call me a perfectionist. When I get an assignment, I don't waste time. I get right to it, I evaluate it, and say, 'This should be done in two days or two weeks. That's the target date.' If I have to work twenty-four hours a day, I'll do it to get the job done. That's what I expect of people who work for me. When people work for me and I've a job to do, I'll ask them, 'How long will it take?' They may say, 'A month,' and I'll reply, 'Gee, I can't pay for a month.' If they say, 'Maybe two weeks, then,' I'll tell them, 'Fine. I expect it done by that date, no matter how many hours per day you have to put in.' "

What's your title here?

Kozanis snorts. "For what it's worth, it's CEO of the Division of Engineering and Construction. Before we went into bankruptcy, that meant something. I was responsible for all the plants we designed, built, and operated under a contract with some third party: generating plants, steam plants, resource recovery facilities. Prior to filing bankruptcy, we had several. Since then, we've been liquidating them. Now, I've only two plants left. Every time we'd liquidate a plant, I'd have to fire people I hired to operate it. I hate that."

Do you own a lot of stock in this company?

"Plenty. Since bankruptcy, it's not worth the paper it's printed on."

What caused the bankruptcy?

"We had invested an awful lot of money in new technology. When interest rates went up, we were faced with bank problems. We were behind with our latest project. We had debt-service payments to make. People said we were obligated to pay them. The plant wasn't completed, so no revenues were coming in; we had to finance the debt service from internal funds. We had invested a pot of money in our subsidiaries. Anything they paid into the corporation went back into new technology, so the money stream dried up. Something like the federal government, only we couldn't just raise the ante on the debt."

What happened to the stock?

"From a high of forty-two"—Kozanis points his thumbs down—"to five-eighths. Quite a drop," he notes dryly. "They stopped trading it. We bounced from the New York Stock Exchange to the Over-the-Counter to the Albanian Rug Market. Nobody's trading it. Nobody wants it. I can't blame 'em. It's not worth much."

There's no way for it to come back?

"I doubt it. In the reorganization plan, they may recapitalize and issue new stock, maybe one-to-one. I wouldn't count on it." He grimaces. "I don't."

What will happen to your position with this company?

"I don't know. My job now is to keep the two remaining entities alive and well, to help the cash flow, to maintain profitability. All the nonprofitable properties are liquidated. Just sold off." He spreads his thick stubby fingers. "That's what I've been doing for the past eighteen months."

Before and after your Bypass?

"I had the MI in January of '81. I was forty-seven. We filed bankruptcy in October '80."

Your heart attack was three months after the bankruptcy proceedings?

"Right. I'd been working twenty hours a day for over a year to keep this thing afloat. Five days before Christmas, I had to fire 2,500 people, people who trusted me not to let them down. That's a lot of burnt-out Christmas trees. We had $100 million invested in that plant, with financing of 53 million through industrial bonds. We spent the 53 million, the plant wasn't ready, and we had no money coming in. Now, we had to finance it ourselves. We went to the banks and borrowed, putting up stock in our subsidiaries as collateral. About 1.5 million was due at the end of '80, unless we got the plant rolling. To meet that deadline, I gathered up a group of engineers as a task force, people from all over the corporation. Working three shifts, twenty-four-hour days, we established a base at the plant site. To catch all three shifts, I had to be there almost all the time. I stayed in a two-bit motel, and came home one weekend in four, if I could. My wife was a teacher, so she couldn't go with me. Last April, they notified her she wasn't being renewed because there are fewer children entering the school system. Her contract's till August. Then, that's it, she'll be out of work."

Seems as though the roof fell in on both of you.

"You survive. You don't crawl into a corner. You come up fighting. It's tough, though. I've always put work first; I don't like to fail. If I take on a task, I want to succeed, not go halfway, then give up."

You're very competitive.

"It depends on circumstances. In sports, I play for enjoyment. I don't care who wins. I coached Pop Warner football. I always made sure every kid, even the worst kids on the team, played every game. I didn't care what the score was. We lost one game eighty-six to nothing, but every kid played. The parents would say, 'Don't put that kid in there. He can't block, he can't catch a pass.' If the kid showed up every day to practice, he played.

"In business, we instituted safety programs for the company—for everything but our money. I'd make my crews win those safety awards, and they would. You have to set good examples, work with the fellows; if something isn't right, you have to discipline them about safety glasses, hard hats, safety shoes, accident rates. You can't sit in an office and expect everything to be done from a distance. It doesn't work that way."

Tell me about the heart attack and the Bypass.

"What happened with the company can't be separated from it. When we were working so hard, trying to meet the big deadline, they'd hear rumors and they'd say, 'Chris, we heard the bank refused to extend the loan,' or, 'We heard the company's running out of money.' I'd say, 'You crazy? You get paid every week, you see we're paying our bills, you see the material being delivered. Don't listen to that stuff. Just concentrate on getting this plant operating.' Then, when I had to fire them, it was like, 'We tried to tell you, but you were conning us.' I felt I had let them down. And I had. That Christmas, I was so depressed. To see grown men cry, to have their wives call and say, 'We've charged presents for the kids and we can't give them back,' you feel like Scrooge himself.

"From May to December, I was trying to do the impossible. I thought I could. Having to terminate everybody I'd worked so closely with day and night, I kind of lost self-confidence. I kept asking myself, 'What could I have done to have avoided it? Could I have done more?' I'll tell you something: this company didn't have to go into bankruptcy. When we were faltering, people were living high on the hog. The management people, especially the guys in marketing, didn't seem to care about the company's problems. They were only interested in making their business trips plush, staying at the best hotels, eating at the best restaurants, even though we were hurting for money, and we knew we were in trouble financially. Rather than going out and spending $150 a night for a fancy hotel room, go to a discount motel, and let the balance of that money go into the plant and machinery, because that's what would keep the company alive. They didn't care. They worried about going first-class, staying at the best hotels.

"If enough people in positions to help out fully recognized what was wrong and tried to pull in their belts, the company would've made it. This may sound corny to you, but I wrote a letter to all the officers and directors of this compay, advising them we were a long way from getting that key plant finished, the plant necessary for the company to stay afloat and sail at full tilt. In the letter, I said, 'Finances are tough; we need every dime to finish the plant.' I suggested we all take a 10 to 20 percent pay cut. No a permanent cut, mind you, but a temporary one. When the company got back on its feet, we'd get that money back in a lump sum in raises or bonuses. They laughed at me. Absolutely ridiculed me. They said, 'You're crazy. Take what you can now. The company's got money. Take it while you can.' I didn't believe in that. I still don't.

"Sometimes I get depressed. It comes in spurts. Over the last eighteen months, we keep liquidating companies. Each time, my areas of responsibility get smaller, smaller, smaller. Each time the final papers are signed at the closing, I realize, 'That's it. I can't go there any more. Those people don't work for us any more.' "

You identify with this company.

"What kind of CEO doesn't feel a responsibility for his men, for their wives and children? I didn't fire only 2,500 men. It was wives and kids and old folks on pensions. What gets me is I didn't realize, because I was so obsessed with getting that plant running, what was happening within this company. I thought I was Hercules, but I couldn't clean the Augean stables. That's what caused the heart attack." He lights a cigarette. "You don't mind, do you? My doctor'd give me hell."

Those weeds didn't help your heart any.

"Doctors say lots of things cause cancer and heart attacks, but not everyone that smokes gets cancer or a heart attack. I'm a numbers guy. I could make statistics show that smoking doesn't hurt you."

Age, sex, family history, the wild tension you describe, and cigarettes are the major causes of heart disease. You can't do anything about the first three, but you can limit your stress and stop smoking.

"I gave up smoking for a whole year. I only sneak a few, now and then. It's better than eating and putting on weight."

That's not true. Some surgeons make patients sign a pledge never to smoke again.

"I never signed anything like that."

At some heart centers, you must promise never to smoke or they won't operate.

He grins. "How do they enforce it? Do they come after you and take their Bypasses back? It's clever psychologically, but smoking does curb my appetite. I was up to three packs a day. It depends what happens around the office. This week, we were trying to close a deal and hit eleven thousand snags. With each snag, I'd go looking for a cigarette, I *needed* a cigarette. When I'm out on my boat, when I'm home with my wife on weekends, I don't smoke. Only when I'm frustrated."

Tell me about the heart attack and how you came to Bypass.

"I didn't have any chest pains. It was Sunday, January seventh, watching the Dallas Cowboys, I felt these shoulder pains, in both shoulders and going down my arms. Not severe, and I kept doing this to my hands." Mr. Kozanis demonstrates how he massaged his hands. "My wife said, 'What's the matter? Are your hands going to sleep?' I said, 'No, I just feel uncomfortable.' All of a sudden, she said, 'You're pale, you're awfully white. Do you feel all right?' I said, 'No, I don't feel all right.' Then and there, she said, 'Come on.' The game was over, anyway. We're Cowboy fans, and they lost. She said, 'You don't look so good. Let's call the doctor.' I said, 'No, it's probably indigestion.' Most people think that, I guess; the feeling is similar. She said, 'Chris, you don't look good at all. Let me take you to Emergency,' and I said, 'No, I'm all right, I'll be all right.' Then, I started getting pains all over, shoulders, chest, down to the hands, as though they were falling asleep, as though all of me was falling asleep. She made me look in the mirror and I could see the difference. There wasn't a drop of color in my face. I looked ready for Petrakis's Funeral Home. I said, 'Okay, come on, let's go to the hospital,' which is only four blocks from our house.

"When I walked into the Emergency, the nurse took one look at me, put me in a wheelchair, took my blood pressure. The resident called my own doctor, who came right in. They took a cardiogram and blood samples, which said only one thing: I was having this MI. My doctor called the cardiologist, whom I'd never even seen before, and bingo, bango, bongo, right into the CCU. I stayed in for ten days, but before I went home, the cardiologist scheduled the catheterization. I don't know why people make such a fuss about that cath. It was fascinating to see him twisting those wires. All of a sudden, he'd wriggle it around corners. Fascinating. Except for the initial injection, the needle for the local anesthesia, I felt no pain. I kept asking the doctor, 'What's happening?' It's like being at a ball game and not knowing the score. When he told me it wasn't good, I said, 'What does that mean?' He said, 'It means Bypass surgery.' But he wasn't the surgeon.

"When I got out of the hospital the next morning, I called the best heart surgeon around. I said, 'Okay, Dr. I-Don't-Remember-His-Name said I need Bypass. When are we going to do it?' He said, 'It takes time. We have to plan. Call my office next week. We'll see about arrangements.'

"At that point, I knew that was it. I needed the surgery; I didn't need to sit around waiting for it. I went over to his office, but he wasn't in. There were three nurses working there. I explained why I wanted to see him. When they said, 'Oh, well, he doesn't make the operating schedule. We kinda—' I said, 'Ah.' The next morning, I went to the best florist in town, I bought three big baskets of flowers, I walked into the doctor's office with the flowers, and said, 'This is for you, girls.' They were thrilled, big beautiful baskets of spring flowers in January. They said, 'What do you want in return?' They were smart. They knew *quid pro quo* is the name of the game. 'I want to be scheduled for Bypass right away,' I said. 'You gals handle all that. The doctor doesn't say who or when. Put me in the hospital and get me Bypassed.' Less than a week later, I was in the operating room. They did it."

How did you know which heart surgeon to call?

"I asked the cardiologist, then I checked around with all the guys who'd had Bypass. It's not hard to pull an ability-rating on a doctor. You just have to pay attention.

"When I was wheeled into the operating room, before they put me under full anesthesia, I saw a status board on the wall with blood type, name, age, and other vital statistics. My name was spelled incorrectly. They'd written 'Kozanitsky.' I remember hollering to someone behind a surgical mask, 'Hold it! I'm either in the wrong place or my name is spelled wrong. I want to see my surgeon unmasked to be sure we're all in the right room, for the right operation, and that my name is spelled properly. If I don't come out of this operation, at least my name will be spelled correctly in the obituary columns.' The operation was delayed ten minutes while things were made right."

Why do we care so much when people mutilate our names?

"Because our names symbolize who we are, what we are, where we came from. I'm not anti-Semitic. I've worked with Jewish people for years, but I'm as proud of my heritage as they are of theirs. Right? People call me Kozanitsky all the time. Jews have been good to me, but there are Greeks out there, too. There's not many Jews or Greeks in the world of big business. When you get up high in corporate structures, you don't see many Greeks, but you see almost no Jews.

"The hospital was Catholic, but we're Greek Orthodox. The nuns and priests from the hospital, and the Greek Orthodox priests from the two Greek churches I support, visited me constantly. When the priests read a prayer over me, I had to remember which way to make the sign of the cross, because Greek Orthodox and Roman Catholic make the cross in opposite directions. The priests were good sports. They said I had both sides pulling for me. If I'd only left my name on the operating status board as 'Kozanitsky,' they'd have sent me a rabbi, too. I liked that.

"My old Navy buddy's rabbi came to see me a couple of times. I covered all bases. I don't have many friends—I'd rather be out on the boat with my wife—but the friends I have, I'd give my life for."

What do you wish you'd been told about Bypass?

"That's easy: that when I woke up, there'd be a damnable plastic pipe in my throat. If they could get rid of that pipe, or shorten the time with it, the operation would be a lot easier. It was horrible. I felt like I was gagging all the time. It was in a whole day. They should take it out, and then, if you got in trouble, they could put the pipe back. Any engineer knows that."

What do you remember most about when you awakened?

"The damned plastic pipe, that they wouldn't let me sleep, and that there were bright lights on constantly, like a B movie about an insane asylum."

What do you remember about the hospital recovery period?

"When I got back to the regular hospital floor, they wouldn't let me walk next door to use the lavatory, even though I could walk around my room. They kept bringing in a camp-type potty chair. I kept putting it out in the hallway. I'd be damned if I'd use it. They'd put it right back in the room. Finally, I opened the window and threw it outside. After that, they let me use the lavatory.

"One night, when my wife was sitting with me, she was exhausted from working all day, coming to see me in the morning before work, staying with me all evening. I let her lie in my bed, while I sat in a chair. We both fell asleep. When I awoke, a technician was taking my wife's blood pressure and saying how well my wife looked and how glad she was to see that my wife was ready to be discharged because she was wearing street clothes. The nurses read me the riot act. We weren't breaking any hospital rules, we weren't even monkeying around. We waited until I got home from the hospital.

"But everything was great. I got flowers and cards and fruit baskets every day from people I hadn't seen in years. My office sent the messenger service every day with paperwork to review, which made me feel I was needed back at the ranch."

After Bypass, how long did you wait to drive?

"One week after I got out of the hospital. Two weeks after discharge, I drove to Boston on business. I was careful. I arrived at ten at night, I left at three in the afternoon, just to avoid the traffic. Not that I was tired. Boston traffic is lousy."

Didn't you have any postsurgical weakness? No fatigue?

"Oh, yeah, I'd get tired more quickly, but I wasn't doing hard physical work. Driving a car isn't physical labor. Sitting behind a desk and talking on the phone or writing reports isn't physical labor. I went back to the office in two weeks, but I wasn't out in the field, climbing up and down ladders, checking plant construction. There wasn't any plant to check. My family overprotected me. They told me I was crazy: 'Don't drive, don't make this trip, don't go to the office, don't lift, call me and I'll move it for you.' Boy, were they overprotective: 'Don't climb stairs. Whattaya need? I'll get it for you.' I didn't want that, I can't live that way. I wish they'd treated me as if Bypass was nothing worse than a hernia."

You've gone back into action more quickly than anyone—

"It's a mental attitude. When people get sick, they don't recover because they don't want to recover. Read Freud. And I know people who enjoy ill health. Not me."

How long after Bypass did you resume sexual relations?

"Two weeks. I'd asked the doctor about it, because God forbid he should talk about sex to a patient."

Were you afraid?

"Nope. Sex is life. Why be afraid?"

Was your wife afraid?

"I don't know whether she was or not. I only know it happened, and we were both glad."

You have a great lust for life.

"All Greeks do. Well, most Greeks do. For me, it's part of what I inherited from my parents. My father was like me. Very much like me. He was a bull of a man. He couldn't retire. We made him retire—and he died. Biggest mistake we ever made. We could see him deteriorate before us, but he'd already sold all his equipment. He'd had a small trucking business. Without 'the shop,' he didn't know what to do with himself, he wasn't enjoying life. I never want to retire. I want to die with my boots on, right here, or"—Chris Kozanis shakes his head mournfully—"on some job. Bury me like the Vikings do: set me adrift in a boat, and set it on fire."

Why did you do so well after the operation? How did you come back so fast?

"All my life, people have asked me similar questions. My folks were immigrants from Greece, from Kasadi, up in the mountains, near Salonika, a very, very rural place. This doesn't meant only that they didn't have refrigeration or lights up there. They had nothing. They had no running water; they never had enough to eat. With such a poor life, my father decided he had to do better for himself and his family. He came to this country all alone, by himself, just a boy with no friends, with no one. Landing at Ellis Island, he talked to the folks at Immigration. Four hours later, he was working as a dishwasher in a hotel. That took guts. I'm not sure even I could do that: pull up stakes, go to a strange country, not know the language. He saved his money, then sent for my mother, who was his childhood sweetheart. She worked helping a pastry chef in the hotel. They got married and worked hard to make a better life. Every bit as much as the early American settlers—the WASP ancestors who those bloodless, thin-lipped types brag about—they were pioneers. All they had was the determination to give their employers a day's work for a day's pay. They did their best in everything. They'd always tell me, 'If you're gonna work for someone and he signs your paycheck, give him the best. If you don't want to give him your best, don't waste his time. Leave. Go find someone else, and let him find somebody else.'

"My father was a great philosopher. He wasn't well educated, at least in book learning, but he was very wise. His advice still sticks with me, and I guess, if I'm gonna do something, I've gotta do it better than anybody else. I keep hearing my father's advice: 'Do your best or don't even try.' "

Even recuperating from Bypass?

"Yes. Most people's problems with Bypass are all psychological. People are afraid to test themselves. You wondered why I went back to work in two weeks. I was testing. I even told the doctor, 'I want to see what my limits are.' "

What did he say?

"He said, 'I can't stop you, but I don't recommend it.' I said, 'But you're not telling me I shouldn't.' Working is like eating: when you feel full, you stop eating. If you're working and you're tired, your body will say, 'Hey, stop.' "

When you felt tired before the MI, you didn't stop working. And you said you smoke to stop eating.

"Since Bypass, I haven't worked as hard." He smiles ironically. "For one good reason: the work isn't there. What's a chief executive officer without any goods and services to execute? We got executed instead. That's why I'm doing so much traveling to Europe. I'm trying to develop something over there. Funny, when I go to Europe, my blood pressure goes up. My pressure started climbing when I came to this company because here no one knew me. I felt, 'Okay, these guys have to know who Chris Kozanis is.' I started pushing myself more, for I wanted to go to the top in my new company. With each promotion, my blood pressure went up. They gave me medication; it'd go down. They'd take me off the medicine; it'd bounce up again."

How long have you been on blood-pressure medication?

"After Bypass, I was off for a while. They started me again about two months ago. I've been on Hydrodiuril for about ten years, off and on."

Why 'off and on'?

"You know." He looks me squarely in the eyes.

Your libido or . . . ?

"Sometimes the medicine makes me impotent. Who needs that? So he takes me off the medication, and when my pressure goes up, he says, 'Start the pills again.' He's tried a million different blood-pressure pills. They're all alike. I see the cardiologist every eight weeks for a routine exam, a fifteen-minute job; every other visit, he does an EKG. He's all right. It's the medicine that's lousy. Doctors are expensive. We don't have annual four-day corporate physical exams any more. There's a lot of adjustment to being the CEO of a defunct company. For the first time in twenty years, I don't have a secretary. I used to get into the office around six-thirty in the morning, before the phones rang off the hook. I'd do all my dictation, list all my phone calls. By the end of the day, the letters would be typed, I'd sign 'em, and they'd go out. What I hate most now is working with lawyers. Lawyers are fellows who say, 'We'll worry about that tomorrow.' And tomorrow, or another tomorrow, when I call with a problem, I get some secretary: 'He's tied up, he's in a meeting, he's in court, he'll be back in a couple of hours, he'll call you back.' They never do. Mostly, I have to call them again. I get impatient. We're paying them, the clocks are ticking away the dollars, and every time we get on the phone, they charge. When you lose power, you're at the mercy of lawyers and secretaries. I can bring flowers to secretaries. Maybe I should bring law books to lawyers."

Since Bypass, have you changed any priorities in your life?

Thoughtfully he rubs his black-bristled chin. "I think so. I'd be satisfied to be a consultant somewhere. I think I've lost my desire to become president of another company, but— I miss being able to challenge myself and other people. I like being in charge. I don't want to control other people; I want to help them become more proficient."

You've done so well since Bypass. Has your chest healed as well as you have?

"Take a look." Quickly, Kozanis unbuttons his blue shirt to reveal a muscular chest thickly covered with black hair, which hides a pencil-line scar. "Pretty good, huh? That scar's healed well. But look at this." He pushes his trouser leg to the knee and shows his leg scars, thick, red, and ropey. "It's a keloid. I've never had one before, I'd never heard of it, and it's sensitive. I asked the surgeon, who said, 'Use vitamin E cream.' Every night, religiously, I put on vitamin E cream. I couldn't see any difference except the druggist now could afford a trip to Florida. The cardiologist recommended a plastic surgeon, who said, 'Well, I don't guarantee anything. It may come back.' I said, 'Then I won't have it done unless you can assure me it'll flatten out or, at least, the tenderness will disappear.' He couldn't. About a month ago, I went to a dermatologist to have a mole removed from my back. When I took my shirt off, he said, 'Boy, you got yourself a zipper. How's it healing?' I told him, 'Fine, but look at this,' and showed him my leg. He touched the scar, and I went like that." Mr. Kozanis winces. "He said, 'It's sensitive.' I told him, 'Oh, yeah, it's very sensitive. Besides, it hurts like hell.' He said, 'I can help you.' I said, 'How?' He said, 'Steroid injections,' which I'd never had in my life. He kept looking at the scar till I began to feel like a girl at her first dance, walking by the stag line. I had one spot like a little snake, all pushed out and brown. The skin was stretched and 'sensitive'—that was the worst spot. 'Tell you what, let me treat that, give you an injection there, and in three weeks, you'll tell me whether you want another injection.' He gave me a needle, the soreness went away, the size diminished by a five-point ratio. I had to go back to him for the mole, so I had another injection in another place. That one didn't go down as much as the first spot, so I'm not sure I'll continue."

Did Bypass make you more aware of your own mortality?

"I was aware I might not wake up from the operation, that people died on the table. I was prepared for it. My wife was all set. She knew where everything was, what to do. When I opened my eyes, my wife was standing there, looking at me. That was great, having her there waiting for me."

I'm sure you're more precious to your wife than knowing where everything is.

"I know my wife loves me and I love her. We've been married thirty-six years, we enjoy the same things, doing things together.

I don't take vacations alone. I don't go out with the boys. She still needs to know what to do if they pick me off."

Nevertheless, did Bypass make you more conscious of your own mortality?

"I never think about it. When my time comes, it comes. If I live to be 60 or 160, it doesn't make any difference. I've no regrets for anything I've done in my lifetime."

Did Bypass make you more alive to the sweetness of everyday life?

"I love life, I always have. I always will, till they come to get me. I sleep like a baby. I take that Hydrodiuril at night. Then, every hour on the half hour, I've got to get up, right? To get rid of the fluids. I go back to bed, put my head on the pillow, and, just like that, I'm asleep again."

Why don't you take Hydrodiuril in the morning?

"It's ninety minutes driving to work. I don't want to get caught on the expressway. At a conference or on the phone, when the feeling comes on, like 'Oh, boy, I gotta go,' it's uncomfortable. It distracts you from thinking straight."

What do you think Bypass did for you?

"It gave me more stamina. To me, it was a plumbing job. The drains get clogged up with grease, the water doesn't run out. You take that pipe out, you put in a new piece, now the water flows. Eventually, it'll plug up again, and what happens? I'll have another Bypass. It's not permanent. It doesn't cure heart disease. It temporarily opens up the lines of fluid flow. What more can you ask? A permanent job? Nothing's permanent. Look at this company."

Do you feel Bypass prolonged your life?

"Sure. From the time of the MI to the cath, even in the week till I got into the hospital for surgery, I could feel myself going downhill. I was short of breath; I don't have that any more."

How long do you want to live?

"I want to live until my time is due; to live a full life and go quickly. I don't want to be crippled, bedridden. My father . . . my father dropped dead—pow!—just like that. He died in my arms. I remember how it happened. We were going to my father's on a Sunday, to leave our youngest boy with him while we went to church with the two older ones. It had snowed. January, it was. When I had my heart attack in January, my wife thought how my father had died in January, my mother had died in January, and maybe it was my time, too. We were on the street. My father was shoveling the snow in the driveway and off the steps, so it'd be easy for us to come in the house. When I saw him, I beeped the horn at him, because we were across the street. Our youngest son adored my father, and vice versa, so our boy kept waving his hands and hollering, 'Grandpa, Grandpa.' My father looked up, he raised his hand, like this, to wave, and he just kept going, falling over in the snow in the direction of the wave. I jumped out of the car, ran across the street, and picked him up in my arms. He was still alive but, you know, when people die, their bodies release. When that happened, I knew, but I didn't say anything. I told my wife, 'Go in the house and call the police.' A passing motorist stopped. The man helped me carry my father. I couldn't carry my father alone." He sighs. "He was a big bull of a man. You think I'm big and brawny? You should've seen my father. We carried him into the house and tried to keep my mother away. When we put him on the couch, we didn't cover him or anything. The doctor came, the police came. Nobody could do anything. My father was dead." Turning his head, Chris Kozanis looks out the window into the middle distance.

"Have you heard that Barbra Streisand song, 'Poppa, Can You Hear Me?' When I got to be president of this company and everything was go, go, go, I'd wish my poppa were alive to see what I'd done. Now that the company is on the skids, I'm glad he doesn't know, but I wish he were here to talk things over." Kozanis blows his nose hard.

Do you believe in God?

"Absolutely. What's a Greek who doesn't believe in God? That's a Greek who isn't close to his family. Greeks are clannish. I'll tell you something else about Greeks. Look at the police records. You'll find very few Greek teen-agers or Greek adults in trouble with the law."

Your generation are the children of immigrant parents who've worked and produced something. Do you think the next generation will do as well?

"Depends on how they're brought up. I've three sons. There's plenty of dope and booze in school, but not one them ever got mixed up with that stuff. They lived at home, we did a lot together, I took them on vacations, I'm really close to my sons. All three are on the Coast, but we talk on the phone two, three times a week."

Is it a disappointment to have them so far away?

"What do *you* think? I wouldn't want them to live with me. I don't want to live with them. Yet I wish they were close enough so, on Sundays, we could say, as my father said to me, 'Come on over for dinner.' If they had to go someplace, we'd say, 'Send the grandson over. We'll take care of him for the day.' I miss that."

It's a deprivation of our society.

"Yes, but we're a mobile society. That's the way it is. Face facts: if you're embarking on a corporate career, the fastest way to advance is to accept transfers, to be willing to move from city to city. My boys did it. In the early years, I did it."

Now that you're a Bypass veteran, what would you advise a prospective Bypasser? What would you have done differently?

"I'd have had no waiting time whatsoever from the catheterization diagnosis to the Bypass. Why wait? Let's do it! I'd tell anybody considering Bypass, 'Don't be afraid. Go ahead, don't let fear make you lose the ability to do everything you like.' "

What's your greatest joy?

"Above everything else, that my MI was mild enough that I could be a candidate for Bypass, that it was mild enough not to bowl me over."

What's your greatest disappointment?

"The other side of the coin. That I needed Bypass, even that I had an MI. Say, haven't you asked me enough questions? Isn't it my turn?"

Sure.

"When's this book coming out? I want to buy it. You know, Bypassers are big at learning about their disease and their operation— *after the fact*. There's a lot of things I want to know. When will it be out?"

In about a year.

"A year! For God's sake, I hope I'll be around in a year. A year!"

You'll be around.

"I'll take that as a promise. There's one thing you've got to put in that book: I've seen friends who had Bypass, and most of them fear the future. Many went on disability. I've seen some sitting around waiting to die. If they were going to push away from the table, what did they have Bypass for? You *must* write, over and over, that Bypassers can lead a normal, productive life, that they owe a good life to themselves, to their families, to the expensive doctors who fixed 'em up, and to society, who helped pay for the operation. End of speech. Now let me show you something."

Chris Kozanis leads me to a small office off the larger one where we've talked. In it, a word-processor is rattling away, spread sheets are everywhere. "This is my inner sanctum. Don't look at the computer," he commands. "Look at this photograph." It is an enlarged photocolor print, framed, of a sunrise. "When I was in the hospital, I didn't sleep so well. Sometimes, when I'd be restless and aggravated, I'd look out the window, and I could see the sun come up. I'd think, 'A whole new day! A whole new life!' Then I'd stop being so antsy. Just before I went home, I had my wife bring in my camera. I photographed that sunrise. I keep it on my wall to remind me. And it does."

2. Stowe Phillips
Gem dealer
Age at Bypass: 30

Wind-burned, handsome, with smouldering dark eyes and black hair, Stowe Phillips strides into his large Dallas office from an adjacent conference room. Wearing jeans and Gucci boots, an open-throated sport shirt, and a leather jacket, his youth and dress belie his status as president of an international gem dealership. His youth and carefree walk belie his status as a Bypass veteran. "Hi. I'm Stowe Phillips," he says, shaking my hand. After pouring us each a vodka-and-tonic, he sprawls in a big leather desk chair and casually places one foot on the broad teak desk.

How old are you?

"Thirty-three."

When was your Bypass?

"Three years ago."

You started young. How did this all come about?

"I had a heart attack on my birthday, June fourth, 1980. I'd been lifting weights at my health club. Either I pushed myself too far or the instructor pushed me too far, but I reached burnout."

Had you ever had any heart trouble before?

"Nothing."

Is there any heart trouble in your family?

"My brother's thirty-six and fine. Both my parents are living. Neither has any heart problems." Phillips sighs. "Everybody asks me the same questions. I smoked for a couple of years in college to prove I was cool. I never liked the taste or the smell, so I stopped. I never had diabetes. Oh, yes, and I'm not married. Anything else?" Phillips asks in a tired voice.

Go on with your story. You were lifting weights?

"By the time I began feeling poorly, the instructor had left. I felt so terrible. When I tried to leave the weight room for the lobby, my arms and legs felt as though electric current was shocking through them. I crawled—literally—to the lobby and fell onto a couch. Nobody paid any attention to me. Finally, a girl came over and said, 'Are you just resting or do you need help?' I said, 'I need help badly. I'm having a heart attack.' "

How did you know?

"I used to be a high-school biology teacher until I decided I couldn't live on a teacher's salary. My anatomical background from teaching biology made me suspect a heart attack because my arms and legs felt so weird. In four minutes, the Emergency ambulance arrived. Their speeding to the call probably saved my life. They rushed me to the hospital; there I stayed for two weeks. It sounds strange, but I enjoyed my recovery. The next day, I felt fine. By the third day, it was as if *nothing had happened.* I was alive. As far as I knew, there was no damage. In my mind, I walked away from it. I thought,

'Nothing's wrong. It's much ado about nothing.' All my friends came to visit. I sipped wine with them in my hospital room. 'La-de-da, I had a heart attack, I can't believe it, where are we going tonight?' "

Then what?

"From lying around in the hospital for two weeks, I was absolutely knocked out. The day my parents brought me home from the hospital, I went for a walk to a neighbor's house. When I got to the bottom of their hundred-yard driveway, I was exhausted. I barely made it back to our house. I recovered very slowly from what I thought was not a devastating anomaly. Very slowly. In the three months from the heart attack to the Bypass, I kept experiencing chest pain. No matter what I did, I'd have that funny, burning sensation some people confuse with heartburn. So I knew it wasn't just la-de-da. Something was wrong. I'd better quit hiding my head in the sand.

"Two months after the heart attack, I had an angiogram, which showed the rear wall of my heart was damaged. Heavily damaged. Nothing could be done about that particular injury, but the blockage needed to be repaired. I hated the angio. The day after, I went for an interview with an international gem cartel. They offered me the job, but the money was a joke."

Did the angiogram affect the interview?

"I'm not sure whether my weakness and pallor made them offer me less or whether having had the angio influenced my attitude towards them. I could make more in a month than they offered me for a year. That year, 1980–81, was the boom year in the history of gemstones. It wasn't a good year to take a salaried position. That angiogram toughened me up for business and for heart surgery. Having suffered through that angiogram, I was gung ho for Bypass: I told the doctors, 'Just give me the operation. Whatever you have to do, just do it and let me get on with my life. If I get through this heart operation, I'll expand my business.' My attitude towards Bypass was tremendously positive."

Why were you so eager to have Bypass?

"Because I thought it was the panacea, that it would fix all my problems. I was convinced my coronary artery disease, which I didn't understand as such, was purely physical. I thought it could be cured. I said, 'Okay, cure me. I'm ready.' I wasn't afraid of the operation. I worked on thinking positively. Because of Dr. Terry's team, with its full-time CABS social worker, I felt confident. They interviewed me, and I interviewed them. I was sure I'd gone with the best team possible."

Before the Bypass, how much time did Dr. Terry spend talking to you?

"About thirty minutes in his office. Maybe longer. I never felt rushed."

Even though you'd hated the angio, you still wanted Bypass?

"Sure. I had the Bypass, I recovered, I tied the hospital record—the next day, I was up walking. I was discharged in eight days. I wanted to leave sooner. That was my attitude. Mentally, I was prepared for a heart operation, and then for building an even better life. That attitude is extremely important."

Before Bypass, what were you concerned about most?

"Going for the second interview. On the eighth day after the Bypass, I was in New York. I was trying to work out a deal. When they upped the ante a little, I knew I'd remain an independent gem dealer, that I'd go big time. I was right. Business is stronger than ever. I've been to Europe nine times since January."

How did you feel when you awakened?

"Time seemed to last forever. Every time I passed in and out of consciousness, I'd wake up and ask, 'What day is it?' I must have asked four or five times in one afternoon. I was intubated; I couldn't speak. I desperately wanted to know what day it was. How come I was still in the ICU with a tube in my mouth? How much longer do I have to go with this thing?"

Would a clock on the wall have helped?

"If the clock had the date, with both night and day, and was in full view, it would have helped a lot. Then I wouldn't have had to ask, or to try and ask. With that tube, it's difficult to communicate."

Did you have a pencil and paper?

"After I enacted these crazy charades, they understood and brought me pencil and paper. I tried to scribble, but it's tough to write legibly with I.V.'s in both arms. I was out of it. All I remember is asking the nurse over and over, 'What day is it? How long have I been here? When does the tube come out? When do I get out? What day is it?' "

What was the worst part of the operation?

"The extubation—the actual taking out of the tube—and the day afterwards. It was excruciating. With the tube down my throat, I thought I'd gag to death between the time he took it out and the time I could take a breath. Yet removing the abdominal drain in the stomach is even worse. He was hauling out a corrugated tube, hand over hand. I couldn't believe how much tube had been in me. That horrendous pain only lasts about five seconds. I wish somebody could figure a way out of it, because you've got to be conscious; it's the last bad part. I was anxious to have everything over with in a hurry. The largest gem show in the world is held in California the first two weeks in February. I had to get ready for it."

Did you go to the gem show?

"Sure. My brother took time off from his job and flew out to help me. Every time I sneezed I looked as though somebody had belted me, but otherwise, everything went fine. Well, sort of fine."

What do you mean by 'sort of fine'?

"After the Bypass, they gave me medicine for the pain, while the sternum was healing. Percocet or Percodan. I abused those. If they told me to eat one every six hours, I'd eat one every three hours, just so I wouldn't have any pain. I abused it, because I liked the way I felt. I'm from the sixties generation. We had to try pills for everything before we found out they were good for nothing. I ate up my scheduled drugs before the pain went away; I had to ask Dr. Terry for more. As luck would have it, my landlord downstairs had bottles of these Percodans for severe back pain. He gave me thirty of his. When I went to California, I had a drug attitude: I was short with people, arrogant and sarcastic. I was right; everybody else was wrong. If I behaved poorly, I never apologized. That was beneath me. My behavior was attributable to the drugs. I think. All through the gem show, I was eating Percodan. When I started counting how many were left in the bottle, I became afraid I was addicted."

How did you stop using Percodan as a crutch?

"When I realized what was going on, I knew I had to get off them; I knew I couldn't get any more. Besides, I didn't like the person I became on Percodan. I wanted to get away from that person. Between Percodan and Inderal, my speech was slurring badly. I didn't like that."

When you quit Percodan, did you become more irritable?

"No. My personality leveled off. I came back to my old self."

Did you become depressed?

"I'm still depressed. I'm young. I want to do things. I find it difficult to excuse myself from my friends' activities. If I'm invited to someone's house and am served a big red-meat dinner, I'll eat it. I hate to explain. I know I shouldn't be eating all this fatty food; there's a conflict continually warring within me."

How does your depression affect you? Does it make you withdraw?

"My tendency is to internalize my feelings, to mask what I don't want people to see or know. To a certain extent, I was withdrawn. I wouldn't discuss my depression with anyone, including the girls

I was seeing. I kept it to myself. I'm the kind who likes to figure everything out by himself. I don't like to need people, to have to rely on people. My state was such that I needed to rely on people, but I wouldn't. I couldn't reveal my vulnerability. What bothered me most after the Bypass was having everyone say, 'How are you feeling? Tell me, how are you *really* feeling?' You don't want to be reminded every minute. You want to forget what you've been through. Last night, I saw a guy who hadn't seen me for a long time. He'd heard I'd had a heart attack. He said, like everyone else, 'How are you feeling?' I said, 'Fine. How are *you* feeling?' I was bitter and angry at him for asking me. I designed a button that said, 'I'm fine. Don't ask.' "

Most of the time, do you feel bitter and angry?

"I think so."

Do you feel bitter and angry at the universe? Do you ask, 'Why me?'

"No, I don't feel that. Unless it's deeper than I know, and it may be, I don't feel that."

About 30 percent of Bypassers experience depression as an aftereffect. Do you think you're depressed as a consequence of the operation itself? Or are you depressed because you're a young guy and you feel singled out?

"Choose one from column A and two from column B. I'm depressed because my body was violated and opened up, because my chest was cracked open. I'm depressed because I was like a frog on the table. I related to that frog on the table, because for six years, when I was a biology teacher, I'd cut open those frogs for my students. That's me, the frog prince, only more frog than prince. I feel terribly violated. Still."

Does the scar bother you?

"It did. For a long time. Not just the way it feels, but the way it looks. Now you almost can't see it. I never liked these gold chains for guys, but they cover a multitude of sins, or of scars.

"I never knew about the internal mammary artery. They used it on one of the grafts. In removing the internal mammary, they damaged the mammary nerves. This whole section is numb. I'm always conscious of an odd feeling there. If I strike it accidentally, it hurts. It'll always remain so. That bothers me. As though my body never returned to its normal state. They tell me the internal mammary remains open longer. I hope so, because I paid a price for its use."

You were working out when this happened. Did you ever feel your body had betrayed you?

"I'm not smart enough to think like that."

Did you ever feel life isn't fair?

"No. I'm pretty lucky. My life-style's pretty rich for a high-school teacher. I can maintain that life-style, even though I've had to alter it somewhat. I've done a lot in my life. Once, I was a professional mountain climber."

Did Bypass make you feel old?

"It made me feel old*er*, and long before my time. Right or wrong, I'm the kind of guy who sifts through what people say about me. That's how I find out about myself—from the things they say. Like 'Aren't you too young for that? A Bypass! *How old are you?*' "

Why don't you reply, 'Seventy-seven'?

"Sometimes, I do. I never know which roils me more: answering sharply or swallowing my bile."

Since Bypass, have you changed much?

"When I was in college and graduate school, I was an idealist. I was going to change the world, or at least teach high-school kids how to know their world, so they could change it. The years of teaching, the administrative hassles, eroded my idealism. When I quit teaching and went into the gem business, I became a realist overnight. My values shifted radically. It's not that they were better in teaching. They were less realistic. In those days, I looked at the world and saw what I wanted to see, not what was there.

"Bypass confirmed what the business world had taught me. Now I need to set my life in order and stop this fooling around. I've had a lot of relationships with women. It's time to settle down. I'm thirty-three. Probably, I'd have realized those needs without a heart attack and Bypass. I've been having fun. Life as a big-time gem dealer is on a faster track than life as a small-town high-school teacher. Bypass has forced my recognition of time's passing." He smiles ruefully. "Bypass is a kind of tuition."

Is there anybody whom you like a lot?

"I'm living with a girl now, but I'm just so unhappy." Tears spill down Stowe Phillips's tanned cheeks.

Why?

"Just because we're not . . . She's wonderful. She loves me more than anyone has ever cared for me, yet I can't see spending the rest of my life with this girl. She's twenty-five; she's stunning. We look great together. I'm dark, and she has long blond hair, blue eyes, high cheekbones. She's always dressed in the latest styles; clothes look great on her. Yet she's not my type of girl. I made the decision for her to come live with me, oddly enough, when I was on Percodan. I met her in California; I asked her to come back here and live with me. Some of it was the Bypass. I felt so alone. 'How long will I live?' I wondered. What kind of life was I living, traveling the world, making big killings? She didn't think twice. She left her job and came back here with me. For a while, we were very close. But it was a bad decision. It's difficult ending the relationship because she's been through some tough times with me. She's given 200 percent of herself for me; now I'm the one who wants to break up. When we began, she was the gorgeous California girl; she was, in a sense, doing me the favor. Now she's weak and insecure. Her job here is minor-league compared with the big time she gave up to go with me. I'm the heavy. But I'm so unhappy. I told her so. Thinking that she's doing something wrong, she's getting counseling. She's not doing anything wrong. People grow apart." Phillips sighs. "Perhaps, from the beginning, I was apart.

"It's terrible, because I've a tremendous need—more so than most people, or so it seems to me—for companionship. Yet I'm not happy with my live-in companion. I tell you, it's been awful for me."

Have you ever lived with a girl before?

Phillips pauses, fiddles with his Gucci belt buckle. "Yes."

Who broke off that relationship?

"She broke it off. I had my heart broken. I didn't want it to stop—ever. It did stop. I had my heart broken less than a year before Bypass patched my heart for me. I'm sure the breakup had something to do with my heart attack. I'm absolutely sure of it. I was so anguished. I wanted to die. She had children whom I loved. It was like losing a family."

Why did she break up with you?

"She started going out with somebody else."

When you were living with her, did you go out with other people?

"Yes. But do you know how that is? You think you can make the rules, that it's all right for you, but not for her. It doesn't work that way." Phillips shakes his head, looks out the window at the bars of rain crossing the sky. "Lately, I've seen her a couple of times. She talked about us getting back together. I've had some good fortune financially, which may have influenced her feelings towards me. When we were together, I was always neither here nor there, traveling, building the business. Once somebody breaks like that, I could never go back. When she suggested it, I wanted to. I still yearn for her, but I've reached the point where I can't trust her again. I don't think I could rebuild my trust. It's not the money I've made. I worry about what role Bypass plays in her desire to return to me. I don't want pity. Maybe I don't know what I want, maybe Bypass compounded the felony, but I can't take the pity!" Stowe Phillips pounds his fist on the desk. "No way!"

What do you think Bypass did for you?

"It bought me time. I'm assuming I reduced my inherent risk factor by half. They told me I needed Bypass surgery. Right away. Without Bypass, I'm sure . . . I think . . . I might not be alive today."

How long do you want to live?

"I'd like to live a full life span. Just like everyone else. Why should I be any different from the rest of the gang? The doctors say they don't know."

The doctors don't know whether you'll get hit by a truck this afternoon.

"That's nice of you to say, but there's no way to know about my heart. Dr. Terry sectioned my aorta. He said mine was the worst he had ever seen in a young person. You want them to level with you, and yet, when they do, a part of you wishes not to know. If my aorta is so bad, then the disease is still going on. Oh, I know, everybody's disease is progressing. If you're a philosopher, an occupation I gave up, you believe everybody's disease of life is progressing to that final end point. But that's different. Metaphysics and Bypass aren't in the same ball park. With heart disease, with *my* diseased heart, it's a matter of time. How much time? The doctor doesn't know. Neither do I."

Are you in a cardiac rehab program? Are you learning to modify your diet, to exercise, to modify your stressful responses?

"They've got a good program at our hospital." Phillips stops. "But I didn't join. It's all old guys. Maybe not so old, but a lot older than I. Their problems are not my problems."

Did you ever work with a psychiatrist about your Bypass, your stress, your depression?

"Not on stress per se. Six months ago, I saw a psychiatrist for the first time, to get help about this girl."

Was he helpful?

"*She* was exceedingly helpful, I thought. I saw her every week for about eight weeks. I don't think her help was permanent." Phillips smiles a sour smile. "What *is* permanent, I wonder?"

Why did you quit?

"I travel so much. I was always breaking appointments. I had to go to Brazil, to Africa, to Israel, to Arizona, and, afterwards, to Germany. Then, something else happened. My uncle died of a heart attack. He was my mother's kid brother. He was my best friend. Just like me, he had a heart attack at thirty. But *his* father died of a heart attack at forty-five. When I was a young boy, very young, my uncle Stowe was always there. We had the same name. We looked alike. Last December, after I returned from my overseas buying trip, he died suddenly in a Ping-Pong tournament. He was playing only a block away from the hospital. He never had a chance. He and I had been struck by heart attacks at the same age. It was like losing a big brother. He was only forty-five, which kind of gave me a timetable. Losing him devastated me. It still does. Not only that he died, that I'll never see him again, but that I have the same problem, maybe the same limited life span, the same fate."

Did your uncle have Bypass?

"He was one of the first Bypassers." He sighs deeply.

"We were very close. We'd talk about it a lot. We never wanted to expose our vulnerabilities to other people. He was adamant about exercise. Every morning, he'd be up at five-thirty, exercising on his stationary bicycle. He'd ridden cross-country and back on his bike. He was always after me to exercise more, to watch my diet more. He and I and his family were being studied at University Medical Center; we have extremely high cholesterols. When he died, I became bitter.

"In my case, a little knowledge is a dangerous thing: because of my studies in genetics, I know the genes were passed to me. I know I'm a carrier of coronary disease. It's been proven. I have the phenotype and the genotype of the problem. I'm bitter because I look at my uncle, who did everything he was supposed to, who was faithful to his regimented exercise program, who watched his diet, and what happens? *What happens?* He dies. Right before he died, only a week before . . ." Suddenly, Phillips's body shakes, wracked with dry, painful sobbing. Struggling for control, he apologizes, "Sorry. I'm really sorry. A grown man crying like that." As he explains, the tears stream down his cheeks.

Sometimes it's good for a man to cry.

"I want you to know about my uncle Stowe. A week before he died, we made a deal. He would go for another angio. That was our deal. Just to be on the safe side. Now he's gone." Phillips covers his face with his hands and weeps.

Did he have children?

"Yes. I keep thinking, 'I don't want children. I don't want to do that to them.' If I don't have a long life span, I want to continue to have fun, especially to be happy, I don't want to leave a family, like he did, because I see what his family is going through. I see his kids a lot. It's tough for them. If I've got a timetable, I want to break up with this girl, because I want the years left to be good ones." Phillips sighs, his voice trembles.

Would you like to be married?

"I think so. Society has said, 'You ought to get married.' Society also says, 'When you get married, you should have children.' I don't know why I care what society says, but I do. Have you interviewed anyone my age with Bypass? Are they married? Do they worry about the same things I do?" Phillips blows his nose. "I want a wife, I believe in having a family, but I'm convinced I won't live long. While I don't want to leave a family as my uncle did, I'm sure he wouldn't have done it differently. I wish I could ask him. That's what nobody understands. I wish I could sit down and talk to him."

If you worry about passing on the genetic trait, you could adopt children.

"I could have my own children!" Phillips answers angrily. "I don't want them left exposed to the world's dirty tricks. If I were here, I could take care of them. If I'm not here, it's over."

Did your uncle have a good marriage?

"Oh, yeah. Great. That's what I want." Again, he sighs.

When you travel on business, does this girl travel with you?

"Not any more. I wish I had a traveling companion, yet . . . I need the space, the time to be by myself."

When you travel to places like Africa, do you ever worry?

"About my health? When my heart is skipping or jumping or missing, I worry all the time. I worry I might drop dead somewhere. And nobody'd even know. That constant worrying isn't a healthy attitude. That's what I need to work on. Maybe it's a realistic attitude, I don't know. I don't want to dwell on the dark side—and I have been. Peering down the long corridor doesn't make life better. It makes it worse."

Are you on any medication?

"Nothing. I can't take the beta blockers for my arrhythmias; they confuse me. I lose my memory. In my business, you're through if you can't remember what you paid for a stone or how much a stone is worth. I buy rough stones. I go to the mines. I have twenty cutters working for me. If stones are the right quality and the right price, I buy parcels of ready-cut stones. I deal in stones rarer than the garden variety of diamonds and rubies, emeralds and sapphires. Stones like tourmaline and morganite."

Don't you have stress in your business?

"All the time. My cardiologist said, 'Get out of that business.' Unfortunately, I love what I do. I won't get out of it. The business is going great guns, but the inventory alone is stressful. Six months ago, I was robbed of $70,000 and six hundred stones."

Were you insured?

"They won't cover people like me, on the road, carrying all those stones. I had a million dollars with me in stones. I was with a client. It was a physical impossibility to bring everything in, so I had it all in a locked trunk. They got into the trunk. Fortunately, they didn't get it all. Many times, when I travel, I can't go out at night. I have to baby-sit my stones in the hotel. That's not only stressful, it's lonesome. God, but it's lonesome. You'd think a young cardiologist who'd had Bypass would be more sympathetic, but he isn't. Maybe he can't be. I think he hates what he does, because, every day, it reminds him." Phillips stares out the big smoked-glass window. "I guess I do need help.

"Hilary has no one but me. Her whole life is me. She'd never go back to California, because she hates her family. She doesn't have many friends here because she's been living my life-style. This morning, I played golf. As I was hitting balls, I was rehearsing ways to tell her: 'You have to move out. I'm not happy. You're crowding me. Please get away from me. Please.' She's never told her mother we weren't getting married. She doesn't want to believe it. She's good at sweeping things under the rug."

If you had it to do all over again, would you have had the surgery?

"I would have researched other treatments first. Right now, I'm feeling fine physically, even though psychologically I'm in Chapter Eleven. I'm on a macrobiotic diet. My cholesterol is down to 350, but those are still dangerous numbers. Somebody told me about experimental plasmophoresis, where they remove your plasma, wash it clean of fats, and recirculate it again. It sounds like a good idea, but that, too, requires a commitment of having it done every two weeks. On the other hand, it couldn't be as devastating as heart surgery. I don't want to need another Bypass. Did you see that program on TV? It made me sick to my stomach. If I'd seen that, I wouldn't have let them operate on me. I never would have let somebody touch my heart."

Does it bother you that somebody took your heart out and fiddled around with it?

"Absolutely. I don't think that the heart is the seat of consciousness or love. I'm not sure why it bothers me; yet knowing someone was there upsets me."

After Bypass, how long did you wait to drive a car?

"Right away. But I was weak."

How long did you wait to climb stairs?

"Right away."

How long did you wait to have sexual intercourse?

"As soon as possible. That was BH—Before Hilary. I was seeing a few girls."

In the beginning, were you afraid?

"I was a little worried. I'd think, 'I don't want to die on this girl. It would be embarrassing.' The girls I was seeing had known me for a while. I would wonder if they worried."

Did you ask them?

"In jest, I'd say something; they'd give me a joking reply. You can be so close in bed and so far apart. Only the heart surgeon got inside me."

Sexually, is your desire the same, less, or more?

"The same." For the first time, Phillips grins. "I've always been a horny guy. I like it that way."

What about when you were on the beta blockers?

"I took them for such a short while that I couldn't answer you. I didn't realize I was in a fog. When I took beta blockers, I was also popping Percodan. I took myself off the beta blockers because I didn't like what was happening to me."

Did your cardiologist ever try to reinstate beta blockers after you stopped the Percodan? Did he ever try a different drug?

"No, but that's not his fault. His brother died and my uncle died. He never knew about the Percodan; I don't want all these lousy drugs. They make me feel like an invalid.

"Funny, the cardiologist himself had a Bypass at forty-five. He treated my uncle for years. That's why I went to him. I don't think he knows all the waves hitting my shoreline. He's too worried about himself. His brother just had a heart attack and died. Anybody who's had Bypass and gets a flip-flop in the chest has to think, 'Is this a heart attack? Am I going to die?' "

What questions would you advise someone, especially someone young, to ask his internist, his cardiologist, and his surgeon, before and after Bypass?

" 'Will there be side effects you haven't told me about?' Like the weird feeling I have from the internal mammary artery. 'Will my body feel the same?' Everyone should ask, 'What about chelation therapy?' and see what the doctor says about it. Dr. Terry thinks it's a joke, yet I bet I've read more about it than he has. Afterwards, ask: 'Am I all right? How long will I be all right? How did the operation go? Were you able to do as many Bypasses as you planned?' Some surgeons are slow. They can't do as many as you need. Oh, they'll give you all kinds of reasons why they couldn't do the three or four or five planned. Before people sign up with a surgeon, they should find out how fast he is, as well as how good. They should ask, 'What's your average time on the heart-lung machine?' The depression, the memory loss, are closely connected to the pump time." Mockingly, Phillips laughs. "First and foremost, they should ask, 'Do I absolutely need this surgery?' I didn't get a second opinion. I'm sorry and not sorry."

*How could the Bypass, the hospital stay, the convalescence, and the
present time have been made easier for you?*

"Regardless of what you're in the hospital for, they don't tell you
what your real condition is. *That is a direct slap in the face.* Right
after my heart attack, I was afraid I was going to die. I wanted to
know how much of my heart was damaged. I wanted specifics in
terms of enzyme levels. I couldn't get an answer. The doctors'
slipping out the door, never looking at me, never listening, never
answering, added frustration and stress. They made a bad situation
worse. I kept thinking, 'Are they telling me the truth? What are
they holding back?' I'm a guy who likes to know. Who *needs* to
know. Some people don't want to know. But doctors have to read
each particular patient. Did you ever read Freud? He talks about
menschenkenner, people who *know* other people, who read faces
and gestures. I doubt many doctors do. Partly because they're not
trained, partly because they don't take the time. They need to ask
themselves, 'Is this patient going to freak out with the knowledge
we give him? Can he accept what we tell him? Should we tell him?'
If they don't ask themselves those questions, they should. They
shouldn't hide from the answers. They need a totally candid review
of each person's position, both after the heart attack and after the
Bypass.

"Before Bypass, I wish I had known just to know. It wouldn't
have stopped me from the surgery, but I wish I'd known about the
numb chest, that my body would never be the same. When I got
out of the hospital in six days, I was so excited: 'I'm going to be
100 percent again, maybe 110 percent.' Mr. Big himself. It would've
made it easier to know, 'Yes, you're Bypassed. No, you can't ever
come back to 100 percent.' "

When you had Bypass, were you glad or sorry you weren't married?

"When I had my heart attack, I wanted to tell the girl who'd broken
up with me, but I never did. I ended up keeping it from her. She
didn't know about the operation till long after. When I was in the
hospital, I had a distinct feeling that I didn't want people to visit
me. It's like when a dog gets hit by a car. He goes and lies under
a bush and nurses his wounds. I didn't want to be sick and white-
faced around everyone. I remember so sharply *not wanting to see
people in the hospital, not wanting anyone to see me weak and vul-*

nerable. When I came home, I wanted to remain by myself. I stayed at my mother's house for a couple of weeks. I didn't want to see people until I was prepared to see them. I didn't feel good about letting anybody see me so pale and sickly. I let my uncle Stowe come to see me, but I was upset because he brought his family. Some weeks after the operation, his wife said, 'God, you didn't look like the Stowe we knew.' I knew that. Consequently, I refused all visitors, except for my family. It was tough enough having my family come in."

In the last six months, this hospital has adopted the policy, pioneered by Cleveland Clinics, of not permitting anyone to see you for three days after Bypass. Do you think that's a good idea?

"The immediate family should be allowed to look in. It's unfair to keep a mother and father out. Nobody else."

With your uncle Stowe gone, do you have any other close friends?

"There's a couple of guys who are close. I don't like to *bleed* on my friends. Men frequently don't have that relationship with other men. From that standpoint, I don't have an outlet to say the things I've said to you today. It's been good for me to talk like this."

Men do themselves harm by—

"By being men," Stowe Phillips finishes. "By thinking it's weakness to talk about what's eating at them inside. Some of my good friends are extremely insensitive to personal feelings, so I don't discuss my feelings with them. Either they're not able to handle it, or they don't want to hear it, or they turn off their hearing aids, like 'What are you talking about? Where are you coming from?' Rather than go into that, I work it out myself."

A real friend is interested in your feelings. You don't have to be afraid to show him your weaknesses.

"That's true. My closest friend—now—is in Vermont. I don't see him very often. I get there on business about once a month. He came to see me after the heart attack. Not after the Bypass. I always wondered why, but I never asked him."

Before your uncle died, had you begun to break off with this girl?

"Yes. Then she went through the crash of my losing him. It was one more place she supported me when I needed it. I feel terrible, I'm breaking her heart. But the bottom line is that my own happiness is more important. I have to become selfish and look after me. The long slow tearing is more painful than one sharp cut. This relationship can't be mended. She's got the looks, but she doesn't have the mind."

Phillips looks at his gold watch. "Say, it's getting late. Trade cards with me." When I hand him my card, he laughs, " 'The Bypass Lady.' That's funny. Too bad you're not younger. That's a good thing for a lady to be!"

3. Tom Fouretier
IRS supervisor
Age at Bypass: 50

Tom Fouretier looks like a younger edition of Paul Newman. On the tennis courts in Nassau, his curly blond hair, dimpled wide smile, impeccably capped teeth, bright-blue eyes deep-set beneath ash-blond brows, sexy laugh, all suggest a film star on holiday. So much for appearances. Tom Fouretier is a senior executive with the Internal Revenue Service, a Bypasser who, because of a tropical rainstorm, consented to be interviewed on his brief vacation.

How did you find out you had a heart problem?

"One day, while playing tennis, I noticed pain chewing at the marrow of my chest, burrowing down my left arm. When I stopped playing for a few minutes, the pain eased off; but when I returned to the game, the pain repeated itself. Because Morgan, my partner, insisted, I went to the hospital, where I had a normal EKG and normal— I'm sorry, I can't think of the word."

Enzymes?

"Enzymes, yes. Everything was normal. Morgan is an internist. He didn't care what the tests showed. In his experience, pain like that indicated serious trouble. He said, 'Get a stress test.' I was dead set against the stress test because, six years before, in the middle of the night, I'd had the same kind of pain. I'd gone to the hospital, gotten Jody—my wife—all excited, spent the entire night warming my rear in the Emergency Ward, and everything was negative. The following day, a stress test had shown nothing. We'd been in the Caribbean, and I'd been scuba diving every day. Their diagnosis was a torn breast-shoulder muscle.

"When I got this pain on the tennis court, I was convinced this was a repeat of that episode. I fought my friend tooth and nail, but he won, even though the resident at the hospital had said, 'When I'm your age, I hope I have heart sounds like yours and a cardiogram like yours.' The next day, kicking and screaming, I consulted Jody's boss, Bill Fisher, a cardiologist. He did a thallium stress test, which indicated an 80 percent probability of blockage. The question was: which artery is blocked? My doctor doesn't believe in heart surgery. He thinks too much of it's being performed. He said, 'You need an angiogram. But unless the left anterior descending is severly blocked, I don't recommend surgery.' They did an angiogram, which showed three blockages, the worst in the left anterior descending. It was 98 percent obstructed. For Valentine's Day, Jody gave me a sketch of my angiogram. 'Here's a real heart for you,' she wrote on the card. Hardly any blood could get through those major arteries. Except for that one time on the tennis court, I hadn't had any symptoms. That's frightening. The week before, we'd been skiing in Vermont. I rode my bike to the thallium scan. I've always been an active guy. They went ahead and did the surgery. Here I am today, as good as new. It came out fine." He looks at his watch. "Two years and five days ago, I got my zipper."

Are you looking at your watch for any reason? Do you have another appointment?

"It's a calendar watch. I like to be accurate about facts and figures."

To what did you attribute your heart disorder?

"To my diet and to my diet only."

Why?

"It was loaded with saturated fats."

Do you smoke?

"I stopped smoking twenty years ago. I'd smoked about a pack and a half a day from the time I was in graduate school until the Surgeon General's report."

Does anybody else in your family have heart problems?

"My father had a heart attack at fifty-two, just my age now. He died of a coronary at sixty-nine. My mother's still alive and well in her mid-seventies." Forrester grimaces. "The women live. The men work and die."

You're very brief about the surgery itself.

"I can talk more about it. My first feeling, on hearing I needed this CABS, was anger. I was enraged. I was furious at my body for betraying me, furious at the timid medical advice I'd received, furious most of all at the milk and cheese, butter and eggs, which my mother had stuffed me with when I was a kid. It was good for me, she'd say, heaping my plate with poison. I was rabid at myself for corned-beef sandwiches and hot-fudge sundaes after theatre, for lunches of hamburgers and french fries, for breakfasts of eggs and sausage. Now, too late, I began looking at the fat content of foods. I realized what I'd eaten and what I'd put my body through. My blood boiled at the American food industry, at my parents, at myself, at my wife, because, after all, she does cardiological research. She knew it was bad for me, and I didn't know. I thought I was immune."

How long did you have to wait for your Bypass?

"Three weeks, but that was because we decided against the home team. Jody had worked with the cardiac surgeon, who'd been recruited from a university. I'm sure you understand medical economics. An open-heart operation is worth at least $25,000 to a hospital. They recruited this guy pretty much as a baseball team would recruit a new pitcher. He would be the star. Just before Christmas, the star lost three people on the table, people he shouldn't have lost. Then, Dr. Fisher, Jody's employer and our friend, told me he couldn't take care of me. He said he was sorry, but I was too close to him."

How did you feel when Dr. Fisher said he couldn't take care of you?

"Relieved. I knew it was too much for Bill; fortunately, he knew it himself. Bill said, 'I don't want you operated on locally. Go to Alabama.' My friend Morgan, the internist, agreed. I owe my life to Morgan, because he took me by the scruff of the neck off that tennis court when I wanted to go home and take an Alka-Seltzer. When they said, 'Don't go to the local guy,' I was delighted, even though at home I could've had it done immediately. Alabama entailed a wait. I wanted to be the first Bypass of the morning. It's not as if we moved into this cold. With Jody's work, I've been close to the medical profession for years. The early-morning slot I wanted took time. As long as I didn't ride my bike or play tennis, I was in no immediate danger. I worked half-days and sat around wishing the time away.

"The worst part about waiting was deciding what to do about my daughter, Maggie, who was spending her junior year abroad. For people like us to send a child to school in Europe is a big deal. She was enjoying it. We were enjoying it vicariously. One of her friends had been called home because her mother was dying of terminal cancer. The girl never went back. I couldn't do that to Maggie. But a friend of ours had been away at school when her father was dying; she hadn't been called home. She always said, 'Why did they do that to me?' Before the Bypass, we agonized whether to tell Maggie or not to tell her. We talked to anybody who'd listen. We made a list of do's and don'ts. Finally we decided we'd send a letter to arrive the day of my Bypass. Then, when I came out of the operating room, Jody would call and tell her, 'Everything's okay.'

"The night before surgery is a long night. They shave you completely, which leaves you feeling vulnerable to the invaders. That last night, I sat down with a tape recorder for about three hours and dictated to her. I talked about everything on my mind and heart. I explained why we didn't tell her before, so that if, God forbid, something did happen, it would be a last conversation between us, just Maggie and me. Thank God, she never heard it. I destroyed it. It was intended just in case . . . I don't want to hear it ever again. I've never told anyone except Jody about the cassette. Nobody else knows."

Does Maggie know?

"Yes. She wept when I said I'd erased the cassette." Fouretier wipes his eyes, clears his throat.

"One significant influence was Bill Fisher. I've always had a rotten gag reflex. Even when I go to the dentist, I gag. Fisher said, 'The operation isn't bad. Unlike abdominal surgery, the pain isn't horrendous, but be sure you're sufficiently medicated. Don't try to be a hero. Knowing you, the endotracheal tube will drive you nuts.' Earlier, a fellow had called and said, 'I've been through it. Can I help you?' I said, 'Tell me everything you can remember. I want to know as much as I can.' He told me about the thirst, the need to drink water, how they put ice on your lips, how you can't speak or communicate, about the tubes everywhere in your body, in every orifice. As he talked, I wondered how I could stand all that. Fisher is a great believer in self-hypnosis. He's not a psychiatrist, but he's made hypnosis a sideline. He spent four hours with me. He taught me how to hypnotize myself, a technique he's used with some success—not as much as he'd like because many of his colleagues look askance at hypnosis. He told me: 'Put yourself out of your own body. Envision yourself skiing or snorkeling on the beach in the Caribbean. Whenever it becomes so bad that you want to rip that tube out of your throat, or you want a cigarette, or a cold drink, put yourself into this trance. You're almost above your own body as your mind takes you to some far-off place.' When I was in the ICU, when the tube jammed down my throat was intolerable,

I'd hypnotize myself for ten or fifteen minutes until the worst was over, until that particular spasm had subsided. An hour later, it might come again; I'd take myself out of my body once more for another ten-minute trip. For the twenty-four hours with that tube, the hypnosis helped tremendously."

A retired Navy captain, who had two Bypasses—

"God, I wouldn't want to do it again. Two Bypasses!"

He said he minded the first one terribly. When he was advised to have a second, he asked everyone, but no one could tell him how to make it easier to tolerate. He heard about self-hypnosis and taught it to himself. Because of self-hypnosis, the second one was, by comparison, 'a piece of cake.'

"It helped me. If you ask me to sum up my Bypass experience, I've had a worse time with extracting a bad wisdom tooth. Other than knowing they've opened my chest and taken my heart out of my body, I don't look back now on my Bypass as really terribly traumatic."

Does the knowledge that somebody was fiddling with your heart bother you?

"It does. Someone actually touches your heart. They actually shut it down and run you through the heart-lung machine. Oh, I knew it was a relatively safe procedure, that they did 150,000 that year, that the success rate is 98 percent. I knew someone like me, without high blood pressure, a nonsmoker for years, without a frank heart attack, had almost a 100 percent chance of coming through with flying colors. But it's still dangerous. If you read any anthropology, for all peoples, primitive and sophisticated, the heart has symbolic meanings."

Since Bypass, do you value personal relationships more?

"Life is precious. I've changed the way I live. I take time to smell the flowers. I didn't before. It was rush, rush, rush. There was no limit to my working day. If I was tired, I blamed it on getting older.

Now, if I'm tired, I say, 'Sit down.' Before, I'd push myself as far as I could."

Is your relationship with your wife, the same, better, worse?

"For a year after Bypass, it was worse. Now it's better. Jody went to pieces completely over my Bypass."

What do you mean, 'went to pieces'?

"She went to pieces. Normally, she's a disciplined, well-ordered, self-controlled, intelligent individual who plans and thinks. She couldn't plan, she couldn't think. She couldn't even react. That first night when I had the chest pain and came home from the tennis court via the Emergency Room, it was 2:00 A.M. before I got home. One of my tennis partners had called earlier and said, 'Isn't Tom home yet?' When she said, 'No, he's not,' he said, 'Sorry to have disturbed you.' That was enough. When I came home, she was up and waiting. She said, *'Where have you been?'* I said, 'I had some angina and went to the Emergency Room.' She said, 'Angina is unexplained heart pain.' I said, 'I had some angina.' She said, 'Angina. You don't even know what angina is. Don't practice medicine without a license.' I explained what had happened on the tennis court. She said, 'There's nothing wrong with you.' Complete denial of the whole episode. I was furious. When a man comes home, you show him sympathy. My mother would have said, 'Tom, what happened to you?' Through this entire Bypass experience, Jody was beside herself. She felt, I guess, that I'd betrayed her, because I was supposed to be young and strong, all this nonsense. It took us a while to work it out together. When we went to Alabama, the business of my changing the cardiac surgeon was murder."

Why?

"Jody worked at the local hospital. Bill was senior cardiologist there. The stress test and the angio were done there. Then, I went someplace else. He said, 'Don't tell anybody I sent you out of town. If they hear, it'll go badly for me. I could lose my hospital privileges.

Jody would be out of a job, and so would I.' This pressured me. He was our friend, *but it was my heart*.

"Once we got to Alabama, there was some admissions foul-up. We waited forever for a room. By the time we got to the room, it was dark. We had to turn on the lights. Fiddling around with the bar on the back of the bed, Jody accidentally pressed the code blue. Everyone and his brother came running. When they found it was a false alarm, they chewed her out. She started screaming back at them. I was very upset. I said to her, 'I'm supposed to be having heart surgery, and *you* are upsetting me. Get the hell out of here and leave me alone!' I lost faith in her. I was terribly aggravated; it took some time to restore my trust in her."

What's 'some time'?

"Probably a year to sort through all this and understand what was going on inside her. She suffered more than I did. She works in ICUs. She knew what I'd look like, she knew everything that could go wrong. What she didn't know is: it looks worse than it is. It's not as bad as the family thinks—or fears."

You said you lost faith in her. What do you mean?

"I thought she'd be able to deal with it better than she did, that she'd be stronger than she was. I thought selecting the doctor, choosing the hospital, and taking me into the hospital wouldn't be a problem for her. After all, she's got a doctorate in physiology. She knows all about it. I didn't understand how helpless she'd feel."

After Bypass, did you become irritable?

"Nope. I didn't go through any of the afterevents people talk about. I didn't have any depression, any memory loss, any loss of concentration. I was just so happy to be alive."

Yet it took a while to nurse back your marriage?

"I never said a word to her. I don't think she suspected how I felt, how my feelings for her had changed, how my confidence had been eroded."

Did that confidence in her return?

"More. More than before. Now I recognize Jody's a human being. If you cut her, she bleeds, she cries, she feels the same emotions I do. Sometimes I've let her down. Nobody's perfect. I'm not. I can't be."

Since Bypass, have you changed your work pattern?

"I work for a big outfit; I'm one of Cincinnati's top men. I used to work all kinds of hours, because I thought they were dependent on me. Now I let my subordinates hustle more, take more of the blame. Every night, I'd bring work home. Now, I only bring it in an emergency, not routinely."

Did you ever make lists for yourself?

"I still make lists, but they're different. I list things I want to do before I die, things I want to *do* with my wife and kids, things I want to *say* to them, to experience with them. Since Bypass, I realize life won't go on forever. It has to end. That end could be tomorrow."

What's on the lists?

"I want to ski in Utah. I want to go back to the Caravanseri in St. Martin. I want to go to certain hotels and restaurants, usually the ones the IRS keeps checking out. I want to ski the Alps with my older daughter, to experience that with her."

Is that daughter Daddy's Girl?

"No. She's her own person."

That's different. Is your daughter your favorite child?

"Sometimes yes and sometimes no. When Maggie lives up to her potential and does the things I want her to do with her life, she's my favorite. When Sue does what I want her to do, she's my favorite. When they're both doing other things, I don't want to be anywhere near them."

You seem exceedingly conscious of what you want from your own life and your family's lives.

"I'm a little more selfish now, because I want to take time out to do what *I* want. I'm not the kind who goes drinking with the boys. My life is pretty much centered on Jody, the kids, our friends. But 'our friends' usually are *her* friends. She runs our social calendar. I used to give in to her about where to go, whom to go with. Not now. I want to see my daughters properly launched on their careers, with their own houses and cars, with the possessions they need in life. Seeing them settled is on my list of things to do before I die. The list comes and goes. If I see antique earrings or a necklace Jody would like, I want to buy it for her. While I'm still here. Better from a warm hand. That's a big change. No tax shelters for me. Those are for the suckers who think they'll live forever or, if not, can take it with them."

Did Bypass make you aware of things you wish you had not done with your life?

"Yes. Eating all that junk. Nothing else. I'm pretty happy with my life. The IRS has been good to me. When I was at the London School of Economics, I never planned a career with the IRS, but it was a good choice."

Did you ever think, 'Why me?'

"No, because I knew why. In one sense, I thought myself extremely lucky: I had chest pain; my friend Morgan was there to push me to the hospital. I didn't have a heart attack, so I don't have any real heart damage. Talk about ambivalence! At the very moment I'd be thinking, 'I'm the luckiest guy in the world to have caught this and fixed it,' I'd be burning with fury. Every emotion has its dark underside. When I dictated the tape to Maggie, I was the saddest man in the world. I thought, 'If she ever hears this tape, I'll be dead. I'll never see her again.' I churned with mixed-up emotions."

But you didn't put the tape away. You destroyed it. Why?

"Since then, I've said most of it to her. So she knows. There's no need for a rerun."

Now that the operation is over, do you think much about the Bypass?

"I seldom think about its physical aspects. I do dwell some on the psychological. Especially now, because it's my anniversary. It's the second anniversary of that three-week period between the tennis-court pain and the Bypass. I think about self-hypnosis, and wonder why more people don't know about it. I think about everyone who helped me. I think about Morgan forcing me off the court. I think about Bill Fisher and his unrelenting honesty about the state of Bypass at our hospital, about his help with the self-hypnosis. I think about those guys and what I owe them, but that's the extent of it. I don't want to make myself a bother. I don't want to call these guys every year, on my Bypass anniversary, and say, 'Thank you for saving my life.' After the Bypass, I said, 'Thank you,' I wrote them each a note. More would be self-serving. It's important to me, but it's just another day for them. Whenever I speak about it to Morgan or to Bill, they act embarrassed and look past my shoulder, even more than doctors do routinely."

Physicians like thank you's, just like everyone else.

"That's what Jody says. When I went to Emergency that night, the woman resident said, 'I've no medical basis for urging you to have a cardiological work-up, nothing except woman's intuition. Nevertheless, promise me you'll make an appointment for a stress test.' After the Bypass, I called her. I was sure she wouldn't remember me, but she did. I said, 'I wanted to thank you.' She said, 'You're the first person who ever called me back.' I said, 'You were right. If you get somebody else in there like me, the knowledge of my outcome will reinforce your medical judgment.' "

Since Bypass, how well have your family and friends supported you?

"I surely couldn't ask for better support. Jody watches me like a hawk."

Does that bother you?

"No. It's difficult to watch every forkful for fat, to concentrate on keeping the HDL up, but the LDL down. I couldn't do it without Jody. She knows almost as much about it as I do."

Has Bypass changed any of your work relationships?

"It has to. My boss said, 'How do you want to be treated? How do you feel?' I said, 'What do you mean?' He said, 'Are you a wounded bird?' I said firmly, *'I'm fine.* I can do anything around here that has to be done. I may do it differently from before, but it'll get done. And I am *not* a wounded bird.' But if you have to ask such a question, it's affected you. Men don't like to be considered wounded birds, not for an instant."

When you were scheduled to be promoted, were you promoted?

"I'm high up in the organization. There are only two levels above me. The first time there was a promotion in the office, I didn't get the job. For political reasons. The fellow who asked me about being a wounded bird got the position. He lasted ten months. When the job opened again, I didn't even apply. I didn't want the pressure of a sixty-hour week. When *I'm* sixty, I'll retire. The government's a funny place to work. You can only make a certain amount of money. I'm already earning the maximum."

Then a promotion wouldn't matter.

"Just an increase in status, to the next level up, but no more money. If I didn't have a Bypass, I'd be scrambling for that job. I'd want it for the prestige."

Does a part of you still want it?

"Sure. It's just as easy to go in and be top man as it is to be . . . the next guy down. Easier."

Before your Bypass, did the surgeon talk to you at any length?

"Twice. Each time, we chatted for a couple of hours."

That's great.

Fouretier laughs at my enthusiasm. "People are funny. They say, 'Oh, *you're in the IRS.*' Then, they have a million tax questions, a million tax angles. We talked for 5 minutes about the operation and for 115 minutes about the IRS. After the Bypass, I saw him very infrequently. I supposed everything was going well, but I would have liked to have heard it from his lips. Most of my contact was with residents and paramedics. I wanted to tell the surgeon about self-hypnosis, that it should be taught to all prospective Bypassers, but I never had a chance."

What was the worst aspect of the convalescence?

"In the hospital, the coughing. When I got home, the terrible weakness. I had no strength. I felt beat. I couldn't walk from here to there."

How long did the weakness last?

"About a week. It seemed an eternity. The first day you go out, you walk from your door to the end of the block. And you return. It took me half an hour to do it. I walked like a little old man. Such tiny, tiny steps. I thought, 'My God, this is terrible. Is this the way I'm going to be?' If I'd known weakness was a normal aftermath of Bypass, it would have helped."

How long after Bypass did you resume sexual relations?

"Six weeks. Bill Fisher took care of that. He didn't wait to be asked. He came right out and said, 'What are you waiting for?' He was nice to Jody. He said, 'Don't be afraid. You can't hurt him. It hurts more not to begin early.'"

The first time, were you afraid of hurting the incision or having a coronary?

"No. When I came home, I worried about how I'd navigate our house. We live in an old town house with seven levels. It goes straight up. I asked him, 'How the hell am I going to manage the stairs? Will I be stuck on the top floor all the time? Will Jody have to stay home from work? Will I need a nurse?' He said, 'You can walk those stairs. Come down in the morning and get your own breakfast and lunch, then walk up once at night.' That was the turning point. Once I knew I could climb all those stairs without dropping dead, I didn't have too many fears about wearing out these Bypass grafts."

What were your hopes for life after Bypass?

"I wanted to do what I'd been able to do before. I was scared to death that I couldn't engage in all the physical activities I'd done before, that I'd be some kind of invalid. To me, it's a miracle. I go out on the tennis court, the sun is shining down on me, I look up at the sky and feel like laughing and hollering with joy. I could never have been a Barney Clark or a William Schroeder. The quality of life matters too much to me. I wouldn't subject Jody and the children to seeing me suffer that way. I wouldn't want Jody to do that to me either; I couldn't stand to see her suffer with a series of operations until you're so weak, you die anyway."

What helps you get through tough times?

"My family—my wife, in particular—my belief that I'm a lucky guy. And some of my father's gutsiness. My father and my wife are much alike. You've heard of a boy marrying someone like his mother. Well, I married my father. Those two loved each other dearly. They both see life as it is, which is a terrible curse, because they see it without frills. They call a spade a spade. People like me say, 'Okay, it's raining today, but it'll be nice tomorrow.' They say, 'It's raining today. I'm losing this time from my vacation. I'll never make it up.' They see things as they are. They think in todays. I think in yesterdays, tomorrows, and todays. They're realists. I'm a romantic realist. They think in numbers. I think in metaphors, which, I suppose, is a strange thing for an IRS man."

If you should need Bypass again, would you have it? Would you do anything differently?

"Sure. A guy like me has to go to the same doctor, the same hospital. You can't quit while you're ahead."

Now that you're a Bypass veteran, what are your greatest fears?

"I'm not afraid of anything. I'm not afraid of dying, because I've had a great life. My greatest fear is losing my job. That would be a terrible blow. Not to be able to provide a good living for my wife, not to have enough money to live in the style we've grown accustomed to."

Is losing your job a possibility?

"It's always a possibility. The government's always reorganizing. A region could be abolished. It could be mine. It's a stressful job, even though I try to de-stress it."

Since Bypass, do you have more fear about being abolished from your work place?

"All my life, I've been afraid of losing my job. Ironically, one reason I cast my lot with the IRS was for more job security. Like a mailman, I was willing to sacrifice earnings for job safety. Afterwards, I found the government doesn't offer a heck of a lot more career protection than the private sector. Nevertheless, I'd rather be near the top of the IRS than scrounging around the middle of some big corporation."

Now that you're a Bypass veteran, what are your greatest joys?

"Living. Just living, even on a rainy day like this one."

What's been your greatest disappointment?

"My children, I guess. Susie isn't progressing the way I wanted. She's an assistant store manager. She's not married; she doesn't have social graces or social contacts. She's into pot—and some other things."

Did your having had the Bypass change her attitude towards you or towards herself?

"For a minute, she paused, said she'd change, but nothing happened. Jody couldn't lean on her for support. During all this Bypass turmoil, Sue provided no strength or succor."

You said, 'My children.' What about your other daughter?

"Maggie's a disappointment. When she was graduated from college, she couldn't get a job, which wasn't her fault. Nobody wants to hire a History major. I had to put her into the Internal Revenue, because she doesn't have the tools to get started on her own. For us, the IRS is like the family business. She's doing okay there, but her social life leaves a lot to be desired. She goes out mostly with older men, some married or separated. I want her to have a good husband, a family, a career to fall back on. Maggie and I seem perpetually embroiled in conflict. She's twenty-four. She's working full-time. She wants to lead her own life, but we want her to lead the kind of life we consider productive."

Does she live with you?

"Yes. I'm ready for her to leave. I'd be happier about my daughter's life if I didn't know everything that was going on. Besides"— Fouretier manages a crooked grin—"grown-up children are like duennas in the house. They inhibit your sex life; they inhibit intimacy."

Why does she stay with you?

"A matter of economics. The IRS doesn't overpay green History B.A.s."

What would you advise somebody who's been told to have Bypass? What questions would you tell him or her to ask?

"Everyone should get another opinion, because there's much needless Bypass surgery being performed. After that, I'd warn them of the dangers of the postoperative time, and what they'll feel before the operation. That's a lonely time. I know how a condemned man must feel sitting in his cell the night before his execution. Your whole life flashes before you."

Is there any way to make that night before not so tough?

"Just knowing it's going to be a tough night should help. If you know and you're not of a reflective bent, then you take a sleeping pill and go to bed. I couldn't do that. Not having Maggie there, not knowing whether to tell her or not to tell her, not knowing if we were doing the right thing, was rough. Later, when I asked her, 'Did I do the right thing not to call you home?' she said, 'Yes and no. If you'd told me, wild horses couldn't have kept me from coming home to be with you.' That's exactly what I wanted to avoid. 'If you'd died, and you hadn't given me that last chance with you, I'd have been devastated for the rest of my life.' I said, 'Maggie, I did not die. I'm here.' I told her about the tape, which alleviated some of her resentment. There was no right answer. I did the right thing, because the Bypass turned out all right. But when I see what Maggie's doing with her social life, dating all these older men, I wonder if she's seeking something from them that I failed to give her, if that seeking isn't the aftermath of my Bypass."

What questions should be asked?

"I don't know. In order to ask questions, you have to be informed. Before I went into the hospital, the surgeon's secretary insisted on making an appointment for me to spend two hours just talking to her."

Were you glad or sorry for the briefing?

"I was happy. I wanted to know. She had a list of things to tell me, much of which I knew from talking to people who'd gone through Bypass, and much of which I didn't know. She was exceedingly frank. She didn't cut me off. She said, 'Do you have any questions?' I had seven or eight in areas where I wanted more detail, or places she'd omitted. Because I was coming from far away, she was extremely patient and talked to me after office hours over the phone."

Would it have been better face-to-face?

"The phone was better, because she has a warm soothing voice. I felt like I was in a cocoon. Like Scheherazade, she cast a spell for me. I still have my notes from that phone conversation. If we'd talked face-to-face, I'd have been embarrassed to take notes. I wish she'd been around the night before the Bypass and, certainly, after the operation. Because the surgeon seemed to ignore me after Bypass, because I only saw him once afterwards, I felt he had let me down. I was a little bit dissatisfied. Many surgeons are cold fish. Every day, the cardiologist came in and inspected me minutely. He communicated with the surgeon. Maybe that's routine. But I wanted the surgeon himself to come in. I don't like truth at two removes."

Describe yourself emotionally for me.

"Reasonably stable. Given to fits of anger and temper. Introspective. At peace with myself. Recognizing the difference between the two. I'm grown-up emotionally, I think, but I still have some of the little boy in me."

In what regard?

"I like to have fun. I like to play tennis, to water-ski. I like to see people laugh and to make them laugh. I enjoy laughing at myself. I'm the funniest person I know."

Since Bypass, do you get misty-eyed more readily?

"After my Bypass, for a time, I got misty-eyed at everything. Maybe that was an unrecognized depression. I'd cry very easily, at movies, if someone was sharp to me, if somebody did something nice for me. My face always shows what I am thinking. All my life, I've had to be careful about my face showing my thoughts, especially to the people who work for me, even when I really don't know I'm doing it."

Describe yourself intellectually.

"Curious, intelligent. I like to look different from the average person, to think differently. I hate TV. I hate any kind of stereotyping. I want to be an individual, to deal with things on a higher plane than the average person. I like the philharmonic, opera, theatre, good restaurants, the pastimes of the reformed liberal."

What's a 'reformed liberal'?

"We used to be liberals, believers in civil rights and all the other fairy tales. Now we're fairly conservative."

Socially, are you a loner, or are you gregarious?

"I'm a loner. My wife is my friend. Then, there are friends whom we both have. I think of them as 'our friends,' but there's no one who is *my* friend alone, somebody not also Jody's friend. None of my childhood friends remain. *We* didn't get along with *my* childhood friends, so we dropped them. All our current 'friends' are *our* 'friends.'

Do you resent this?

"Somewhat. But they weren't the kind of people *we* would have been happy with."

Are you a perfectionist?

Fouretier laughs. "Only semi."

Are you comfortable with what you accomplish in a day or a week?

"As I get older, I'm less comfortable with the quantity and the quality of what I do. Time is getting shorter. People can express time only in terms of how long they've lived. If you're one year old, you see a day as a fraction of 1/365. As a ten-year-old, you look at one year compared with ten; the fraction has become 1/10. If you're fifty years old, it's 1/50. The numerical value involved means it's moving five times as fast. A minute or an hour isn't an absolute amount of time. As you get older, it speeds up on you, and you don't get as much done. Probably I'm slowing down, too, because I definitely feel I don't produce as much as I'd like."

Since Bypass, in what ways have you changed?

Fouretier smiles. "You're assuming Bypass warns people. You're assuming that once warned, people will change. Most Bypassers I know haven't changed an iota. But I have. I appreciate life more. I'm more relaxed, although it may be hard for the naked eye to see. I can turn myself off, stop my accelerator's automatic revving. I enjoy looking at the sky and watching the cloud formation. I'm glad to be alive. It's nice to be able to walk, and not be imprisoned in a wheelchair." Fouretier looks out the window. "The sun's coming out. Why don't we call this thing to a halt and I'll go out on the beach.

"But before I go, I want to tell you a story which shows how little other people know what's in your heart. When I was under the thallium scan, Bill Fisher came down with the results of the stress test. He put his hand on my shoulder and said, 'It doesn't look good. There's an 80 percent chance of blockage. An angiogram will be much more exact. You'll probably need a Bypass.' I thought it was terrible. I was so agitated. He started to lecture me as though I were a kid. 'Don't get so upset. The CABS success rate is high. We've done 150,000 this year. Next year, we expect to do 200,000. You're a healthy specimen.' He started talking about my muscle structure, my blood pressure and all those goodies. He kept repeating, 'Don't worry. A million Americans Bypassed since 1968. It's all routine procedure.' In his best professional manner, he delivered all the calming, soothing verbal nostrums a good doctor brings to a worried patient.

"Three weeks later, on a Thursday, I went through Bypass. A week from the following Friday, I came home from the hospital. Saturday morning at seven-thirty, I was sitting upstairs at the desk in the front room when the phone rang. An extremely distraught

Bill Fisher was on the phone. He was much more distressed than I was when I heard about the surgery. He was stammering so, I could barely make out the words. I said, 'Bill, calm down. What's the trouble?' He almost wept into the phone, 'I-I-I'm going to be audited!' As true as I sit here, he was that wrought up! I said, 'Don't worry, Bill. We do 100,000 audits a year.' In my best professional manner, I told him all the things that the IRS tells people, that doctors tell people: 'You don't have a thing to worry about. It's all routine. It won't hurt you a bit.' Everything came out fine for him, too. But everybody fears the unknown. The professional doesn't have to be concerned, because he's been through it a thousand times. For the individual, it's the first time, and he's scared to death. Funny, there are tons of books published about 'How to Live Through a Tax Audit.' There's so little on 'How to Live Through a Bypass.' I wonder why.''

4. Jed Anderson
Business executive
Ages at Bypass: 54, 58, 59

In Elyria, Ohio, "everybody" knows Jed Anderson, chief executive officer of the town's largest employer, White's Metals Works, one of this country's largest manufacturers of heavy tools. While a few other third time–arounders were interviewed, Jed Anderson has the distinction of being the only Bypasser talked to after *each* of his three Bypasses. Tall, attractive, tanned, with bright-blue eyes, a shock of white hair, a remarkably unlined face for a man of fifty-nine, Anderson, ten weeks after his third Bypass, still looks like an ad for Hart Schaffner and Marx in his beige suit, white shirt, and brown paisley tie. The only son of a small-town hardware merchant killed in an automobile accident, as was one of Jed's two daughters twenty years later, just before his first heart surgery, Anderson, an engineer, went to work for the then-faltering White's Metals Works to settle his father's debts. White's Metals and Jed Anderson's career flourished. Today, his company is listed on the New York Stock Exchange. Jed Anderson had his first coronary at forty-eight, his first Bypass at fifty-four, his second at fifty-eight, and his *third* at fifty-nine.

After his first two Bypasses, Anderson didn't change much. He remained impatient with ineptitude: "I never tolerated fools gladly. I won't stand in line. I'd rather tip somebody and get a seat right away." He'd never honked at the driver ahead of him: "In Elyria, that's impolite, especially from me. But I beeped the horn in Boston. Everybody does it in Boston." After his second Bypass, he'd talked about getting stuck in Boston's Callahan Tunnel on the way to Logan Airport: "My daughter's old car went kaput, right there in the tunnel. Just plain quit. I picked up my bag and said, 'I've a plane to catch. I'll have to leave.' I walked out of the tunnel, found an airport bus up ahead, got the driver to open the door for me by waving a ten-dollar bill in the window, went to Logan, and flew home. That's where I'd come apart, stuck in a hot fumy tunnel, with all those Boston drivers giving me the finger and a God-awful old car refusing to run." After his second Bypass, he admitted his impatience hadn't diminished "an iota. It might've gotten worse."

At the same time, we'd talked about the Type-A personality. "How in the world," Anderson had demanded, "could you be the CEO of a big corporation and not be Type A? This country rewards ambition and achievement. As it should. There aren't enough of us around. I like to be competitive. I like to win. I'm not a sore loser, whether in sports or in business, but I don't like to lose. In business, you have to compete, to offer challenges to yourself and to management. As CEO, your standards and goal must be higher than some middle managers think necessary."

Anderson was, he had asserted after the first two operations, "no different. I don't want to be different—just better. Bypass gave me the opportunity to do more. Before the second Bypass, and the first one, too, I'd have trouble traveling. That *A* in Type A must be for airports, the worst places in the world. At O'Hare, if I carried a light valise from one terminal to the other, I'd run out of gas. I'd have to stop. I couldn't make it. That left arm'd shoot me full of holes. The doctors would say, 'Don't let yourself get in that bind.' But if your plane's leaving in ten minutes and you're a mile away from it, you figure, 'If I push a little, I'll make it.' The first Bypass took the trouble away for four years. The second Bypass never relieved the trouble."

Four years after his first Bypass, Anderson remarked questioningly, "I've doctored with Peter Conwell, a sweetheart of a guy. He's famous, but not much of a disciplinarian. Peter never mentioned weight. Never mentioned diet. Never mentioned exercise. I see him once a year; he checks my equipment and says, 'How're you feeling?' That's a little strange." Clearing his throat, Anderson added, "I had my heart attack in '73, a Bypass in '79. I'm still walking around with the rest of the people, so I can't fault him too much. Despite what I read in *Time* magazine, he never told me not to salt my food, never warned me about cholesterol and fats."

Recalling the second operation, Jed Anderson claimed, "I fully recognized what happened. I don't try to analyze who's to blame, whether I was singled out. I've never felt sorry for myself. Who're you going to blame? Some people have cancer. Some people are born with birth defects. I had heart trouble. When I lost my daughter right after my heart attack, when my second daughter ran away and we couldn't find her for a month . . ." His voice catches. "Since Bypass, I've noticed I've less control. I'm less resistant to—emotion. When I was a kid, my sister'd sit in some tear-jerker movie with two boxes of Kleenex. And I'd razz her. Now, I'm liable to use up a box myself." Yet after Bypass, Anderson says he was never depressed. After his first heart operation, he had commented, "I wonder how realistic I was, because I never worried about the operation or about coming out okay. I decided, 'It's not exploratory surgery looking for some tucked-away incurable cancer. It's done every day. Why should I have a problem?' "

Just before his second Bypass, before Jed Anderson knew he'd need a second Bypass, White's Metals had to lay off a thousand workers. Living in Elyria, seeing people struggling with the company's layoff was hard on Anderson: "It's not like living in Chicago or New York or Boston, where your neighbor works for somebody else; they don't participate in your problems. Here, everybody knows what's going on. They all know who's in charge of what. You get used to that. I've lived in Elyria for years now. It's a small town. You've gotta keep your mouth shut. It's tough to hold a secret. You go into a store and buy four pork chops, two steaks. The following Tuesday, somebody says, 'Gee, I saw ya over at the A & P. How were those chops? Having pretty nice company if you bought those thick steaks.' I mean, nothing's sacred."

Following his first Bypass, Anderson reduced his corporate responsibilities, brought in somebody else to be president, although Anderson remained CEO. When we first talked, he didn't like discussing his anticipated yielding of the CEO's position. Pushed to comment on the loss of power, he frowned: "If you think about turning over the CEO's reins to somebody else, you have the same feelings as when some big outfit aims at an unfriendly takeover. So far, we've been able to fight off those buzzards.

"The professional 'management' boys may be good businessmen, but their attitudes towards this company and its workers are different from mine. They didn't grow up with it as I did. I'll miss the hurly-burly of the CEO's job. Anybody like me, in the operations side of business, feels a little robbed when he's no longer the honcho. But it happens every day."

Done with his second Bypass, he'd noted: "Everything went according to Hoyle, as expected. The only unexpected occurrence was the second Bypass itself.[1] I thought, 'Only one to a customer.' Shows what I knew. The pain from the second Bypass didn't bother me so much. I was prepared for the pain. Actually, number one and number two weren't so different. Each time, I needed Bypass, I had it, it's over." He'd stopped, carefully examined his father's gold pocket watch, then added, "I hope.

"The second time, they had me practice with that Triflow gizmo, had me practice blowing up those little balls. The first time, we used the same device, but without any preliminary practice sessions. The practice helps. This time, they suggested hugging my pillow when I coughed. That helped. A firmer, fuller pillow might be better insulation. Even the tube didn't bother me so much, believe it or not. I knew the tube was part of the postop program. Knowledge is strength.

"After the second time around, I became less self-involved, more sensitive about family situations, more appreciative of what we had, of my wife and my family. After each Bypass, I became very sensitive. When the Marines' coffins came back from Beirut, I cried. Almost uncontrollably. Some of that wears off; not all. As a result of Bypass, especially this one, the sensitivity to human relations is awakened. Sometimes, the world goes by, and you're so busy, you don't even notice. After two Bypasses, you get more involved with your own little world."

At the time, Jed Anderson didn't have much advice for somebody

---

[1] The average number of years for grafts to remain patent (open) and the "redo" rates vary with the surgeon, the hospital, the patient, and the location of the Bypass. Because of the growing ranks of Bypassers now five to ten years after their initial Bypass surgery, the number of redo's obviously is increasing. While this book is not a statistical study, many Bypass verterans were still doing well ten to fourteen years after their first heart operation.

who'd been told to have a second Bypass: "If it's indicated, if the patient has confidence and feels sufficiently troubled to have a second go, if the cardiologist recommends it, he should proceed. In my case, they did a good job. I'd like not to be in the hospital for three days before the operation. That's unnecessary.[2] Teaching hospitals have all these fine, young, inquisitive, pain-in-the-ass, arrogant kids coming in for long drawn-out interviews. Over and over, they ask the same questions. They don't read the file, because they're supposed to build their own files. The patient feels like a broken record. Enough's enough. Let them teach on somebody else.

"The second time, there'd been some improvements in the postop program. There was a new exercise regimen. A physiotherapist lined everybody up in the hall. She put the whole crew through these exercises. She asked the gang to continue these light exercises after discharge. But they didn't put any of us into a formal exercise project. Even though I'm a guy who hates being given orders, if they'd prescribed a group exercise program, I'd have gone for it. One of my buddies went to Alabama for his Bypass. In the hospital, they set him up with special exercises, then more for the first six weeks, then more for the first six months. It was carefully structured, what fellows like me need."

Asked what he thought the second Bypass had done for him, Jed Anderson had replied slowly. "I hope it extended the use of my repaired heart, my once-repaired heart. To the best of my knowledge, it fixed my cardiac problems. I won't say Bypass gave me a new lease on life. I hope it extended the lease. I don't have any fixed ideas about how long I want to live. I don't want to be a cardiac cripple. I'm no Barney Clark. In the interest of pure research, he has to be commended. If they want to try some noble experiment, tell them not to call Jed Anderson. When it comes to tubes and machines hooked up to every orifice, I'm no hero."

While our talk four years after the first Bypass had been triumphant, our conversation in Anderson's newly redecorated corporate offices that spring day three months after the second Bypass had seemed troubled.

"I haven't played racquetball yet. I've been out playing golf a few times, I walked around the course. One thing bothers me. After

---

[2] Many hospitals now are trying to have patients admitted the day before Bypass.

I got home, I began feeling some symptoms like before the operation. Not pain, but that tightness. That bothered me a little bit, because I said to myself, 'I wonder if this set of grafts has taken? I hope I'm not in Failure Corner again.' When I saw Howland for my six-week checkup, I asked him, 'How do you know if the operation is successful? What evidence do you have?' He said, 'The only way we know is your ability to do things without pain. We no longer take angiograms after the operation, so we have no objective evidence. If the patient feels better, the Bypass is successful. If the patient's in trouble again, then it may not be successful.' What they're saying is, 'Why do that diagnostic test? Why not ask the patient how he feels? If he isn't feeling good, then the operation wasn't any good; if he is, you got the job done.' Even though the argument sounds like my grandmother's reasoning about spring fever, I accepted it. But if I walk at a certain pace, I still have this slight problem. When I told Howland, he didn't say a word. When I went to see Dr. Conwell, he was disappointed and concerned. He said, 'You ought to have a stress test.' Because I had to go to Texas and he had to go to Jiddah, because he's a big-shot cardiologist, we had a timing problem. He said, 'Just jump up and down for two minutes right here in my office.' I did; he checked me. My blood pressure was up, my pulse rate was up, and I was sweating. He said, 'Do you have any pain?' I said, 'None.' "

Did he take an EKG?

"No, but he was standing right there, checking everything. He said, 'I'm satisfied.' If Conwell is good enough for a sheik, he's good enough for me."

How's it been since then?

"Better, I think. I still have it, but it takes more effort and more exercise to produce the tightness. The situation's improving. Don't ask me why and how."

Since you jumped up and down in his office, have you seen him?

"Yes, because I had the problem again in Mexico City, where the elevation is 7,800 feet. There, when you tell somebody you've got chest pain, they say, 'Everybody does.' They don't worry about it. But everybody *doesn't*. This tightness in the throat, a symptom before my second Bypass, still bothers me, but it may be waning. You don't understand. I *have* to feel the operation probably went okay."

Because you needed Bypass number two, did it make you feel old?

"Nope. I'm the same young guy I always was."

Did it make you feel life isn't fair?

"No, but here, my religion helps. Lots of people are put in this world for various reasons. Lots of them don't deserve what they get, but it happens. I'm not a fatalist. I don't have a persecution complex. When it happens, you get it fixed. If it breaks down, you get it fixed again. If it works after that, you go on from there and try to help others. You keep pressing me whether I've changed, especially the second time around. My one trade-off has been less concern for the company, less fire about doing a perfect job. I'm not sure that's due to Bypass. With this executive transition, some-body else is supposed to carry the ball. If I butt in, it's dirty pool. Still and all, it might have something to do with the operation: I got through this thing twice. Let's enjoy the present and not worry about the future."

You waited no time in driving a car. How long did you wait to climb stairs?

"Right away. They said, 'No problem, if you walk a certain way.' The first time, you had to slide up and down on your rear, like a little kid, only once a day. This time, go up one step at a time. Step up, pull your other foot up, and continue like that. Sounds philo-sophical, doesn't it?"

How long did you wait to have sexual intercourse?

"About three or four weeks."

Did anybody talk to you about sexual activity?

"Not the first time and not the second time. Doctors don't like to talk about things like that. It's like death. It makes them nervous."

Were you afraid the first time after Bypass?

"I don't think so. She was more concerned. We're a little older, our children are out of the house. It's gotten down to her and me. If something had occurred that was other than satisfactory, she might not have felt comfortable about it. She was more uptight than I, but she masked it pretty well."

Now that you've been through Bypass twice, what are your greatest fears?

"It's not a great fear, because I can't dwell on it too much, I just can't. Yet, I wonder what will be the outcome of the second Bypass. The benefits of the first Bypass terminated in four years. Since the second Bypass, I've had minor recurrences of this tightness. It's, it's subsiding; I don't know if it's gone. I wonder what is the second operation's life expectancy. If I hadn't had the second Bypass, I'd probably be able to work and play in moderation, maybe find some acceptable pills permitting me to live quietly. I wasn't willing to do that. I don't like pills. I'd do it if it were my only option. But they offered me the option of another operation, and I said, 'I'll go for it.' You wonder whether or not the benefits will continue. One consideration's a comfort: technology progresses. In the last two decades, it's improved immeasurably. If you can hang in there long enough, they may find something more advantageous in the future, something a lot easier to tolerate."

What explicit questions would you advise people to ask their internist, their cardiologist, and their surgeon, before and after the operation?

"For the cardiologist: How do you know you're going to need an operation? Or a second one? What kind of improvement can you expect in your life-style after the operation? What kind of limitations might you be subjected to? What's the future? What's the life span?

"For the surgeon: What is he doing and how does he plan to do it? What methods and procedures is he using, in what kind of time frame? What are the odds for success or failure? What is his view of your chances? He's the technician. He's putting the hardware together. What other techniques might be considered? Is there any alternative to basic Bypass surgery? You read about this balloon technique and the laser research. How is it going? What are the options?"

Since Jed Anderson and I last talked, a year had passed. Still strikingly attractive, only ten weeks after his third Bypass, he seems muted, weary. The flames of his Type-A fire are embers of his earlier self. Nevertheless, his marvelous smile is brighter than it was a year ago.

What were the events leading to your third Bypass?

He grins ironically. "You mean, three times up at bat and out? Well, following my second Bypass at University Hospital, I questioned the operation's success. I had the same difficulties as before surgery. Every three months, I'd be checked. By nine months after number two, time enough to have a baby, I'd worsened badly. If I exercised, if I dashed through an airport to catch a plane, my throat would choke, my chest felt like a pressure cooker. In three or four minutes, I'd get shut down. I talked to Peter Conwell, my cardiologist: 'Peter, what d'you think?' Peter tried beta blockers and calcium blockers and nitrates, and varying combinations of the above. I never seemed to get any relief. Finally, I went back to him: 'It's not getting any better. The medicine doesn't do any good; it only poops me out, clouds my thinking, kills my sex life. I'm a young guy. Relatively. Do I have to finish out my life limited like this?' Peter said, 'The only alternative is another Bypass.'

"After number two, I swore I'd never have another Bypass. I'd said, 'I'll use a gun first.' But I thought it over, and decided, 'I'm a realist. If I want to get better, I'll have to consider another Bypass.'" Anderson winces. "With all due respect to Peter Conwell and University Hospital, with two outs and bases loaded, I thought I'd better get another opinion. I know a lot of heavy-duty metal manufacturers; I don't know many cardiologists around the world. I got a recommendation from Dr. Conwell; he sent me to a fellow in Virginia who'd trained with him. Dr. Breakers put me through my paces, prescribed medication, essentially the same stuff Dr. Conwell used, and told me come back in a month. I told him: 'I don't think those pills will help, but I'd be glad to go through the charade.' And we did. A month later, I went back. This time, I walked the treadmill for five minutes, rather than four and a half minutes. Dr. Breakers said that kind of 'improvement' meant drugs weren't much use. He sat down with me, covered a lot of bases. Finally, I interrupted him, 'What's the bottom line?' 'You ought to have another Bypass.' I was surprised, yet not so surprised. 'If you were me, would you go for it?' He didn't fudge: 'I would. Even though it's number three, even though it's no picnic, you're in good shape; your problems are fixable. The chief of vascular surgery here is excellent. He's reviewed your case. If you want, he'll be glad to take the assignment of fix-up number three.' I thanked him and asked him to send a copy of his reports to Dr. Conwell.

"When I went back to Peter, he said, 'You've got two opinions. What are you going to do?' 'I'm resigned to having an operation, if they can determine that biological failure isn't causing my trouble. If it's a chronic biological rejection, why bother? It's just gonna happen again, kinda quick.' Peter didn't think it was biological, but added, 'If you intend to have another Bypass, and I recommend it, I don't think you should come back to University Hospital for the third one.' " Anderson drums his fingers on the desk. "I said, 'University Hospital never was under consideration. Enough's enough. But I don't know where to go. Can you suggest anyone special?' When I'd asked Dr. Breakers, he'd suggested Virginia, Hopkins, Texas, New Orleans. Dr. Conwell said the chief honcho at Virginia was more of a transplant man; funny, I've since learned he's a red-hot Bypass guy. I wasn't interested in transplants, so we ruled him out. Peter recommended Cleveland or Washington. Talk about tracking. It's like high school. If people here go out of town, they almost always get sent to Cleveland or Washington, never to Boston, Houston, or Birmingham. Having checked them out, he decided on Washington's top man, Dr. Santos Lento. I later learned Lento had trained at University Hospital. Those doctors sure go in for the daisy chain. I said, 'I'll consider it, but first I want to talk to him.'

"Dr. Conwell sent all the prior angiograms and test results. On a Sunday, Dr. Lento called me and talked for an hour. I liked him right away. Good personality, good approach. I said, 'I'm not willing to undergo a third Bypass unless I'm sure my trouble's nonbiological.' He was very discreet: 'There's a possibility of a technique problem in your second Bypass, maybe even in your first. We'll have to catheterize you. Come out on Monday. We'll angiograph you on Tuesday. If it's needed, we'll Bypass you on Thursday.' So I went. As he suspected, it was correctable." He scratches his head, puts one long leg across the corner of the desk. "But the guy did such a super job. I'd never been exposed to this kind of care. He came up to the room, sat down with Sally and me, got a piece of paper and began diagramming the heart, where the problem is, what they can do. At University Hospital, nobody had ever done this for me—either time. It's important. Then he said, 'That's a general view. But why don't you and your wife come down to the lab? We'll set up the films and run them. They're not that tough to understand.' He ran all three angiograms, after the first, after the second Bypass, and the one taken the day before. We could see the blockages; we could see the crimps in the grafts done in my second Bypass, done only nine months earlier. I said, 'Okay. Let's go for Thursday.' *That* Bypass was a tough one. Really tough." He shakes his head.

Why was number three so much tougher?

"With the other two Bypasses, I got back on my feet pretty good. I was back at work quickly. This time, I couldn't get my head off the pillow. They'd had me on the operating table for twelve hours. That's a long time, by anybody's standards. Because I was down so long, they said I had to rebuild my blood supply. Apparently, the longer you're there, the more time you're on that heart pump. Every time it pumps through, the more damage is done to the blood cells."

Why did this Bypass take so long?

"Corrective action on the old Bypasses, adding new Bypasses, scrounging around for veins, because the veins had been used twice before. I don't know. Dr. Lento told me he's considered a little slow; he was good, but he wasn't a fast surgeon. Before he went into the operation, he said, 'It might take four or five hours.' It took lots longer. I'm not sure why Dr. Conwell sent me to somebody good but slow. Dr. Howland, the surgeon at University, was slow. People say surgical speed matters. They ran into problems. The third time out, Lento hit scar tissue; he had to be more careful. He wanted to be very sure things were definitely improved. He used a special technique—maybe they use it everywhere. I don't know. He puts a magnetic flow meter in the artery before he fully closes and then tests the flow. After the operation, he said, 'You've got 50 percent more flow now than before, when you thought you were fully healthy.' The recovery prblem resulted from the time on the operating table, the deficiency in my blood, and one little bonus"— he laughs weakly—"which made it a bit tough. The day after I came out of Intensive Care, twice I went flat on the monitor. Things stopped. They had a little Chinese fire drill trying to hook up some new monitors and check out the wire extending from my stomach."

You're speaking metaphorically. Are you saying you went into cardiac arrest?

"Yeah. The heart stopped beating. Only for ten to fifteen seconds each time."

Twice?

"That's what I'm told. So they decided to put in a pacemaker. But that was Saturday night. Take my advice: don't get sick in a hospital on Saturday night. Because they don't show up till Sunday morning. The doctor came in Sunday morning and inserted a pacemaker. If I knew then what I know now, I might've argued against it. That pacemaker wasn't necessary. The heart stoppage was a momentary occurrence from the strain of Bypass. That failure wasn't going to prevail. Dr. Lento was surprised I even had the stoppage, but he put in the pacemaker as backup—'an insurance policy,' he said. Once they put in the pacemaker, they make you lie flat in bed for two days. They don't want you to move because they want the lead to get fixed permanently in the heart muscle. I lay flat on my back for two days and two nights; for forty-eight hours, I never slept a wink. When it was all over, I had hallucinations. I had a terrible time. They said, 'Hallucinations aren't unusual after anesthetic and prolonged sleep deprivation.' That was the expla-

nation; it didn't help me any. Some people might think my recuperation was par for the course. I don't think so."

What did you blame for needing a third Bypass?

"From what I'm told, technical error during the second operation.
If you take a piece of copper tubing and bend it, not much is going
to get through. Two arteries were closed; the Bypasses were crimped
when installed."

How did Washington differ from University Hospital?

"Washington's got cherry blossoms and filibusters. Besides that?
The preop was better. The surgeon communicated with me. We
had a lot to talk about: lacrosse and golf, Williams and Yale. He
interviewed at University Hospital, but they didn't give him the
job. Too bad, it might've saved me some trouble. Our personalities
meshed. Although that didn't matter so much to him. He has great
patient manners. He makes you feel as though you're number one,
that he understands your situation, that there's a good chance of
success. Postoperatively, the nurses were well-trained and helpful.
There wasn't a fat one in the bunch. Nice-looking kids, easy on the
eyes. At their hospital, they do so many Bypasses—two thousand
each year, can you imagine that?—that they've developed a cadre
of nurses with real expertise in handling the Bypasser. While the
facilities weren't like some of those VIP floors in Los Angeles hospitals, they were much nicer than those at University. When I was
ready to leave, a couple of people spent a lot of time making sure
I knew what was ahead of me at home. After two previous Bypasses,
they weren't telling me anything new, so I didn't get too excited.
But they didn't just hand you a booklet and say, 'Here. Read this.
Any questions?' They went over each detail point by point. They
encouraged questions. They behaved like professionals, much more
so than anyone at University. The therapist worked with breathing
exercises and outlined an array of home exercises. Like the rest of
the staff, she was so intense about trying to insure that the patient
understood his role in helping himself get better. The level of personnel was excellent. I run a big corporation. Sure, metals are
different from hearts, but a tight ship is a tight ship. At University
Hospital, they didn't batten down the hatches as well. University

had an exercise program, but no follow-through after discharge. University had no real communication program. In Washington, I had to go up and down two flights of stairs three times a day before I could get discharged. At University, there's no stair practice. If you go anywhere, they take you in a wheelchair on the elevator. God, I hated that. A wheelchair is a certificate of enfeeblement."

Did they recommend any cardiac rehab?

"The cardiologist urged me to consider the Pritikin diet. Not to go to the Pritikin Farm, but to eat Pritikin's way. I looked it over. Sally read Pritikin's book. I try, but it's not that easy at dinner meetings and on airplanes. That Pritikin is really strict. After they put in the pacemaker, they offered a telephone service to check its functioning."

How often do you have your pacemaker checked?

"I haven't done it yet. I've forgotten how often they told me. When I got home, Dr. Conwell said, 'We've got the same service. I'll send you the material and get you signed up.' So far, no material. The pacemaker's not necessary, anyhow. It's only a machine working on demand. It's set at sixty beats a minute. I'm running a little faster than that, so it's not called on to work. I'm considering having it taken out. It's a bother. I know it's there. When I scrub up, I bump into it. That area's taking its time in healing."

Did anybody recommend behavior modification? Did you ever read the Type A book?

"Look. There's Type A and there's Type B. You're not going to change your approach to life just by reading a book."

There are group-therapy behavior-modification programs. With a good leader and a good patient, frequently they help you change.

"By the end of the year, I'll be able to do more things outside the business at a more leisurely pace. Sixty's a fairly early age to back away from the business climate, but I've got some other business deals cooking. Probably, I'll have enough on my plate not to get too bored. I'll still conduct the annual meeting, so long as the earnings remain respectable. I'm changing. When I was recuperating, I skipped a directors' meeting. I couldn't lift my head off the pillow. In other days, even though I was bushed, I would've flown back home for the meeting. Now my blood supply's better. Dr. Conwell put me on iron pills, and on Persantine and aspirin. Some Canadian study said Bypassers do better with Persantine and aspirin. Washington didn't give me any prescriptions."

At the hospital in Washington, do they have a house staff, well-trained residents and interns?

"I don't believe so."

When you got sick on Saturday night, you weren't operated on till Sunday morning. What doctors took care of you on Saturday night?

"No doctors." Anderson smiles wryly. "*I* knew I had a problem. Evidently, they didn't think it was that serious."

Did any doctor come into see you?

"Just nurses. Finally I made them call the doctor. I told them to say, 'Get your ass in here.' They said, 'We've got him on the phone.' I said, 'Tell him again, "Get in here!" ' " Anderson shrugs. "No luck."

Did that upset you?

"Sure. At the time, it upset me a lot. Then I fell asleep. Sally didn't know about it till the next morning. It was late evening; she'd gone back to the motel. She was sore that they didn't call her, that the doctor didn't come in. They obviously knew more than I did. Apparently, they didn't feel it was that big a deal. The guys were probably all out going to cocktail parties. They scheduled the pacemaker for ten the next morning. That's when they did it."

When you had two cardiac arrests, no doctor saw you? No doctor was in the hospital?

"Nobody with an M.D. degree."

Did it scare you?

"Yes and no. I didn't know what had happened. They didn't tell me. I knew something was wrong because they were running in and out of there with test equipment. I didn't know till the next day that my heart had arrested twice. It's scary to think that your heart stopped. It's like dying and coming back."

What made you say, 'Get the doctor on the phone. Tell him to get in here'?

"The nurses were running in and out, maybe eight of 'em. They were having trouble getting this monitor thing hooked up in the room. They couldn't connect the wires. Finally, I told them, 'Check if any are broken.' Sure enough, one had ripped. That's what you call a broken heart." He forces a game smile. "They weren't getting the right readings. The next nurse said, 'Let me see if I can fix it.' Those nurses were going back and forth like crazy. When I said, 'What's happening?' they'd say, 'It's all right. We're just checking.' I said, 'Hey, look. Don't give me that. Something's going on. What is it? Whose heart is this?' Like broken records, they'd say, 'We're checking the monitor. Nothing serious.' I told 'em, 'It sounds like you've got a problem. *I've* got a problem. Call the doctor.' 'Oh, no,' they said, 'we can handle this. Don't worry so much.' I watched for a few more minutes. Talk about feeling helpless! I said, *'Look, I want a doctor in here.'* They said, 'Don't worry. We have a doctor on the phone.' I said, 'When you talk to him, tell him to get his cocktailed ass in here.' " Anderson's laugh is falsely hearty, as though he were laughing at a customer's tired joke. "They ignored me."

The next morning, did you complain to Dr. Lento?

"Sure. All he said was, 'They felt comfortable with what they were doing. They have the experience. If there were a real red flag on your condition, you'd have had people there. Don't worry about

it. They probably performed okay.' When I look back on that night,
I guess maybe they did. It's the unknown that you worry about.
Right? You don't find out the answers to the unknown until a day
later. If you're lucky." He scratches his head. "Sally was fit to be
tied. She said, 'If the doctors didn't come to somebody like you,
what would they do with a little guy working on the line?' I just
laughed at her. 'That's democracy, Sally. No special treatment.
They would've done the same thing! Not come in till the next
morning. We'll all go together when we go.' "

Since this third Bypass, are you better?

"Yes, but I haven't tested things much because it's only ten weeks.
I can exercise. I couldn't three months ago. How much? I don't
know yet. Next week, I've a date to play a little racquetball with
my son. Maybe then I'll find out more about how I'm doing."

What did they tell you about exercise?

"They don't tell you anything. This is the damndest operation.
Some places tell you lots. Some places tell you little or nothing.
They said, 'You have an internal barometer. We fixed your condition. Okay? As time permits, as your health recovers, you should
be able to do things you couldn't do. Without a problem. If you
have a problem situation, you will know. You'll get this message.
If you get a message, then we'll talk.' " His laugh is grim. "And I
thought only annual reports and lawyers spoke in generalities."

*Did they specify about singles or doubles, about jogging versus walk-
ing?*

"No limitations. No particular proscriptions—or prescriptions. All
that's left to your 'internal barometer.' "

*Having gone through three Bypasses, what was the worst part of this
one?*

"The recovery seemed to take forever. I had no—what's the word?—
tenacity. After two hours of being up and around, I'd be washed
out and have to sack out for a couple of hours. I wasn't improving.

For four weeks, I was flat. Nothing seemed to get better. The hospital had warned me I'd feel this way: 'This is the third time around. You've got age on you. You had a tough operation. You've got to restore and rebuild your blood supply. Your recovery's going to be drawn out. For heaven's sake, don't get despondent.' After four weeks, I called Dr. Lento long-distance and said, 'You know something? I think I'm going to get despondent. This recovery business is stretching out so damn long.' He said, 'It's not abnormal, hang in there. You'll be all right. Everything's in good shape.' "

Since this third Bypass, do you have a tendency to get depressed more readily?

"I told myself, 'You're not going to get depressed.' I was discouraged that it wasn't improving. I refused to think getting depressed was necessary. My wife was great. Superb. Better than she'd ever been before. She cooked the things I wanted. 'Do you want a drink? How about some ice cream? Let me help you. Let's go for a walk in the moonlight.' When I struggled for the right word—boy, I hate that!—when I took so long to get my strength back, she understood. Even now, I have trouble finding the damn word. Without her, I might have been very depressed."

Did you tell her?

"Only once. I don't want to ruin it."

You had said you'd take a gun rather than face another Bypass. Yet you went for number three.

"Time changes your views. Conditions change all those adamant assertions. I'm a practical guy. I had two professionals saying, 'If you don't want to live with this standard of living, this restricted set of conditions, you don't have much choice other than another Bypass. We'll check it out for you, find out whether you're a good candidate. We'll get the best guys lined up. If they agree you need the operation, you can decide whether you want to go through it a third time.' They looked me over. Dr. Lento said, 'I am a true professional. I can handle it. I can fix the problem. You're a good risk.' That softened the blow in deciding whether to go for it or not. That helped convince me maybe I ought to go through it one more time." Jed Anderson raps on the desk. "Knock wood, so far, so good. After the second Bypass, I never got better. After three months, I got worse. Things deteriorated. Life on those terms was unacceptable."

Since your third Bypass, are you better than you were at this time after your second go-round?

"A qualified yes. I can walk farther and longer than after that second one. Without angina, or tightness in my throat, or a knock in the shoulder blades. To me, that's an indication of some success. Because of the long recovery period, I haven't been equipped with the energy reserves to extend myself. As I keep pushing, I assume everything will be all right. I don't know how much 'all right.' With a little luck, maybe the plumbing leak's been fixed. Don't forget: this time, my business life isn't so pressing."

What made you decide to change your life?

"In these years, I've put the corporation back in good shape, the right people are in the right places. I can lie back and let somebody else run the show. Two years ago, I couldn't do that."

If the company were as it was two years ago, and you were as you are, what would you do?

"This time, I might back off. Even a country boy like me only has to be hit over the head with a two-by-four three times before he pays attention. This is the third time, yet I still don't think the heart problem is work-related. It's not class A or class B. I think it's heredity and chemistry. Whether I work hard or not, whether I eat too much cholesterol or not, isn't going to change my fate. It's in the genes. Whatever minute alterations might benefit the cardiac structure aren't worth modifying. They're not 'cost-effective' for the body's engineering. Why bother?" Anderson stops, scratches a little stain from the edge of his desk, then looks piercingly at me. "I hate being out of the business. Running the company is therapeutic. Those guys on the board just don't understand."

Having been through Bypass three times, do you have particular questions to advise a Bypasser to ask his physicians, before and after surgery?

"What was particularly helpful was being exposed to the process by which a cardiologist and a surgeon make up their minds that you're a good candidate and why. Dr. Lento's taking me and showing me the films, delineating the problem with a pointer, and indicating, 'This is correctable. There it is: here, here, and here. We can do this, fix that.' At Washington they explained the same way. Before my first two Bypasses at University, they didn't give me a chance to know the score. It would have been nice. All people are different. Not everybody wants to know, needs to know. I would query the cardiologist and the surgeon, because I felt more comfortable knowing what was going on. Both the cardiologist and the surgeon should detail what you'll be up against during recovery. They should tick off what's important to watch. Dr. Lento said, 'Look, Jed, when you get home, you're going to sweat a long recovery. Try not to get depressed. If you have any questions, here's my home telephone number. Call me at night, at home. I'm available for answers.'

"Bob Howland, the guy who did the first two, doesn't speak up. He's never been one to come out of the crowd. If everything goes all right, then getting fixed by a nontalker isn't so bad. If questions are circling in your head like planes stacked up for a landing at O'Hare, then the questions get magnified. Because you don't know what to expect, your concerns get blown out of proportion. Skill is the name of the game, but communication can't be discounted. Another doctor in Washington, well-known for his surgical prowess, would sweep into the CCU with his retinue, look at the patient's elbow from the middle of the room, say, 'How are you?' Without waiting for an answer, he'd make a U-turn and be out the door. His patients resented his impersonal manner. He may have been a genius with the knife, but he had zero personality. The last person in the line of Faithful Followers (FFs, I call 'em) would stay behind, his hand on the door, to answer questions. My doctor wasn't like that. Except on Saturday night, when he was out stepping."

When you came home, had you been instructed as to when you could drive?

Anderson laughs. "The second time, nobody had said anything, so I drove home from the hospital. About a hundred miles. This time, they said, 'Don't drive for a month.' Apparently, it takes time for all the anesthesia to escape the bloodstream. The reaction time is slower, the reflexes are down, which mightn't be good for me or the other driver. Besides, Lento had said, 'Don't louse up all my handiwork by cracking your chest on the steering wheel.' "

They told you to wait a month to drive. How long did you wait?

"Two weeks." Anderson's lopsided grin is engaging. "After three interviews I guess you know me better'n most people."

Why did you wait only two weeks, instead of four?

"I wanted to test things a little."

How long did they tell you to wait before having sexual relations?

"They never said a word. Three Bypasses and nobody's talked about sex. Maybe they figure CEOs are too busy making money to make love. I suppose Lento's crew knew I wasn't a neophyte. I'd been down this trail before. When you're in graduate school, you don't need to be taught your ABCs. Although"—Anderson shifts his big frame in the chair—"some people might need a refresher course. Anyway, they didn't talk sex. I waited three weeks. And it was fine. Just fine."

The first time, were you or Sally afraid?

"I wasn't. I don't know about Sally. She didn't say anything."

After each Bypass at University Hospital, you had complained about their cupping you. How was it in Washington?

"They don't do that. The physiotherapist encourages a breathing exercise: a big inhale, expand, and exhale out of your mouth. Once an hour. No cupping, not even one. I said, 'Oh, my God, this is super!' When I was at University Hospital, I tried to bribe the nurse not to cup me. This big fat nurse would come in and say, 'Now you've got to cough.' I'd tell her, 'I can't get anything up.' She'd say, 'Everybody else does.' In Washington, they're forever checking for rales. If people have problems with fluid in their lungs, they revert to plan B, the cupping, but they don't torture you routinely. There's enough to go through without what they call the 'pulmonary toilet.' They ought to flush that procedure down the toilet."

What did your operation cost? All the bills, doctors, and hospitals.

"About $35,000. The first one ran about $25,000; the second one was $28,000. This one was more, but times change. You have to allow for inflation. I had an angiogram out there. And this damn thing, this pacemaker, runs about $5,000. Time-and-a-half for working Sundays."

If you'd had to pay for number three, would you have had the operation?

"Sure, but I can afford it. If I were working on the line, on the third shift and making ten dollars an hour, had three kids at home, was paying off the car and the house and the dishwasher, I mightn't have been able to have a third one. Maybe I couldn't even have had one. I had the money. I couldn't live with a contracted compass. You put your money where your priorities are. I'd have had the third Bypass, even if I had to sell my boat."

Then you're glad you went for a third operation?

"Oh, yes. *Now*, I am."

When were you not glad? For how long?

"I was never too dissatisfied with the third Bypass. Following the operation, I was pretty uncomfortable. Up until about two weeks ago, I had no energy, no ambition. It seemed like forever."

What about pain?

"The physical discomfort only lasted four or five days. Mostly, I hurt from this pacemaker, from the lack of sleep. And my legs were a little sensitive. They cut me from here"—he points to his ankle, and traces a path up his legs—"all the way up to here, in my groin, on both sides, then down the back of one leg. I can't fault his playing hide-and-seek with my veins. I didn't have much left for him to use. He may've been slow, but he's sure. They healed beautifully. Take a look." Anderson slides his trouser legs up to reveal three fine lines up each leg.

How long did you hallucinate?

"A couple of days. Every time I closed my eyes, I'd see animals, I'd see blotches moving around the walls, moving closer to me. I'd see the walls moving. In between, I'd try to kid about it. 'Maybe I'm seeing into the future,' I thought. 'Maybe I'll see ways to extend the business.' I saw blueprints of computer schematics. I saw military hardware I didn't know existed. It was like a trip through outer space. But no new metal formulae, no new uses for metals."

You make it sound like a game. Did the hallucinations bother you?

"Oh, yes. Every time I closed my eyes, I'd see this stuff. If my eyes were open, I was okay. So I didn't like to close my eyes. If you fight to keep your eyes open, you don't sleep. Right? Then, I started hallucinating more from sleep deprivation. I didn't have any bladder control. No control like that." He shakes his head. "Strange, to be helpless like that. So lost. I'd never been there before. It was much tougher than the first two times." Anderson lets out a deep breath. "They took good care of me, but I had to go through that valley. Those events terrorized me. Even so, it's over." He scrapes again at the stain on the desk. "When you're going through all these aftereffects, you know they'll go away. *If*, if you can just last out those few tough weeks or months."

If you were recommending, would you recommend that hospital or would you recommend a hospital with a house staff?

"Sally says I'm a denier, that I defend doctors too much, but the house staff mayn't have been so important."

This time, do you think you're changing your life?

"The changes suit my purposes. Not because another cardiac insult threatens. The heart's finally been fixed. I think. I've got a few bucks. A nice big family." Anderson passes his hand over his eyes. "Not so big a family as I had before that punk took my daughter out for a ride in his junker and got her killed. That's something I can't forget. A life just wiped out. Poof! She was a good kid. Her death was so *undeserved*." He clears his throat, blows his nose in a big white monogrammed handkerchief. "Anyway, the other kids seem to be getting there. Sally and I might go sailing in Greece this summer. We're building a new place in Delaware. I've got things to do. I've got the business settled right. I don't have to be concerned about our shareholders, our management, our employees. The stock will come back. People keep asking about our stock. I can't tell you when for sure, but it'll be better." He drums his fingers on the desk. "I'm not the guy in charge any more. I'm the guy kicked upstairs. It's up to the boys in my office to put the company further on the road."

Clearing his throat, Anderson stands, slips into his suit jacket. "I've got a plane to catch. As always, I've enjoyed the discussion." Anderson's laugh is ironic. "As always, I hope we don't have to talk about another Bypass."

I hope we don't have to do it again either. When one of your directors told me you'd had a third go-round, I was a little uneasy about calling you. I was afraid you'd think I was bad luck.

"No. Your influence doesn't have anything to do with how my heart runs. Nevertheless, it's been an interesting year: going through this mill again, the testing, the decisions, the who, what, when, where. Now it's behind me, it's looking better. The heart's pumping well." He nods his head. "It's been interesting. Sally says the Chinese have a curse: 'May you live in interesting times.'

"Maybe 'interesting' isn't the right word. Since this third one, I've problems with word retrieval. But I say 'interesting' because I learned about myself and the world around me: How do you do these things? First, you've got to decide, to admit, you've got a problem. That's not too difficult. By comparative analysis, you can judge on the basis of facts. Once you get the information. Sometimes, it's a little hard to know how to get the data, where to get it, and how accurate it is.

"I'm keeping my fingers crossed that my new tailor did a better patch job than the old one did."

Now that you've had three Bypasses, how often does your own internist check you?

"I see Peter Conwell about once every six months. He doesn't say anything about when to come back. He still never says a word about diet or exercise."

Do you have an internist?

"Not that I see. The company runs an executive physical on us once a year, sends us over to a big clinic outside Dayton. They go over us for certain things. I guess the lead doctor's an internist."

If you were sick in the night, could you call him?

"Here in Elyria, I have a family doctor. 'Course, he's a surgeon." Jed Anderson grins sheepishly. "I know what you're getting at. I'd never take care of White's Metal Works the way I take care of Jed Anderson. Two of my directors have had Bypass. Their internists helped them get their act together. But finding a good internist who'll talk to you like a human being is as tough as finding a good stock in today's market."

5. Carole Cosby
Part-time sales clerk
Age at Bypass: 42

Carole Cosby is small and bouncy, with sequined red felt hearts appliquéd on her gray sweatshirt and sweatpants. "Valentine's Day is Tuesday," she explains. "I'm wearing my heart on my sleeve." Although she wears a running suit, she's carefully made up, complete with mascara and false eyelashes. Despite her many illnesses, she looks younger than her forty-five years, her mien remarkably cheerful. Her Bypass was three years ago, when she was only forty-two.

"One day, when I was at work, I blacked out for no reason. I have epilepsy. Most of the time, my seizures are controlled. I didn't know if I'd had a seizure or not. Since my Bypass, the doctor stopped the Dilantin, but I haven't had any trouble. It used to be when I'd get upset, I'd have a seizure."

Do you have grand mal epilepsy?

"No, no. Nothing like that. I black out. I can hear, but I can't respond. I get a warning: a little headache, blurred vision, and I know one's coming on. My epilepsy was in perfect control when, suddenly, this one week, I had four or five blackouts. I called my neurologist, who said, 'From what you're telling me, you ought to call a cardiologist.' I said, 'What for?' He said, 'It doesn't sound like epilepsy. It sounds like heart trouble.' I never even called my internist. He was the kind who'd say, 'It's all nerves, Honey.' Whenever a woman calls him, 'It's all nerves.' Before I found out I had epilepsy, I went through the wringer. I called a cardiologist. I got a name from somebody. He found an 'irregularity,' but 'nothing substantial.' Every three months, I went back to him. After about a year, out of the blue, I got high blood pressure. He told me I was in the Stroke Belt area. I wish I were in the Sun Belt area instead." She smiles brightly. "As a matter of fact, when we went to a weight-reduction clinic in the South, I got my first severe angina attack. When I got off the plane, I started with these horrible pains in my chest, nausea, and cold sweats. I have a hernia, but this wasn't hernial pain. It knocked me over. Like getting a shock."

At forty-two, most premenopausal women are resistant to heart disease. Their hormones protect them.

"I had a hysterectomy when I was thirty-six."

Is there any heart trouble in your family?

"My father's first heart attack was at forty-two. Just like me. He died at fifty-three. Neither my brother nor my sister has heart disease. My mother's fine. She works every day." She stops, looks into the middle distance, then says faintly, "Nobody else has epilepsy. Thank God, my children don't have epilepsy."

When you got this pain, what did you do?

"We went to the motel. I lay in bed for two days. I kept throwing up. The pain got worse. Finally, I said to my husband, 'You'd better take me to the hospital.' When I got to the hospital, they put me in Intensive Care for ten days. They said I had unstable angina. When I came home, I changed internists. I'd had enough.

"The chest pains kept getting worse. I flunked three stress tests. Every time I flunked, I got a new medicine. Nothing helped. Not beta blockers, not calcium antagonists. Nothing. Finally, I said to Dr. Bernhardt, 'I can't go on like this.' He said, 'You're right. We have to do something about you.' He got on their backs, the cardiologist and all the muckety-mucks. He forced them to do an angiogram, which showed 70 percent blockage of one of the main arteries. They said, 'Let's wait till it gets worse. Let's try some other new medications. They tried. I tried. Nothing helped. In '81, six months later, my internist pushed for another angiogram. This time, the artery was almost completely closed. In six months, it had shut tight. Two weeks later, Dr. Haku did the Bypass." Her voice drops to a faint whisper "I can't stand Dr. Haku."

As a person or as a doctor?

"You can't separate them. Look, my Bypass was a failure. Maybe it'd have been a failure with somebody else. But Dr. Haku is a failure as a human being. He's a flat-faced, flat-voiced, inhumane automaton. Let me tell you. The night before the operation, Dr. Haku came in. That's the first time in my life I'd seen the man who was s'posed to fix my heart up for me. He insisted my mother and my sister be there. He didn't want to talk to me alone. He walked in with a chalkboard, propped it up on the windowsill, and proceeded to draw all this stuff, the heart and the arteries. One-two-three, he told us everything that's going to be. It's tough when you're a layman. You don't know what questions to ask, like, 'What happens? How long will I be sick? Should my kids come home from college? How long will the Bypass last? Is it guaranteed? Will my arteries close up again? Will I be bedridden?' Things like that. He did say, 'The chances of your needing another Bypass are about three percent.' My sister verified this. She's got a good memory. Then, he erased his chalkboard."

Did Dr. Haku give you a little sketch to keep?

"Nothing, nothing. To me, it's a cold, calculated way of doing business. In fifteen minutes, he was out of there. For the life of me, I couldn't tell you what he said."

Did any of you ask any questions?

"I was in a state of shock. I knew I ought to talk to this man, but he didn't want to talk to me. I wanted to ask him all kinds of questions, but I didn't know what to ask. I guess he plans it that way."

In the year before that episode of severe angina down South, did your stresses intensify?

"There's something I should tell you. I was separated from my husband. We were separated for three years."

When did you get back together?

"Fifteen months ago."

After the Bypass?

"Right."

Didn't you go to the weight-reduction clinic with him?

"We were still married." Carole Cosby lifts her chin defiantly. "What's so wrong with that?"

I didn't mean that. You were still friends.

"Good friends. We loved each other. We couldn't live together."

What made you come back together?

"My heart surgery helped a lot. For the first time, you realize life is very short. Even without heart surgery, you haven't got much time around here. Things you were picayune about ten years ago don't matter. What's important is caring for somebody and having somebody who wants to take care of you. When I found out the Bypass didn't work, I was pretty frightened. That's scary. Two months before my Bypass, my husband told me he'd met a woman he wanted to marry. He asked me for a divorce! Two months before Bypass, we went to a lawyer. I didn't want to give him a divorce. We couldn't live together, but I loved him. At that point, I hated him. His timing was so unfair."

What happened?

"I held off on the divorce. After the Bypass, my recuperation was terribly slow. Every time I went to the doctor, I'd say, 'I still have pain. I have the same chest pain, just as bad.' He'd say, 'You've got to wait. This is healing pain. You've got to give the muscles time to heal, the nerves time to knit. Give it six months.' After six months, I was just as bad. My internist said, 'Maybe you're a slow healer. Give it another six months.' At the end of a year, he said, 'We should have another angiogram.' Funny, the way they all say 'we' when they mean 'thee.' '*We*' had another angiogram. The Bypass had closed. Completely. They were supposed to bypass two vessels, but they only did one. It had shut down tighter'n a union shop during a strike." Carole Cosby sighs. "So there I was with a broken marriage and a broken Bypass." She sighs again. "If I'd been better prepared for the Bypass and its aftermath, I wouldn't be so downhearted now."

Tell me about your Bypass preparation. Had you been told beforehand that you'd have a tube in your mouth when you awakened?

"No, no. When I couldn't speak, I thought I'd had a stroke. Nobody gave me any preliminary instruction. Most places take you on a tour of the surgical room, show you the machines, the life-support systems, the procedure, so you and your family won't be so frightened. I didn't see anything. I didn't know anything. When I couldn't talk, I got so frustrated. They gave me a pencil and paper. I couldn't see what I was doing. I could only grope around."

Was your husband there?

"He wasn't there. I wanted him to come on his own, because he wanted to, not because I needed him. He knew I was having Bypass. Afterwards, he wanted to visit me, but I wouldn't allow it."

Why?

"When I had Bypass, who knew whether I'd live or die? If he couldn't be with me when it was most crucial, coming in when it's all over to say, 'Hey, I'm glad you came through,' is unnecessary."

After Bypass, did you become irritable?

"Not irritable. Depression was my big problem. As soon as I went home to that empty house, I sunk into such a blue funk. I had no one to take care of me. I didn't know what would happen to me. I wanted to stay in the hospital for a couple of days more, but they insisted on sending me home. They make you wait five or six weeks in that hospital just sitting around keeping your place in line for Bypass. Afterwards, they ship you home before you're ready. Being alone after Bypass is frightening. I got weepy and despondent. Dr. Bernhardt put me on some antidepressant which freaked me out. I got horrible nightmares. I'd wake up shaking, in a cold sweat. I stopped the medicine. I couldn't understand why I wasn't getting better. Bypass was supposed to alleviate all that chest pain. I had as much angina as before. They kept saying, 'Just be patient.' "

Did you tell anybody, 'I'm afraid to be alone'? Your mother? Your children?

"Only my doctor. When he said, 'You could have a visiting nurse,' I decided against it."

After all that, how did you and your husband reunite?

"Our reconciliation is the only beneficial result of my Bypass. I was at my cousin's house for Thanksgiving dinner. My kids were home for the holiday. At that time, I wasn't talking to him. When he asked me for a divorce before my Bypass, I stopped speaking to him. He'd been pushing me to go to court. He wanted to get married to her. My doctor wouldn't let me go to court. The only time I'd call him was when he was late with the check. He walked into my cousin's house. When I saw him, I thought I'd have a heart attack. My heart started pounding. I could hear it beating so fast, I couldn't catch my breath. I started crying. I didn't know where to hide; I ran out the front door. My son grabbed me and said, 'Mom, where are you going?' I said, 'Leave me alone.' I didn't hate my husband, but I felt so abandoned. When I needed him most, he had forsaken me. I couldn't greet him as though nothing had happened. It would be like forgiving him. He came over and kissed me. I thought I'd pass right out. Finally, I left.

"He called me and said, 'We should be friends. We should talk.' I said, 'You only want to get me to court.' He said, 'No, let's be friends.' Then, we both were invited to an anniversary party. When he asked me to go with him, I said, 'Good. You can pay for the anniversary gift.' That night, he said, 'When I saw you on Thanksgiving, I knew I always loved you. You're so beautiful. I want to embrace you. When I see how beautiful you are, I can't understand why things changed.' After two months, he told his friend, even before he told me, 'I'm going back to my wife. I'm going to ask her if she'll take me back. I like you, but I love her. I want to be with her.' After that, when we went out, he'd sleep over at my house."

When you went home from the hospital, did anybody talk to you about when you could resume sexual intercourse?

"Seeing as I didn't have a husband around, I guess they didn't bother saying anything. When I went for my six-week checkup to the surgeon, I asked. He kind of pursed his lips." Setting her face censoriously, Carole Cosby mimics her surgeon; " 'If you feel well enough, if you feel you *need* it, then go ahead.' That's all."

Is your desire and your ability to come to orgasm the same?

"My desire is the same, maybe better. I don't have the same steam. I liked making love for a long time. Since Bypass, I can't do that. I get so tired. You can't imagine how tired I get. Sometimes, I feel as though I'm 102. It embarrasses me. The foreplay tires me out. Intercourse itself exhausts me. I used to go on for a long time. I could come six or seven times. Not any more. I like to make love just as often, at least two or three times a week, but long, lingering lovemaking wears me out. That's a loss. If my Bypass hadn't closed right up, I bet it'd be different. Since Bypass, my ability to sustain physical exertion is more limited. Bypass made me feel so old. Thank God, my husband is understanding."

Does he know?

"Oh, yes. He knows. Since we've gone back together, we discuss everything. No more faking. I open my mouth; I tell him my most intimate feelings."

Does he speak as freely to you?

"I try to make him. I'm more open than he is."

What if a physician said, 'Mrs. Cosby, I think you should have another Bypass'?

"Dr. Bernhardt just said it. After this last angio, my third one, they called me up to University Hospital for a conference. When I walked in, there's three doctors sitting there, each one with a long face. I didn't know what was going on. They simply said, 'Carole, we're sorry. The Bypass has closed, along with the graft. Your body rejected its own saphenous vein. We can't explain why.' I said, 'What's next? What do I do now?' They said, 'We don't know.' I said, 'What do you mean, you don't know? Am I supposed to walk around like this until I drop dead?' The surgeon said, 'We don't know if the same thing would happen again. We wouldn't want to use your saphenous vein again, because the first one was rejected.' I said, 'Hey, okay. Use somebody else's. I don't care.' Use a pig's or a plastic one. As long as it works, I don't care. The cardiologist said, 'We can't do anything for you. We don't feel University Hospital is the place for you.' I didn't even ask, 'Why?' I was in shock. What does a patient say, when a doctor says, 'Go away?' What would *you* say?"

Did they suggest some other hospital or medical center?

"Nothing. When I walked out of there, I said to Dr. Bernhardt, 'What the hell's going on?' He said, 'They don't want you, Carole. It's as simple as that. They don't want to be responsible for you.' I said, 'Can a doctor do that?' He said, 'They think they can do whatever they want, because they're University Hospital. Even though Bypass didn't help you this time, I'll send you to another cardiologist.'

"The new cardiologist has scheduled another angiogram; then we'll decide where to go. Out of town for sure. I couldn't be talked into having another one here. This town's medicine has left a bad taste in my mouth. I even wonder about the epilepsy. I've been off Dilantin for three years. Once I started taking heart pills, I never blacked out. Not even once. He sends me for a CAT scan every year. They do it next-door to his office."

In a few hospitals, there's a full-time Bypass counselor. Would routine hospital counseling have helped you?

"Definitely. There were all men on my floor. Every day, the 'therapist' would come in and say, 'Okay, it's exercise time.' I'd go out in the hall with these four guys. Their wives were there. I'd think, 'Those exercises couldn't possibly be good for me; they're all explicitly for men.' It was like I was there, but not there, as though, 'You should do what the other guys are doing.' I'm not one of the other guys. I'm me. I'm not even a guy. When I realized their exercises were geared to men, I asked for exercises for female Bypassers. They got very huffy. 'We're not prepared for female Bypassers. We don't have anything special for women. Most Bypassers are male.' I couldn't believe my ears. Twenty-one percent of Bypassers are female. That's forty thousand a year.

"When I was in Intensive Care, all that separates the beds is a little sheet half-hanging. That's fine and dandy. But I'm a very private person. Most women are. If the ICU were all-female, that public nudity wouldn't bother me. With a man to the right of me and a man to the left of me, it's embarrassing. The ICU is not a place to win friends and influence people."

What should hospitals do particularly for female Bypassers?

"Women should have a separate unit. At a few hospitals there's a separate unit. When I got sick, I had a room, a beautiful nice room, with a camera, monitors, the works. The danger of infection is less; they can see you. Not every hospital can afford that setup, but women should be given privacy. They shouldn't be treated like lesser meat."

What about seeing your family? Some hospitals won't let you see your family for three days after Bypass.

"That's fine. For the first couple of days, it's better for the family and better for the patient. When my family came to see me right after Bypass, I don't remember it. Afterwards, when I was better,

I wanted them. Even then, visitors aren't the main thing. For the longest time, I had to go to the bathroom in a bedpan, which I detested. Especially with a male audience. When I was able to get out of bed, I said, 'May I go to the bathroom?' She said, 'You're not allowed.' 'Why not? I'm allowed to walk.' 'You can't go to the bathroom because we have nobody to go in there with you.' I said, 'If I get in trouble, there's a string I can pull. When you're in labor, after the enema, they send you alone to the bathroom. That's lots more dangerous.' She said, 'We can't be responsible for something happening to you.'

"They brought in this chair, this commode. You're supposed to sit on it. I raised holy hell. 'In no way, on God's green earth, will I sit on this potty chair with a man over there, and a man over here. I want privacy.' They said, 'You can't go to the bathroom.' I said, 'In that case, I won't go until I explode.' They brought in everybody, all with the same slogan: 'Carole, you're so unreasonable.' I told them: 'I don't care. Did you ever think how unreasonable hospitals are? First of all, I feel as though I'm in a zoo. To me, this Grand Central Station is second only to hell. This is the worst place in the world to try to get better.' With all that hullaballoo, I got chest pain; my heart started beating fast and loud, the machines started going haywire. After they got the heartbeat quieted down with medication, I conned a nurse into letting me go to the bathroom. It was heaven."

What explicit questions should people ask their internist, their cardiologist, and their surgeon, before and after Bypass?

"Only my internist ever answered my questions and talked to me. Because he thought the surgeon had explained everything, even that talk was after the fact. The whole surgical process should be explained in detail. They should show every procedure, what it's for, why they're doing it, what its purpose is, how long you'll be on it, whether it'll hurt and where it'll hurt, what to expect. They should tell you how many days you'll be in the Intensive Care zoo, what to expect in Intensive Care, what you can and cannot do.

"What I resent most about doctors, hospitals, surgery, institutional behavior, is their attitude. When they examine me, they don't see me as a whole human being. They put me in a category with a hundred other people. I'm not a hundred other people. I'm me.

My innards don't work like a hundred other people's. Obviously, mine didn't, or my Bypass would've been a success. I don't like being treated like an animal in a stockyard, where they're putting me through one of those little gates, stamping me, and getting me ready for the slaughter. I don't like it at all. The doctors don't tell you anything. They think they're too busy and too important. They figure the nurses will tell you what you need to know. The nurses don't tell you anything. Whatever you ask, they repeat the same line—'I'm sorry. You'll have to ask your doctor.' Everything is hurry, scurry. While they're scurrying, they're screwing you around."

Should hospitals have an ombudsman, somebody who investigates your complaints, and tries to ameliorate them?

"Definitely. When I was in the hospital, the surgeon never saw me. He sent his entourage, another thing I don't like. I'm not a groupie. The cardiologist was so stiff and distant." She makes a frozen face. "I don't mean to disparage him. When you talk to a doctor, he should volunteer information. You shouldn't have to pull teeth. They should recommend rehab classes. When I said, 'How much should I walk?' they said, 'Walk at your own pace.' They've got this one liner: 'Do what you feel you can do.' How do you know what you can do unless you push your limits? How do you know whether you're pushing too much? Or not enough? I'm a middle child. Middle children give more love, but they need more love. They don't ask questions."

Did Bypass make you aware of what you wished you'd done with your life?

"That's why I patched it up with my husband. Bypass made me realize I was all alone. Bypass made me wonder how I'd make it financially. How long could I work? I'm a sales clerk. That's no big-deal job. Mostly, they call me during rush season. Bypass made me want someone who cared about me and what's happening to me. My mother loves me dearly; there's nothing my mother wouldn't do for me. But my mother's getting older; she's been through so much heartache. It breaks my heart to tell her what's happening to me. How much can she take?"

Even though Bypass hasn't helped your heart disease, has Bypass changed you in other ways?

"I'm more mellow. I don't lose my temper so quickly. My husband says I've come a long way; that's only because *he* has. One thing complements the other. We've both come to understand that life is short. My heart's gotten progressively worse. After I have that next angiogram, my new cardiologist predicts Bypass will be in the cards."

You've had three angios and you're having a fourth. Do you mind the angiogram?

"Never. While they're doing it, I talk to them. They put me at ease. They're great. It doesn't hurt. Nobody should be afraid of the angiogram. I've heard people say, 'Oh, it's horrible!' It's not horrible. No way. They keep you tranquilized, but alert. The pain is nothing. The flush is no big deal. A kidney x-ray, an IVP, give the same flush. I'm allergic to the dye; before and after, they give me steroids. Even the sandbag isn't much. Because they explained it all, I understood the whys and wherefores. If I have another Bypass, I want it soon. I don't want my heart trouble to interfere with my life. We're going abroad for the first time. I'd never go before. I'm deathly afraid of flying."

You've been through all this and you're 'deathly afraid of flying'?

"We all have our weaknesses," she notes acidly. "Some of us don't like to go to the bathroom in front of men. They defeated ERA with the fake issue of unisex bathrooms, didn't they? Hospitals should have special facilities for women, no matter what. They get paid enough. Hospitals should consider the woman patient. That's part of recovery. Another thing: look at this." She lifts her sweatshirt to reveal a red, ropey keloid between her breasts. "Isn't that horrible? It's the grossest thing I've ever seen. It hurts. I bought out an alcohol factory, practically. Alcohol helps some, but not a lot. I tried to have plastic surgery; they said, 'No, you can't.' It's painful. In the hospital, my breasts would pull on the incision. If they'd told me to wear a bra, the wound itself would've been much less painful. It would've healed better. The bra would've held up my bust. When I got home, I put on a bra. I didn't stop wearing a bra for months. I wore it day and night, just a loose bra, like after you have a baby. A Bali Flower bra.[1] I never wear a low dress. I used to have such a nice bust, with a lovely cleavage. Now, all I have is a hollow wasteland with an ugly snake burrowing down the middle. Women tend to be vain about their looks. Maybe men make us vain, I don't know. But doctors should tell women about the possibility of keloids. Women get them more than men. My cardiologist said, 'It's ridiculous to be self-conscious.' How would he know? He's never had one. I sleep with a little tiny down pillow between my breasts. Even though it rubs the scar, it's soothing. It separates my bust, so one boob doesn't pull over the other. When it's hot and I sweat, the scar burns." She stops and looks piercingly at me. "Did anybody ever tell you about the hands? Since Bypass, I don't have strength in my hands. I can't even open a ketchup bottle. If you're used to counting on your own strength and suddenly it's gone, it's hateful. Like everything is slipping away."

Since Bypass, have you had any memory loss?

"My memory is terrible since my heart surgery. It's strange you should ask me that."

Memory loss is a common aftereffect.

"You're kidding me. I thought I was getting senile. Since Bypass, I'm so forgetful. I can be talking to somebody and forget his name. My mind goes blank. I double-check my accounts. I worry about epilepsy, but it's not a seizure."

Is the memory loss better or worse?

"Worse. Don't forget, the first year, I only thought about myself. After that, my husband and I put it together. Going into marriage and becoming responsible for two people puts more strain on my memory."

[1] As noted in Comfort Station (p. 412), another woman Bypasser recommends the Mary Jane Sleeping Bra.

Perhaps you yearn to go back to being the same girl you once were.

"I don't want to go back. I'm not so dumb. I know I can't go back to the same girl I was. Who wants her? But I don't remember what I do with things. I used to have instant recall. I had a fine memory. Forgetting bothers me. I get so frustrated."

Does it make you less upset to know that memory loss happens to other Bypassers?

Regretfully, she makes a little *moue*. "To be honest, that's no consolation. People only care what happens to them. That's the truth about all of us. Would *you* care? When people make generalizations, I don't like it. We're not all the same. I am me. I'm an individual. I like to be unique. If I were running a hospital, I wouldn't let it be such a big institutionalized zoo. I'd try to make people feel they counted. Otherwise, why try to make them better? Unless it's to keep the zoo in business." She giggles.

"When my Bypass failed or never took, my doctor suggested I try biofeedback. First, I had to come to terms with myself, to see if I was ready to delve into those dark places that I've closed off. I don't know if I'm ready now. I'm preparing myself. In my own life, I had a lot of things to forgive, but not forget."

It's a good idea to forget, too. Until you forget, you don't forgive.

"It's not easy to forget. Now we can joke about the past, a sense of humor is life's saving grace. I say, 'You never paid forty dollars for a bottle of perfume for me, all the years we were married, but you ran out and bought her a keg of Joy.' Little things. He often says, 'How long will I have to pay for this . . . little lapse? The rest of my life?' I say, 'Perhaps so.' "

Weren't you tempted to find somebody else?

"I didn't have time. He asked me the same thing. When I came back from that trip down South, I was sick at heart, then I had Bypass surgery. I waited a year to find out my Bypass didn't work. Before the two operations, my kids were still living at home, like a pair of live-in chaperones. My husband said, 'You're my mother. Mothers don't do that sort of thing.' "

Your husband said that?

"I mean, my son. What a Freudian slip! My son said, 'It's all right for Daddy to have girlfriends and go out. It's not all right for Mommy to have boyfriends.' Even in divorce, there's a double standard. He made me so mad. I couldn't believe he felt that way. But he did. And he let me know." She drums her enameled nails on the desk.

"Patching a marriage is like having a Bypass. You never know if it'll work. I only hope my marriage works better than my Bypass. With my second Bypass, I hope it'll work as well as the new marriage we're trying."

6. Jordan Bredely, Ph.D.
Headmaster, boy's preparatory school
Age at Bypass: 37

With his rusty-brown hair, red beard, and bushy red brows, his large bay window covered by an old-fashioned waistcoat, and suitably chained by a gold pocket watch from which the requisite Phi Beta Kappa key dangles, Dr. Jordan Bredely, headmaster of the Governor Hay School in Asheville, North Carolina, towers over me. As he settles me and my tape recorder on a damask-covered Queen Anne love seat in his house near the exclusive boys' school he governs, he explains, "I didn't want you to come to the office. Too many people, trustees of the school, parents, even erstwhile 'colleagues' who want my job, are eager because I've had Bypass to categorize me as 'sick.' I'm only forty-one; I was thirty-seven when I had my Bypass. The job market is not as fertile as the gossip mill for men like me. I don't want to jeopardize my position here."

Tell me how you came to Bypass, what problems you had with your job and with Bypass's aftermath.

"Before I came here, I was director of placement at the Coolidge School in Las Vegas, an exceedingly competitive prep school. Out of 120 students, even kids in the bottom half of the class were successfully applying to the Ivy Leagues. Most of the Ivy application deadlines are January first. My coronary was December twenty-ninth, two days before all the Ivies were due. There was *tremendous* pressure on me in the three months preceding my infarct. At the time, I'd been at the Coolidge School for fifteen months."

Why were you under so much pressure? Weren't the students the ones in the pressure cooker?

"The first year, I got my feet wet, learned the ropes. If not everybody made the grade, I was the new kid on the block, so it wasn't my fault. By that second year, I had to demonstrate my ability. There wasn't enough staff to handle the paperwork and phone calls. I had to write all the school recommendations, the heat was on to recommend 120 kids, most of whom I hadn't known and hadn't worked with until just that September. I had to get to know them and their talents well enough to write valid, convincing recommendations. At the same time, I was dealing with colleges, fielding balls from juniors and sophomores who were antsy about college, having to do guidance programs for them and for their parents. It was a high-pressure job, sixteen to eighteen hours a day, seven days a week. Fortunately, or unfortunately, depending on how I feel in the midnight hours, four years before, I had been divorced. I had no family pressures on me to be home for dinner at a regular hour." Dr. Bredely sighs. "My divorce's rawness, the scalding inside, had eased. You look quizzical. By '79, the divorce was no longer a causal factor in my having a coronary." He sighs again. "At least, I don't think so."

Why did you go to Las Vegas?

"How do the computer people phrase it? I wanted 'hands-on' experience to decide whether I wanted to be a headmaster or a college-placement director, whether I wanted to teach, whether I'd be willing to starve in a garret and write. As you can see"—Bredely pats his broad belly—"starving isn't my métier. Before I went to Coolidge, I'd looked around for three years for the right school, not just an interesting job in itself, but a launching pad if I wanted to be a career headmaster. The Coolidge School seemed to have everything, at least on paper. When I got out there, I discovered I didn't want to be a headmaster. Ever, ever, ever. I made that discovery shortly before I had the coronary."

About your marriage, how long had you been married?

"Two years."

Not long.

"We had known each other for fourteen years before we married. We were the 'perfect couple,' everybody said at our wedding. I'm afraid I'm one of those old-fashioned people who believe there is only one marriage for each person. I still feel sad about the marriage breaking up, yet we were destroying each other in the marriage. You can't go on like that." Bredely lights a cigarette. "Or so she said. And yet, and yet—she's never remarried either. We're still two people wandering around looking for each other, and not able to find each other when we were there."

Tell me how you learned you had heart trouble.

"The thing was so strange. Like many people, I didn't know the signs of a coronary. For someone my age, I was completely stupid. With all the big neon signs posted for me, I should have been more conscious about the potential for a coronary. But I wasn't."

You weren't that old. You were—

"Thirty-seven, but when you get towards forty, you should be aware of what the hell is possible. Particularly if you're overweight and have a tendency to high blood pressure. For a week or two before the coronary, I felt logy, so listless and draggy. It was Christmas. A dear friend from Cardiff, who, since my divorce, has been the great love of my life, was coming to visit. Because I was in the throes of getting the students squared away with college applications, we decided we'd wait till January first for our time together. I'd worked until midnight that particular day, snapped on the TV to see what was happening in the world, and immediately had fallen asleep.

"I came to, because I was very uncomfortable. I couldn't figure out what the hell was the matter. It felt like indigestion, but my arm was numb. I couldn't get comfortable, no matter what I did. From two in the morning until noon, I kept getting up and taking showers, using a heating pad, everything to make myself more comfortable. I was charged up with the work, so I attributed the discomfort to tension. I couldn't think of anything I'd eaten to give me indigestion. Believe it or not, I hadn't eaten much either, because I wanted to get some weight off before my friend arrived from London. I didn't know what to do. I tried to think of somebody I could call who wouldn't laugh at me for being a hypochondriac, because a little voice inside me began insisting, 'Maybe this is a heart attack.' The only person I could think of to call was my sister back in Mississauga. From Las Vegas, I called her and told her how I was feeling. Talk about long-distance advice. She said, 'I would go to the hospital Emergency Room, and I would get there as quickly as possible. It might be heart, it might be gall bladder, but it's important for you to go. And right away.' Then, she said, 'And don't get smart and ride your bicycle to the hospital.' I drove myself to the Emergency Room, where they treated me with great speed, care, and urgency." Bredely laughs hollowly.

Did you have a doctor?

"Of course not! What did I need a doctor for? I was thirty-seven, in the best of health." His laugh is self-mocking. "In the Emergency Room, I lucked out. There was a very good, very unusual resident on duty, who was candid about my condition. He suggested an internist who worked out of that hospital, someone he respected. The internist came in and took over. He recommended a cardiologist for me. Between them, they took good care of me. I was only in the hospital for ten days."

What made you have Bypass surgery?

"As we neared the point where we'd agreed I'd go back to work, my cardiologist thought it made sense for me to be catheterized first. My sister was against the catheterization. I agreed with the cardiologist. As I lay on the catheterization table, he showed me those three major blockages on the screen. Let's see, where were they? The left main, the left circumflex, and the left anterior descending. How's that for a fellow who got his one D in high school biology? It ended up a quadruple Bypass. 'So long as you're in there,' they said, 'you might as well fix everything that needs patching.' "

Did you go back to school that semester?

"Not for any teaching, just for graduation, which was my responsibility. By the time they did the cath, it was St. Patrick's Day. By the time they did the Bypass, it was Shakespeare's birthday. That's April twenty-third," Bredely instructs. "When it's *your* job at stake, *festina lente*—make haste slowly—seems to be the name of the game. In some ways, you collude in the doctors' dilatoriness. After the angiogram, even after Bypass, you fantasize, 'Maybe this is all a medical ruse for the doctors to make money. How do *I* know I had a heart problem?' All I endured, apart from the pain of Bypass surgery, was mild discomfort on one occasion. But seeing the blockages on catheterization is a reality which shoots down these denial fantasies. You don't deny consciously; you consider yourself too intelligent for such game-playing. Yet if you're called upon to do something you know you shouldn't, you think, 'I'm all right. I feel terrific. The problem doesn't exist.' That kind of wishful thinking persists, especially with someone my age."

Bredely lights another cigarette. "Everyone wants to lump you with all those people who've had heart Bypasses. If anybody discovers you've had Bypass, he immediately knows someone seventy or seventy-five who's had it. There's this age thing that bugs the hell out of me, in terms of what other people do, how they deal with me. There's the syndrome where people say, 'If you've had Bypass surgery, obviously you still have terrible angina. In case of emergency, where do you keep your pills?' All this hyperreactive response to a Bypasser contributes to his desire for denial."

You don't like being lumped with all those other Bypassers? You want citizenship in the World of the Well?

" 'The World of the Well'! What an obnoxious phrase. It's not a yearning for 'the World of the Well'—necessarily—but everybody is different. You can't huddle every bum heart into some Bypassers' concentration camp. I want to be treated as a unique individual. I get very angry when people start categorizing me by my Bypass." Bredely blows a perfect smoke ring, obviously the result of practice. "I got pretty sore at my family, too, for the way they behaved with the Bypass.

"They decided somebody should fly out from Mississauga. 'You're having major surgery; you're all alone in Nevada. Somebody's got to be with you.' They were all solicitude and honey. I didn't feel someone had to be with me.

"My mother would've been more trouble than it was worth. My sister is petrified of flying. My brother was out of a job; that's his specialty, unemployment. Suddenly, he became the epitome of devotion, calling me, telling me how he'd take care of me. It turned out he wanted a free trip to Nevada, which I'd pay for. When I nixed the deal, he was incensed at me because I'd ruined his trip. Of course, when I moved back from Nevada to Toronto, everyone was much too busy to help lifting boxes, or getting cupboards in order. My family was great at pious platitudes by long distance. When I returned to home territory, they were absent from school the day they taught familial help. When I came back, I particularly needed emotional support. It wasn't there. These are ancient family crystals of nonallegiance, which the Bypass precipitated out. That's a pretty mixed metaphor, isn't it?"

When you had Bypass, was your friend from Cardiff there?

"She had to go back. She's a history professor; classes were beginning. After the heart attack, she postponed her return for three days, until the doctors said everything was under control. She can only afford to come to the States once a year. I go there in the summer. It's a helluva way to conduct a relationship, but that's the way it is." Bredely lights another cigarette. "She's another reason I feel guilty about all this Bypass monkey business."

Why would you feel guilty?

"Guilty that I've wasted time. Guilty that I've not been able to work towards goals I'd set for myself. After Bypass, I spent two years finding a full-time position. The sifting-out process became exceedingly onerous to me. At the Coolidge School, I had job stability going for me; I had a future. Suddenly, it was like starting out all over again, only you're not young any more. Not old, mind you, but not young. I feel guilty about time wasted until I get to a secure level where I have the freedom and the wherewithal to do things."

Many people say they feel guilty. It's hard for me to understand why.

"It's as though somebody came in and stole time away from you. Yet you feel guilty because you caused the theft."

If I stole from you, I should feel guilty. Not you.

"I know, but I'm not the only one who blames me. When I moved back to Mississauga, I said to my mother, 'This saga of heart attack and coronary Bypass certainly has reversed the course of my life. It's like a tornado struck my whole world.' She said, '*Well!* I don't know why you think that way. You brought it all on yourself.' I said, 'What do you mean by that?' She said, 'You're the one who didn't eat properly, didn't exercise, got divorced, ran around with women.' She made me feel anew that it was my fault for having a heart attack. I wanted to say, 'What about those hereditary factors? We don't know all the causal factors, but I don't think you can safely assume it's a question of immoral living.' She sees life, especially my life, through a puritanical lens. She made me feel so guilty, so damned depressed."

Did you feel guilty and depressed immediately after Bypass?

"Not until I came back to Mississauga."

What made you return to Mississauga?

"Because I had family there. Foolishly, I thought family was an important draw. I'd been wanting to write this novel for years. I figured, 'I can write anywhere. I had this close call, this brush with death. It's time to appreciate my family more, be with them more.' Quickly, I discovered I was the only one who wanted to give. Everyone else thought, 'To hell with him. Who is he, anyway? Box him up and ship him somewhere else.' "

Did the Coolidge School offer you a contract for the next year?

"They did. With a fair-sized raise, to boot. I turned the contract down. I wish I'd had some counseling. Occupational counseling ought to be a must at every hospital performing Bypass. I figured, 'Everything's been good until now. Why shouldn't it continue to be?' I didn't see changing jobs as a big deal. I'd made a good recovery. Everything would be just dandy." Bredely lights another cigarette from the lit tip of the last one. "A lot of my troubles were the shifting nature of the job market for academicians, the demographic decline of students in Canada and in the northeastern United States, but something else tipped the scales. My headmaster had written me a terrific recommendation, but in it, he mentioned my leaving Nevada because of a heart attack and Bypass surgery. Schools look at the most recent letter. Here's this glowing recommendation, but all the school sees is 'heart attack.' If you're the headmaster, and you see this balloon coming in for an interview, you say to yourself, 'God, he's only thirty-seven. He looks like a linebacker for the Green Bay Packers, and he's had a heart attack. No, we don't want to hire him.' I know for a fact, several schools turned thumbs down because of the coronary and the Bypass. The decision to leave the Coolidge School, to leave Las Vegas, where I had stability and friends, where I had everything going for me, was incredibly naive—and self-destructive.

After Bypass, did you have any routine psychosocial counseling?

"Not from anybody trained. The doctors are concerned with the short-term aspects: to get you through surgery and the immediate in-hospital recovery. Then, you're on your own. No one said anything about job implications. The closest anyone came was the cardiologist, who said, 'When you're sending out your résumé, make no reference whatsoever to Bypass surgery.' I was astonished. I asked him, 'Why?' He said, 'It's better to omit such details.' Nobody discussed job problems. I've thought a great deal about the need for routine psychological and occupational counseling. It's absolutely mandatory, but I'm not sure how it should be set up. Bypassers range from their twenties to their eighties. Their occupations differ markedly. If you're already retired, your problems are different from someone who's younger and working, who's feeling shut out of career opportunities. A lot of Bypassers I've talked to felt stranded afterwards, alienated from their families, their work places, the goals they'd set for themselves. Patients need to be made aware that these estrangements might occur, what actions or strategies could help avoid these roadblocks. Someone my age should have had counseling about the realities of employers and their attitudes towards damaged goods like me. It never occurred to me that my Bypass would be an issue. I'd never gone for a job and not been offered it on the spot. Never, in all my life."

Before opting for Bypass, did you consider trying medical management?

"After the angiogram, when I called my sister, I asked, 'Should I have the Bypass?' She said, 'If I were you, I'd lift nothing heavier than an unsalted potato chip for the rest of my life, and I'd not have the surgery.' Her choice of metaphor seemed exactly right for me. I wanted to do everything in my power to ensure *not* dropping in my tracks. The prospect of going without Bypass scared the hell out of me—more than the operation did."

Did the prospect of Bypass scare you?

"All my life I've been scared of doctors, terrified of cutting my finger and having to have a stitch in my hand. But when faced with the reality, I thought, 'To be well, I can endure anything. It seems to be worth it. I'm petrified, but I'm more petrified of not doing it.' From the physical point of view, they fulfilled all my high expectations of life after Bypass. For my long-term emotional health, they did a lousy job. I don't think they're interested in the aftermath. I've not received even one follow-up letter, yet all they do is cardiac surgery."

What kind of preparation and strategy might have helped you?

"Talking things over with people who've experienced heart surgery, not just the Heart-Menders or Broken Hearts,[1] but social

---

[1] Dr. Bredely means Mended Hearts, the various Zipper Clubs, Heart Beats, or other volunteer support groups of Bypass veterans.

workers, psychologists, trained to say, 'Okay, maybe you've not encountered job difficulties before, but you'd better think about it, because it's important.' When my mother was widowed, she made all kinds of quick changes: she sold the house; she sold the car; she moved to an area where she didn't know anyone. Later, I read that one of the most important rules for the newly widowed is *not* to make any big changes for a least a year, not to act on any snap judgments. That kind of advice is what I needed. No matter how well you do with Bypass, you're still newly bereaved: you've lost that wonderful sense of yourself as young and indestructible. If I had been able to talk to people who'd gone through the operation, who could tell me what they'd encountered in the work place, the last three years would've been entirely different. At the anecdotal level especially, their experiences would have helped.

"When I came to Mississauga, I was in despair. I didn't think I'd ever have a full-time job again. Not because I couldn't handle a full-time job, but because I couldn't find one. Every time someone heard anything about the heart, he'd drop me like a hot potato; someone else would get picked. Finally, I told my cardiologist in Toronto. He said, 'When you first came to me, I didn't want to say anything. You seemed to have so much going for you. I thought perhaps your experience might be different. But the pattern with patients' jobs is that nobody much wants them after a heart attack or a Bypass.'

"Before my Bypass discharge, somebody should have told me, 'Getting a job might be a problem,' should have said, 'How are you going to deal with obtaining a job? What are your strategies for job-hunting? What will you say in a job interview if they ask about Bypass?' Should you be truthful or should you just not mention anything about a heart problem? I'm one of these people who'd feel terribly guilty if I'm not completely honest about my medical history. If I glossed over this great hole in my transcript, I'd feel as though they were coming after me for the lockup. I needed somebody to say, 'Buck up. That's naiveté. Nobody tells nothing-but-the-truth.'

"And not just job-market advice, but family advice. What are a family's likely reactions to a Bypass? I read someplace that wives are very supportive of husbands who have Bypass, but husbands are completely unsupportive of wives who have heart attacks or heart surgery. I don't know how other families behave towards a divorced family member. Is my family the only family to behave so cavalierly? I doubt it. But it'd help to know, help in dealing with them and with myself. I felt unworthy and unwanted. Was I the only one? The psychological counseling should have dealt with family, with intimate relationships, with present and potential employers, with strategies in the job market, with avoiding job-market exposure unless it's necessary. All kinds of people meet me and assume, because I've had heart surgery, 'Oh, my God, he can't lift that book, he can't go on that trip, he can't maintain that relationship.' "

Has there been a shift in some of your relationships?

"There's been a physical shift because, like a jackass, I moved from one coast to another. I'm stuck here, while most of my friends are in New York or Boston. Phone conversations and letters are inadequate. With some friends, I detect a response which I don't particularly like. Whenever I open my mouth, they feel they have to ask me about my health. I keep saying to them, '*I'm fine.* Let's get on to a more interesting subject. If I need your help, I'll let you know. If necessary, you can send flowers to the hospital.' With certain people, when I hear their voices, I know the first thing they'll say is, 'How are you? Be honest with me,' as though I'm lying. In that sense, there's been a change. I'm now numbered among those who are ill, about whom they must worry every time my name comes up, or when they hear my voice on the phone."

Do you think some people try to keep you out of the World of the Well?

"Absolutely. The two dread diseases, maybe because they're the biggest killers, are heart disease and cancer. If either of those words come up, *eeeee*, some people go ashen, as though it's catching. Immediately, they feel impelled to tell you about somebody they knew who had heart surgery, 'But, of course, he's no longer with us.' " Bredely chuckles. "Had I been married or had a close daily relationship with someone right here, my return to that World of the *Nearly Well*—because we're all walking wounded—would have been easier. I had no children, my love was in Cardiff, I didn't have anyone else but this family of mine, which was no family of mine, but I didn't realize it until I returned to Mississauga."

Did anybody on the hospital staff talk to you about when you could resume sexual relations?

"A nice gal from physical therapy casually said, 'If you can climb two flights of stairs, you can have sex again.' Her manner was great. She laughed lightly and said, 'We're both young people. You can carry on sexually; we young people always can.' I wondered what they said to over-forties."

When you resumed sexual relations, did you worry the first few times?

"I worried, 'Am I going to be different somehow? Has this operation changed me somehow?' I don't mean physically, or in terms of performing, but, 'Am I suddenly going to be outside watching myself and asking myself, "Can I cut the mustard?"' There was a kind of anonymous, neurotic, Woody Allen worry eating at me, but it was at a low level of consciousness. I didn't worry, 'Oh, no, am I going to meet my Maker?' I knew my heart would make it. I just hoped the rest of me would. And it did."

Did you worry that your having had Bypass would affect your sexual partner?

"Not really."

Cardiologists say, 'You can have intercourse with someone who's been a spouse for at least twenty years,' implying that twenty-year sexual relationships remove self-consciousness.

"In some ways, the casual . . . uh . . . experience is easier than intercourse with someone who cares about you a great deal. Because this therapist spoke freely and easily, sex was not an area where I worried much. I was dreadfully self-conscious about the scar. And I'm not the only one. Three men in my apartment complex all confessed to me they didn't go swimming because they didn't like to bare their scars. Maybe it's a sunshine syndrome, the emphasis on the body perfect."

Some men consider it a macho sign.

"The Purple Heart for fighting the War of Ambition? No way! For me, it's worse than a mastectomy scar must be for a woman. I said that once to a woman who'd had mastectomy; she got sore at me. But that's the way I feel. It's not the mark of macho, but the mark of limitation. We all have it, but we don't all have to emblazon the scarlet letter on our chests."

What do you think Bypass accomplished for you?

"It improved my life, it may even have lengthened my life. I hope. But I worry, 'After ten years, will I need more surgery?' Right now, we've about fifteen years of Bypass history to go on. Will they find out that these gaskets don't hold up? Will they have to do a repair job? The long-term prospect is unknown, although the technology and procedures are improving every day. If I behave the way I should"—Bredely lights another cigarette—"am I good for ten or fifteen years, or am I good for the rest of my born days? If I get hit by a car tomorrow, yes; but if I don't get hit by that hypothetical car for forty years, will the Bypass still be okay?"

How long the grafts last depends on a number of variables: the surgeon's skills, the location of the grafts, the progression of further heart disease. Holding back the heart disease is, in some measure, your job. Did they talk to you about diet, about exercise, about not smoking?

"For God's sake!" Bredely explodes. "Don't you start in on me! An interview is not a license to nag!"

Since Bypass, what's changed for you? How has life improved?

"Economically, until I got this job, I've been through some hellish times. Financially, Bypass was one grand disaster. I went from earning $45,000 a year to scrounging rent money from friends. I even had to sell a couple of paintings, a lovely Chippendale chair, and a Japanese Samurai chest. It was a tough comedown. This job's okay. I hope I can keep the board of governors, the students, and their parents all happy."

You said you liked this woman in Cardiff.

"Very much."

You've had a heart attack and Bypass surgery. You see each other twice a year. What are you waiting for?

"Maybe to be old enough!" Dr. Bredely laughs hoarsely. "She's widowed; her husband was the longest surviving transplant patient in Britain. While we're close, she says, 'I don't want ever to go through that again.' She's bound by her job in Cardiff. I've avoided letting relationships get too serious. I don't want to hazard getting scorched again. In Mississauga, my life was a fight for survival, without room for relationships. If you don't have money, it's hard to meet people. As the headmaster here, I have to be careful about letting myself go. It's a small town. I'm a demonstrative man who wandered into a singularly undemonstrative family. I'm a touchy-feely type whose mother and sister haven't kissed him in twenty years. Maybe I'm leery of establishing a family of my own. Sometimes I wonder if families aren't an anachronism. In relationships, I catch myself holding back. I say, 'What's going on? Normally, you're touchy-feely-warm. Why are you building this wall?' I can't blame heart surgery completely. It's Bypass and it's divorce working together. If 'working' is a properly chosen word." His laugh is harsh.

Do you believe in God? Do you believe there's a design to the universe?

"I'm pretty much an Anglican, although since they took away the Book of Common Prayer, I've seriously thought about turning to the Society of Friends. But I don't think God says, 'Now for Jordan Bredely, we've got this mess. Let's see how he gets himself out of it.' His filing system and His index cards may need a better computer. Maybe He needs to go back to MBA school. Yet my youthful skepticism has softened. I've begun to see the validity of my father's rock-hard principles."

Were you close to your father?

"Only in the last twenty-four hours of his life. Until then, my father, at eighty-two, never had a real conversation with any of us, surely not with my mother."

During Bypass, was religion a comfort to you?

"It's hard to say. When they took me out of the ICU to the general hospital floor, a strange thing happened. In the ICU, I was doing terrifically well and moving faster than they thought I ought to. When I'd push myself, they'd say, 'Don't overdo,' which annoyed me, and I'd say, 'I'm fine, I'm fine.'

"In the move from the ICU, I got a little tired. It was time for lunch. The orderly brought some God-awful mess, the worst hospital food I'd ever seen. I said, 'I don't want this. Take it away.' Some nurse came in and began berating me: "You *have* to cooperate, you *have* to follow my directions, you *have* to do this, you *have* to do that.' I felt I was doing bloody well. I didn't need her giving me orders. I caught her accent and her intonation. I said, 'I don't need some Jewish American princess telling me what to do, thank you. Why don't you go back to the Bronx, where they appreciate your so-called virtues? I don't. You leave me alone and I'll be fine.' She went out in tears, as well she might have. The orderly said, 'She's a good nurse and was only doing her job. That was undeserved.' I said, 'I know. I feel bad about it already.' Later, when she had to come in to take my blood pressure, I apologized. She took the apology very graciously. After that, we became very close; she was terrific. I owe her a big debt for my recovery. If either my father or my mother had been so barbaric to a nurse, I would have been wild, yet there it was, lurking beneath my supposedly liberal façade.

"This business of outsiderhood gets in the way between people. When I lived in England, I longed to be back in America. Not in Canada, but in America. James Baldwin once said that most white people will never understand what it means to be black; but if, as Americans, they ever live in Europe, they might begin to understand."

It's not unlike being Jewish.

"Oh, that's different. One is either Jewish or Episcopalian or left-handed or whatever. In England, I was accepted, but I was always the *American* friend. In Nevada, that Yo-Yo land, I was the Canadian friend, yet I was less the outlander than in Britain. Here"—Dr. Bredely gestures towards the Gothic buildings whose outlines appear through the leaded-glass casement windows—"I'm a *novus homo*, a newcomer, but I think I'm settling in. I hope so. I'm sick of wandering. If Bypass can just help me get my citizenship papers in your 'World of the Well,' I'd like to live out my days working here."

7. Sven Thorgesen
Television weatherman
Ages at Bypass: 35, 35

Sven Thorgesen is the Weather Man on television. Every night, at six and eleven, Sven predicts tomorrow's weather. With his charts and pointer, he prophesies how many inches it will snow, whether the sun will break through the clouds, if the rain will turn to sleet. Only thirty-five years old, a one-time linebacker in professional football, Sven Thorgesen himself has been dogged by stormy weather. At twenty-seven, he was struck by Hodgkin's disease. Five years after, told he was cured, he married, later had two children. Then, chief of a television weather bureau in Merrillville, Indiana, he believed he had it made. Telling his story, Thorgesen adds, "Or so I thought. Until one evening last spring, while watching television in my chair, I had chest pains. Not severe. More of an ache than a pain. I mightn't have thought a thing about that achiness, except my brother had the same little twinges two years ago. He got Bypassed at thirty-nine."

Is there any other heart disease in your family?

"My brother and I were the lucky ones." Thorgesen grimaces ironically. "My mother's a great old girl at seventy-six. My father died of cancer at sixty-four."

What did you do about those chest pains?

"Nothing. But a couple of days later, while I was doing some yard work, those aches returned. Every time I stopped working, the aches would go away. I got a little worried, and made an appointment with our family doctor. Nothing was wrong. My resting EKG was perfect. Because of my brother, and because of my history of Hodgkin's disease treated by radiation therapy, he sent me that same day for a stress test. I lasted three minutes. The cardiologist pulled me off and said, 'You've definitely got heart disease. The questions are, How should we treat it? How extensive is it?' He scheduled a catheterization for the following Monday. After the cath, he said, 'You need Bypass. Your left main coronary artery is 90 percent blocked.' He recommended several Bypass places, was very straight about who he thought was the best man. I took his advice. I got done with surgery, recuperated, and went back to work in six weeks. Everything seemed to be fine."

Did you have a stress test before you went back to work?

"Sure. It was fine. I was like that old Dorothy Parker story, 'You Were Perfectly Fine' except I wasn't fine at all. I'd been going to work, I'd felt real good. One evening at work, while I was on camera, I felt a rub, an inflammation from the surgery. They treated me for it. The rub went away. I had no more pain. Then I began getting a sharp knife-in-the-chest pain, different from angina, like somebody shoving a switchblade in and giving it a hard twist. I called my family doctor, who said, 'It should be checked out,' and gave me an appointment for later in the week. I went to work, but I felt so terrible. I had to leave work, which I'd never done before. I couldn't go in the next day; I saw the doctor, who thought it was that rub returning and put me back on medicine. Within a day, the medication cleared the pain and I went back to work. By this time, it was the weekend. Out of the blue, I started having those old chest pains again, not the sharp rub pain. The doctor told me to go to Community Emergency, where they did a thallium stress test. The thallium scan showed I wasn't getting enough oxygen to the front part of my heart. If I promised to stay in bed, they'd let me go home. Even in bed and taking medicine, I still had pain. Monday, on my own, I went to University Emergency. They admitted me and catheterized me. Both Bypass grafts had closed completely. No blood was flowing through. They scheduled me for a second Bypass on the following Monday." Thorgesen breathes heavily. "That's my story. One Bypass on Memorial Day. The second Bypass on Labor Day. And a third baby born in-between."

How've you done since your second Bypass?

"Pretty well. The second time wasn't as pleasant or as easy. After the second Bypass, initially I recovered much more quickly. Once I got home, things slowed down to a crawl. I couldn't walk as far, I couldn't walk as long. I've had troubles with fluid building up. I've had to see the surgeon twice now. He's inserted a needle through my back and drawn off fluid. Next week, they'll x-ray me again. The fluid's coming back again, because I can't walk down the hall without getting short of breath. They're talking now about putting me back in the hospital"—Thorgesen sighs—"and inserting a chest tube. They want to drain this fluid off again and insert medication. Lots of aches and pains this time, but it's all minor. Nothing worse than a toothache."

How's your spirit?

"Good. Once in a while, I'd like to scream, 'Enough!' I get over that quickly. I keep telling myself, 'At least you're alive. If this second Bypass and the chest tube work, and apparently they will, you'll go back to a normal life and forget all about this crazy year.' "

How's your wife doing?
"Real well. The three kids drive her nuts." He laughs.

Before either Bypass, did you get a second opinion or consider medical management?

"With a surgeon, a cardiologist, and an internist, I figured I had enough opinions. I asked them about medical management, but all three didn't think it would work. I asked about angioplasty, but they thought Bypass was the only way to go. The location and the size of the blockage said, 'Bypass—and quickly.' "

In the year before your first Bypass, did stresses or your responses to stresses intensify?

"I was put under more pressure because I'd gone from being number-two person in the department to being boss. It's my ball game. We'd moved to a new city, to a more aggressive weather-news channel. What was right and what was wrong were my responsibility. This channel had paid a lot of money to get me out here. I was grateful for the chance, but I felt I owed them. As far as home pressures, the only home stress was another child, first on the way, and then here."

What did you blame for your heart problems and your need for Bypass?

"My family history—my brother's had it. My medical history—the Hodgkin's or the radiation therapy, one of the two. My surgeon feels strongly that my cancer and its treatment played a role. He thinks I'd have had heart trouble, but not for ten or twenty years. When they opened up my chest, he said the vessels didn't feel normal. They felt rubbery, changed, brought on by some unknown factor. He's operated on one other person who had Hodgkin's disease. They had to redo him, too, because of scarring much like mine."

How did you feel when you were told you needed Bypass?

"The first time, I didn't worry that much. I don't know if it was the drugs they gave me, but I wasn't too concerned. I've a lot of confidence in the medical profession. Granted, they screw up once in a while, but everybody does. I never doubted this would be successful. I knew that they'd go into my chest, that I'd hurt for a few days, that I'd be out of work for a few weeks. Afterwards, I'd go back to work, and everything would be better than before. I justified my reasoning by telling myself, 'You can't live a life where you can't do things because of chest pain. You don't have any choice.' Once in a while, sure, I wondered whether I'd die during the surgery, whether somebody would goof up and something would go wrong, whether I'd have a heart attack. But I didn't think about it much. When I'd gone through the cancer treatments, I'd read up on Hodgkin's disease. I knew positive thinking played an important part in getting well. I figured it was the same with Bypass. I tried not to let doubts hang around too long. I listened to the doctors' advice. If I had questions, I asked them. I expected them to be answered truthfully. I think they were. I hope so."

How about the second time around?

"The second time, I worked hard to have that same positive attitude. Obviously, I had a few more doubts. I wondered, 'How many times can you do this? The second time, is there a greater risk?' They'd told me that the second surgery would be a little longer than the first, but the risks were the same. I wondered, 'If the first one didn't work, is the second one going to stay open? If I have the second one, how will I feel if ever I need a third? What's going to happen in ten or fifteen years? Will I have to go through this again? Once or twice?'"

Would you be willing to have a third Bypass?

"I think so. Obviously, both times, I felt I had no choice. When you're given no choice, well . . ." Thorgesen's voice trails off.

What's helped you face two Bypasses at thirty-five?

"My wife and I are totally different. She likes to talk things out, to get her feelings out. Like my family, I tend to keep things in. After all, I can talk to my wife, I can talk to the doctors, but when push comes to shove, I'm the guy who has to go through it. If she wants to talk, fine. I'd just as soon say, 'Let's get it over with, get it done, and not dwell on it.' Hemingway was right: women talk a thing to death. I want to forget it. I don't talk about my problems. I don't want support from other people, from my family, from the church. This may sound conceited, but I rely on my own inner strength. All my life, whether it was academics or athletics, whether it was the Army or civilian life, I've been very fortunate. I've been extremely successful. Whatever I've accomplished, I've relied on myself, not on other people. I grew up in a small town in Montana, where I learned self-reliance young. It's stood me in good stead, because that self-reliance is getting me through."

After Bypass, did you take stock and decide to change certain aspects of your life?

"The only change was the decision not to work quite so hard. I used to work six or seven days a week, twelve to fourteen hours a day. I never felt put upon. I love my work. The Bypasses didn't institute changes. The cancer did. Hodgkin's disease made me step back and take a long look at what's important to me. The two Bypasses confirmed I'd better live for today instead of postponing till tomorrow."

What about personal relationships?

"From the response to my being in the hospital, the cards and the letters, I feel accepted by this community, which is a new place for me. As for closer personal ties, that's the same. They may have restructured the roadways around my heart, but I'm still the same loner."

What about your wife and children?

"Unfortunately, I let the kids get away with more. I used to be the disciplinarian. My wife relied on me to be the tough guy. Now, I'm less strict. I figure, 'They're only kids. Let them grow up. They'll be fine. They have to enjoy themselves, too.' I worry less about how they'll grow up." Thorgesen's face clouds. "I wonder why I've laid off on the kids."

After either of the Bypasses, did you become irritable?

"After the second one. For three days, after I got home, I wasn't fit for man or beast. I was yelling at the kids, at my wife, for no reason at all. Finally, I took a big, noisy old fan into our bedroom; I turned the fan on so I wouldn't hear anything outside those bedroom walls; I stayed there for three days. When I came out, I was fine. I was ready to live again, like a human being, with my family."

After Bypass, did you become forgetful?

Thorgesen laughs. "I don't remember. But no, I don't think so."

Did you become depressed?

"I'm not someone who cries easily. But a few times after the first Bypass, and more times after the second, the tears suddenly would come out like the Johnstown flood. I guess that's depression."

Was this in the hospital or out?

"Both. After the second Bypass, it happened more often at home."

What might have helped you fight the depression?

"I don't know. After the first Bypass, I had a lot of visitors after I got home. I got depressed. After the second Bypass, I didn't have many callers. Sickness gets to be like yesterday's newspaper. I still got depressed. Visitors weren't the answer. Drugs might have helped, but my doctor doesn't like to use drugs on Bypassers because of possible arrhythmias."

In a few hospitals, there's a full-time psychological counselor who visits you routinely before and after Bypass and after discharge. Would that have helped you?

"That's difficult to answer. I don't know what brought on these depressions, what got rid of them. A professional might have guided me in understanding *why* I got so down."

Did the Bypasses make you want to extract more from life for yourself alone?

"Since the second Bypass, I've started thinking about what *I* want, I personally versus we the family. I want a boat so bad." Thorgesen laughs embarrassedly.

"I love to go out on that lake and leave everything behind. We need curtains and a rug for the new house. Even with a bigger salary, we've got a stack of bills. We decided we can't afford this boat. I said, 'We'll put off a boat for a year or two.' Yet with this shortness of breath and with their siphoning off this fluid, I've been thinking about *now*, not two years down the pike. When spring comes, and the trout season opens, I may go buy that boat and say, 'To hell with everything.' "

Did the Bypasses make you aware of things you wish you'd done or not done?

"No, I'm extremely happy with the way my life has gone. I've done almost everything I've ever wanted to do."

Did it make you feel old?

"Sometimes I think, 'I'm a young man with an old man's disease. That's a helluva way to run a universe.' When it gets me down, I tell myself, 'You're getting all this garbage out of the way now. When you're eighty, you can chase women and drink and have a good time.' But," Thorgesen adds slowly, "with this shortness of breath, I feel as though I'm a ways from being done with Bypass and doctors and heart disease. I question sometimes whether"— he laughs uneasily—"I'm ever going to be done. It seems to go on and on and on."

When things go wrong, is your surgeon available to you?

"He's got a number we call. I talk to a nurse-practitioner."

What about talking to the surgeon himself?

"When I've needed fluid drawn off, he's said, 'Come in tomorrow. Come in this afternoon.' He's not available to ask, 'How many times will you have to poke around with this fluid? When will I be better?' The man's always so busy. Both the first time and the second time, I felt, 'I mustn't take up his time. He's got more important things to do.' He let's me know he's too busy to talk. These guys check you. They listen to your breathing. They pat you on the back, 'How're ya doin'? Fine! Great!' And *pfft!*, back out they go before you can say a word, ask a question. It's not enough. You feel so helpless."

Does he call you by name?

"The first time, no. The second time, yes."

When he comes into your room, does he sit down?

"He sat down twice, the day before each Bypass, and briefly explained what they planned to do. Just when I'd framed a question, he popped out of the chair like a jack-in-the-box and was gone."

Are you more alive to the sweetness of everyday life?

"Oh, yes. When I had cancer, I'd go out in the woods, tramping around by myself. I'd sit in the dark and watch a fire. I'd get out on the boat and listen to the waves beating against it. I wouldn't catch any fish, and I didn't care. Since the two Bypasses, going out alone on the boat, hiking through the woods, mean even more to me."

Since your Bypasses, is your marriage the same? How's your love life?

"My love life's damn near nonexistent because of my breathing problem, Betsy's having the baby, our trouble with birth control. She's thirty-five, like me, so they don't want her on the pill any more. I'd scheduled a vasectomy, but they said, 'No vasectomies. People with vasectomies may have a higher incidence of coronary artery disease.' They're not sure about the connection, but in my case they're afraid."

What about an IUD or a diaphragm?

"She has an appointment today to have an IUD put in. Hopefully, things will pick up shortly." Thorgesen's laugh is hollow.

Are you on any medication?

"Persantine and Inderal. The usual. At first, the Inderal made me a little tired. Now, I don't feel any effects."

Does Inderal affect your sexual desire?

"I really don't know. Sometimes I've wondered about it, but with my shortness of breath and the new baby, it's hard to tell."

"Does it affect your ability to have an erection or maintain one?

"It doesn't seem to, but we've only had a couple of times to check it out. All these little things need to be talked out with the surgeon. I don't think he's ever spent enough time with me. Maybe I'm a little spoiled. When I had cancer, I was a career officer. I had my spleen removed for Hodgkin's disease at Fitzsimmons Army Hospital in Denver. The Army surgeon sat down and talked to me every day. Before and after the operation, he got books out and explained everything. My civilian heart doctor told me only the basics: 'We open the chest. You're on the heart-lung machine.' That's about it. Both times. The second time, especially, I kind of thought he should have talked more extensively to me, but no dice."

After the second Bypass, how did you know you were filling up with fluid?

"I couldn't breathe. I was having some pain. I saw the cardiologist, who thought he heard a rub again. He got an x-ray, and"—Thorgesen's big hands open helplessly upward—"the x-ray showed a chest full of fluid." He takes a deep breath.

Does it bother you to talk?

"Not much. I'm used to pacing myself for the camera. It bothers me to walk. I hate that."

When you awakened from Bypass, how did you feel?

"The first time, I remember Betsy and her mother beside the bed. Each had a grip on my hand, and I thought, 'I'm awake! It's over! It worked!' It was great. I don't remember the second time. I do remember hearing a guy yelling for his mother. The ICU nurses tried to quiet him down. I'd hear them saying, 'You can't do this. You're disturbing everybody.' After listening to his hollering and their admonitions for what seemed like hours, I had this terrible urge to go over and tell him, 'Shut up! Just shut up! I don't have to take this crap! I have problems of my own!' I didn't want to listen to him. Of course, I had the tube in, so I couldn't speak."

Before the Bypass, did they explain about the tubes?

"They were good about explaining the tubes. A nurse took me to the ICU and showed me a person who'd had Bypass that same day. He still had *all* the tubes in and that gray Bypass pallor. Then they took me to see a woman who'd had Bypass the day before. She was sitting up. She had a little oxygen in, and that's it. She made me feel good. The nurse told me, 'Every time we take out a tube, you know you're getting better.' The first time I counted tubes." Thorgesen laughs. "By the time I awoke the second time, all the tubes were out. Maybe the anesthetic was different, maybe it's because the surgery was seven hours, instead of four. The second time, they put me to sleep much sooner. The first time, they shaved me, took me down, put all those tubes in my arms. I remember them wheeling me into the operating room and saying, 'Somebody didn't show up on time.' Somebody important. Not my chief surgeon, I don't think. His assistant or somebody who was supposed to operate the heart-lung machine. When they wheeled me back out, I thought, 'This is a helluva way to run a hospital.' Finally, they wheeled me back in. The last I knew, someone said, 'Move your head so we can put that tube down your neck.' After that: nothing. Until I woke up and found Betsy gripping my hand. I could've done without her mother there, but I couldn't say anything. In more ways than one.

"The second time, my last memory is of someone saying, 'I'm giving you something to make you sleepy.' After that, I knew nothing till I awoke in ICU with all the tubes out. That was much better. It's the way to do business."

What was the worst part of the surgery, and how can it be alleviated?

"The worst part of the first Bypass was before they started the surgery. They can alleviate that by putting you to sleep a lot earlier. The worst of both Bypasses was the first day in Intensive Care with all the tubes. I felt so dry and hot, so miserable, even though I was on painkillers. I didn't hurt, but I was wretched. The nurse would wipe off my face with a damp cloth and put some stuff on my lips to keep them from drying out. Those little things felt so good. Nurses are there almost all the time that first day. When their shifts change, which is three times a day, they have these eternal staff meetings, which takes almost everybody off the floor for an hour. That's when you need somebody standing by to wet your lips and wipe your brow."

What was the worst part of the hospitalization? Is there any way it can be improved?

"Three things were bad at University Hospital. Number one, and maybe it can't be avoided, is that rotten cupping for the breathing. There's gotta be a better method. Number two is waking up at night and *just aching so bad,* because it's been a while since they've given any pain medication. You hurt so much, you can't move yourself even to ring the nurse for pain medication. There've been some articles about undermedication. The first time, I could've used more painkiller. The second time, I was fine. Because they medicated me more promptly, I think I used fewer pain pills." Throgesen stops. "The third thing can be fixed: the food at University Hospital *stinks.* It's salty and it tastes awful."

Did you complain?

"Only on the questionnaire they gave me at the end. They probably file those in the circular file. Why ask if you don't respond? They make you feel so useless."

What do you think the operation did for you?

"I hope it gave me a leg up on my normal life span, sixty or seventy, whatever I'm entitled to. Without Bypass, I probably didn't have a chance."

Sixty is too young. Even seventy is too young.

Thorgesen laughs grimly. "Okay, sixty-one. Between the cancer and the heart disease, I've a good chance of not living a normal life span. I'm not prepared to die at fifty-five, but it wouldn't surprise me. I've had two Bypasses. Each time, I've said, 'Okay, I'll get through this and go back to living a normal life.' And *bam*, somebody booted me in the rear. Here I am, back in the hospital. I still don't feel as well as I did after the first Bypass, and that one was a flop. I get tired easily, I get frustrated. I missed pheasant season; more'n likely, I'll miss deer season. I say, 'Well, next year. I hope.' The only guy who makes me feel I'm not a number is the cardiologist. Yesterday, I got a letter from him: 'I saw you on TV. Your weather forecast stunk, but you looked great! P.S. Consider joining the Y or the JCC for cardiac rehab.' I intend to, but right now, I can't breathe. I can't exercise, because I can't breathe. Betsy says I should call my cardiologist about the breathing. I gather the surgeon hasn't kept the cardiologist posted."

What helps you get through the dark night of the soul?

"This doesn't answer your question, but it brings up another issue where I'm having problems I don't understand. When I come home from work, I'm exhausted. I finish at the studio about midnight, drive an hour into the country to our house, get in bed about one-fifteen, lie down, and my eyes refuse to close or to stay closed. Many times, at four o'clock in the morning, I'm still lying there watching my Technicolor horror show. The strangest things go round and round in my mind, memories dredged from my past life. Stupid stuff like something my third-grade teacher did to me that I considered terribly wrong, terribly unjustified. I'll think about my football coach in high school. He'll call a play, and I'll think, 'This guy does a lousy job. Why is he doing that?' I'll remember somebody who didn't like me in my hometown, something that happened in college or in the Army. I'll go over it and over it and over. God! I can't stop myself from circling like a scavenger crow over a dead deer. I never think this way except when the lights are out and it's two o'clock in the morning. If our sex life was better, I could put my arms around Betsy and console myself with her. That's what marriage is about. Maybe the IUD will help. I hope so. Breathless as I am, I need it."

What did your operation cost?

"Everything was completely covered, except for the anesthesiologist. Blue Cross allowed $300 both times. He sent a bill for $900 the first time, and for $1500 the second time." Thorgesen whistles. "That's pretty steep, I thought, but I paid it."

Did you complain to the anesthesiologist about the bill?

"What good would it do?"

What explicit questions should people ask their internist, their cardiologist, their surgeon, before and after?

"I've needed Bypass twice, once on Memorial Day, once on Labor Day. Most Bypassers are like me: we read up on Bypass after we have the operation. Afterwards, you find out that Bypass isn't always successful, that a certain percentage have problems, have to be done over again, that a certain percentage have pain for the rest of their lives. Going into Bypass, I didn't have enough knowledge to ask. People should ask, 'What are *my* chances for a *successful* Bypass? Will I ever have problems again? If so, how long do you estimate I'll be feeling well? Given *my* condition now, *my* past history, what kinds of problems will *I* have? Tell me more about the heart-lung machine.'

"That's the one piece of equipment everything centers on: whether you'll wake up afterwards; whether you'll have memory loss; whether you'll be the same person. I want to know more about the actual mechanism of the operation itself, more about the mechanism of the heart-lung machine. If it involves me, I want to know as much as I can. If there's something I can do to make it better, I want to know, so I can control myself and my environment. In Bypass, obviously you can't improve the heart-lung machine, improve the skill of the person preparing the grafts, improve the surgeon's skill, but if I could do *anything* to make it better, I'd want to know.

"After Bypass, the doctors ought to do more to get Bypassers together in the hospital. The first time, we had a little group going. Everybody wanted to be friends, to talk, to compare notes. We enjoyed each other. The second time, nothing. I don't know why. Partially, it was the dynamics of that set of personalities. The hospital people could've fostered connections between people, but they didn't. You'd do your laps around the desk in the central nursing station, and nobody'd be talking to anybody else. The nurses didn't even look up and smile, 'Good morning.' The smile and the surgeon talking more to you *every day*, explaining more, would be easier to live with."

Thorgesen pauses for a long time, sighs deeply, then continues in his mile-a-minute fashion. "If heart surgery comes out from behind closed doors, people will be less afraid of it. Before my first Bypass, I called my boss and asked him if he wanted to do a series on heart surgery, on my personal experience. He refused. If they taped my Bypass, he was afraid people would think my operation was a publicity stunt, just for show, even though that doctor performed Bypass live on PBS. I think people would have accepted its educational newsworthiness, but I couldn't convince my boss." He puts his big hand on his forehead. "I love my job. I can't think of anything I'd rather do. It's exciting. They pay me well. What else could I ask for? But I hate fighting with my boss for extra camera time. You'd think I was trying out for the movies. They give me three and a half minutes for a weather segment. No more, no less. If the weather's bad, you need more time, but you've got to fight for it, tooth and nail." Thorgesen stops, rubs his forehead, pulls on his bushy blond mustache: "It's like my life. The weather's been bad. I've had to fight for more time. I just wish I could get done with the fight and get on with the life."

8. Thomas Windsor
Businessman
Age at Bypass: 60

Thomas Windsor is president of Gulf Wood Products in Carlington. "We do," he notes, drily, "just what the name implies: we manufacture wood products for big companies like Sears and Ward's. We're not a big outfit, maybe a hundred employees, but we're not bad for a black corporation." Windsor is one of seven children. All four brothers have heart disease, although Thomas Windsor, the youngest son, is the only Bypasser. "None of my sisters have heart problems, but all three have multiple sclerosis, which is most unusual. Compared with my sisters, my heart trouble is small potatoes."

How did you learn you had a heart problem and needed Bypass?

"You asked two questions, not one. In 1965, I was enlisted as a participant in a governmental gerontology study. The participants were all ages, both sexes and colors. At forty-three, a part of this study of aging in America, I had my first EKG. Surprisingly, it wasn't normal. Some time earlier, without knowing, I'd had some heart damage. I had been an active man. I never was aware of any problems. Shows how much you know what's going on inside you. My pressure was up. They gave me blood-pressure medicine. In 1968, when the study was over, I transferred to my present cardiologist. He's a Board-certified cardiologist and angiographer, has all the certificates. He's black like me. And successful like me. My pressure was normal, so he took me off all medication."

Do you smoke?

"After the operation, I stopped. I was never an excessive smoker. No more than a pack a day."

How did you come to Bypass?

"I've had ulcers since 1959. Since my Bypass a year ago, amazingly, I haven't had any ulcer problems. Prior to that, I'd been hospitalized twice with a bleeding ulcer, once in 1959 and once in 1969. When I'd get pain, I didn't know which was which: whether it was ulcers or heart. In the fall of '82, during the hunting season, if I climbed a ridge, I'd notice pain in my stomach. Before that, I began noticing pains after I'd eaten a big meal. My abnormal EKG from '65 remained abnormal. It hadn't changed, but that pain was getting worse and worse, from less and less. My level of endurance dropped. I could bring on that pain without much effort.

"On Christmas Day, I was sitting looking out the window. I love to hunt, but it's a family tradition never to hunt on Christmas. It was early in the morning, about seven-thirty. From my window, I could see way across the fields. I don't like being crowded, so I live on the edge between suburbia and the country. As I looked across those snow-dusted fields, I saw a ring-necked pheasant in my neighbor's cornfield. From the house, I could see the top of his head. The garage door was up, but I knew I couldn't open my trunk and get my shotgun out because the slightest noise would alert the bird. I took my rifle from the gun case in the family room, opened the side door, and shot him in the field. He flew up, then fell. Down he plummeted. Dead in the cornfield. They're good eating, you know. From the excitement of shooting him, the exultation of getting that bird, I had so much pain that I couldn't move out the door. So much pain, right in here, I couldn't move. When I couldn't move that Christmas morning, I said, 'This is ridiculous. I've killed

my bird and I can't go get him.' The day after Christmas, I called
the cardiologist and said, 'Okay, Doc, I'm ready to go in and search
out this diagnosis of yours.' "

Did somebody get your bird for you?

"Later, when I felt a little better, my next-door neighbor came
over. We looked everywhere, but the bird was gone. I think a fox
or a cat got it. My retriever dog was down in the country. Normally,
I'd have sent that setter into the field. He'd have brought me my
bird. But he wasn't there. Things have changed out where I live. I
moved there so I could train my dogs in the field across the road.
Used to be two covey of quail in that field. Best place to train dogs
for the hunt. Now that field is gone. The quail are gone. It's all
houses."

*In the year before shooting the bird at Christmas, did stresses or your
responses to stresses—*

"For a few years, I'd noticed excitement could create the pain. It
was like getting on a horse who's trying to throw you. When I think
back, I remember a number of things that'd trigger the pain. In
winter, I seldom wear even a topcoat; when I'd walk out, I'd get
that jolt. When I'd go hunting, walking in the cold, little pains
would hunt with me, but they'd pass right on. Nothing serious.
It'd pass right on."

*Bypassers say heart disease sneaks up on you, little by little. Was that
true for you?*

"Because I had ulcers, I was accustomed to pain. For three years,
I ate soup and oatmeal, with a little baby food for dessert. Some
baby food is delicious. I won't say Bypass cured my ulcer, but I
will say I can eat things now which I could never eat before. I
hadn't eaten fried chicken for thirty years. It tastes mighty good.
I don't eat it regularly, just once in a while. My next test is pigs'
feet. I passed the chitlins and the hog-moss test. After all these
years, I'd forgotten how good they were. The other day, I had fried
lake trout, fresh-caught."

When you learned you had serious heart trouble, that you needed Bypass, what did you blame?

Windsor smiles. "Two questions require two answers. We'll try one. That January, when they did the angiogram, it showed 100 percent in one artery and 80 percent in two others."

Which arteries were involved?

"I've a picture here in my wallet if you'd like to see it. I carry it close to my heart to remind me how lucky I am." Windsor knocks wood. "Every time I think about putting this picture away, I say to myself, 'Tom, maybe you better carry it a little bit longer.' Now, there are other answers to your questions. The life-style causing stomach problems causes heart problems."

Stress?

"What may be stressful to you is not necessarily stressful to me. When you look at groups of people, particularly by ethnic or racial background, as you're attempting to do, their individual and their group stresses vary. If you look at black folks, again there's this tremendous variation under the whole black umbrella. I've learned coping mechanisms as a way of life; for someone else these tensions could create tremendous strains. Black people have a much lower incidence of suicide than nonblacks."

Blacks also have a much lower incidence of Bypass than whites. Why?

"Now you're taking the lid off a whole new kettle of fish. Bypasses are expensive. Because of the expense, the individual needs a strong insurance program. Fewer black folks fall into the economic group carrying good insurance, fewer are even eligible for adequate insurance. We're living in the Age of Specialization. People who go to a general practitioner and die under the care of a general practitioner are not necessarily exposed to the sophistication of catheterization and Bypass. They're not referred for extensive investigation. I'm not saying their doctors aren't as knowledgeable. Because of economics, the doctor can't refer this person to an expensive specialist. The expense begins long before you get to the hospital. Even when the person has insurance, he's unwilling to miss work, so he's reluctant to find out what ails him."

Outside his doctor's office, where we talk, the hospital loud-speaker crackles: "Alert Team, Alert Team, Room 5023." Windsor chuckles. "Now you see what I was talking about. Stress. That voice made you jump. I never flinched, did I? Your pressure jumped twenty points. Mine didn't. Admit it. I'm calmer than you are!" Windsor laughs delightedly.

Did insurance completely cover your Bypass?

"Ninety-five percent. It cost about $15,000, all told."

How long did you have to wait between the decision to Bypass and the operation itself?

"When they said I needed it, I asked, 'When can I get it?' I waited two weeks. That's too long."

When you were told you needed surgery, how did you feel?

"Something had to be done. The sooner the better. I saw the an-giogram with the doctor. I saw the blockage. I couldn't walk around like that."

Are you usually of an accepting nature?

"I try to change things to suit me. If I can. The Bypass was the change, not the as-is."

Do you usually do what people tell you?

"Only if I agree with them. I'm not in politics. I don't want to be enmeshed in the structure. I don't want to be forced to do anything I don't believe is right. Although I am able to go along with authority, I like to be in control."

Is there anything you wish you'd done or done differently before your Bypass?

"When I found out I needed Bypass, my cardiologist told me, 'Stop bowling. Stop hunting. Take a break and be careful. We don't want to lose you before the Bypass.' I was careful. I went to the office every day, but I lowered the flame under the pot. I could be careful for two weeks, but that's not what I wanted for the rest of my days. Perhaps I could have existed without Bypass, but existence is not enough for me."

After Bypass, did you take stock of your life? Did you plan what you might like to do now?

"I'm not all that unhappy with what I've done. Other than not having enough money. At times, I think, all of us look at our lives and say, 'What would I have changed? Should I have done this differently? That differently?' In 1973, I left a business. I had to leave it because I had overextended myself to form a corporation. I had this vision of five black men running a chain of wood-supply stores from Vermont to Florida. We set up a corporation consisting of five of us. Nobody put up any money but me. I used my company to underwrite the whole thing. I didn't leave the business; it left me. I regret that mistake because it bankrupted a viable company I'd worked hard establishing. Oh, well, you can't have the pain of losing a million if you haven't had the pleasure of making a million. Remember that."

You lost a million dollars?

"Sure. My brother was in with me; we could have pulled out. I got tired, I didn't want to harm the other men. I said, 'Let it go.' I went on to another field. I regret not fighting harder to hang on to it, because that would have provided financial security for me, if money was that important. As far as my relations with people, I don't have a lot of regrets."

Are you close to your wife?

"Not necessarily. Not an intimate closeness, but maybe it's closer than we realize. After thirty years, we understand each other. Now that I've had Bypass, I don't feel I have to make up for lost time. When I found I had to go for Bypass, I didn't rush to make a new will and all this crape-hanging. It never occurred to me that the operation wouldn't be successful, or that I wouldn't be back to work in short order. I know it's a very serious operation; not everyone comes back upstairs. I understand that. In some cases, they lose the patient because he's brooding and pessimistic. Fortunately"—Windsor knocks wood again—"worrying just didn't occur to me."

After the operation, did you become irritable?

"No, because I was lucky with my doctor. He laid out exactly what I'd have to do, every step of the way. Number one, stay in the house for two weeks. Number two, go driving in the car, but with my wife at the wheel. I couldn't drive for six weeks. I may have cheated a few days on the driving. With my house set in the country, I could walk right outside, around the house, sit on the patio. I could look outside at the hills beyond the fields. I couldn't shoot any birds, though. The confinement didn't make me irritable, because I could talk on the phone, I had visitors."

Did you become depressed?

"Oh, I had low moments. But I've had low moments before Bypass, before any heart trouble. There are times when a person isn't as emotionally keyed up. You can't sell the Brooklyn Bridge every day. There isn't always a buyer."

Did you become forgetful?

"I didn't notice anything. Maybe that's because my doctor gets you off the heart-lung machine fast."

Did you change your work pattern?

"I work fewer hours and I don't work as hard. The business is different. I'm the pivotal person, the man in charge of buying, purchasing, managing, the whole bit. For the past year, the business has been more dependent on me to make it go. The economy has been bad; business has been bad; with Reaganomics, business is going downhill. I voted for him. 'The businessman's President,' I thought."

Is it stressful for you with business doing poorly?

"No more than normal. As you get older, you get bored with the same things day after day. Halting this downhill slide has been a challenge. If I'm not successful, that'll be a stress. That dream of black entrepreneurism won't let go of me."

Since Bypass, have you changed much? You stopped smoking. What else?

"I smoke a pipe now and then. Years ago, when I'd stopped smoking cold turkey, my normal weight, 194 pounds since college, zoomed up to 208 pounds, which on my frame has to be called fat. For two years, I fought this weight battle, trying to get under the 200-pound mark. Even though I was much younger and more active, even though I was drinking bouillon cubes and working fifteen hours a day for sales, I couldn't lose that weight. Because of that weight gain, I deliberately started smoking again. The minute I went back to smoking, I dropped right back to 194 pounds, where I belonged. When I went into the hospital for Bypass, I had a fresh pack of cigarettes in my pocket. I put them on the table beside the bed as a challenge. I'd look at them and not smoke. Eventually, I got this craving for sweets, especially chocolate. I love chocolate. To counteract the chocolate, I fill a small pipe in the morning; that lasts a whole day, and I don't blow up like a balloon."

Before the Bypass, did you have any fantasies or nightmares?

"I only had five or ten minutes of apprehension. That was the night before the operation. They took three of us down for a tour, which was good for us to see, but when I got back to the room, I felt fearful. Just a little. It passed off quickly. The next morning, I noticed one guy had a priest there, and another guy had a rabbi. The father was praying and the rabbi was praying. I didn't have anybody because they'd said, 'We prefer not to have the family there before you go down for surgery. Sometimes, the family gets upset and their alarm frightens the patient.' I didn't want my minister or my wife. I was just glad to get it out of the way. I can't even tell you why my misgivings vanished so quickly. I read a lot of Shakespeare in the hospital. Maybe he helped. I was a math/engineering major in college, but I took a second major in English. I wish I had more time to read."

Before Bypass, did your surgeon talk at any length to you?

"A lot of doctors don't tell you much, but this one was great. He tried to prepare me physically and emotionally. I did better than I expected. I didn't lose my voice as many people do. I didn't even have a sore throat. When I woke up, I started talking to the nurse. Maybe I talked well." Windsor smiles. "She said, 'Let me check to see whether you can breathe on your own.' She tickled my throat, I started breathing, and she got the doctor to remove the tube."

How could you talk with the tube in your mouth?

"You can talk some. You can nod your head. Maybe I did well, because I didn't lose the whole day. I don't like to sleep my way through life. When I woke up, my eyes were wide open, she talked to me. Twelve hours after Bypass, the tube was out. When the tube comes out early, that's a big plus."

What was the worst part of Bypass?

"The constipation. The pain medication is constipating. I had one hell of a time. They unblocked my coronary arteries and blocked up my intestines. When I talked to the doctors, I told them, 'If you can tell me *why* I was constipated, you should do something to prevent it. When you stop the heart blockage, you should stop the bowel blockage.' They agreed that people should be given a solvent prophylactically in the hospital."

What was the worst aspect of the convalescence?

"Trying to adjust to the weakness. You can't lift anything. You're incredibly weak. When people would come to the house, I felt I had to entertain them. When they'd leave, every muscle would be vibrating in my body. Walking fifteen times around the outside of the house gave me a mile. I measured it. In the beginning, walking five or seven times would be too much. Afterwards, I'd have to lie down on the sofa; my whole body would be quivering. The physical exhaustion from very little exertion made my muscles shake like Jell-O. I couldn't control my muscles. As I got stronger and stronger, it'd happen less and less, but if I overdid, those muscular shivers would kick up. If I'd known about the weakness, it might have been easier, but I guess there are different levels of tolerance for different people."

Did you have any complications after Bypass? Any inflammation or chest pain?

"Nothing. I used only one pain pill, because I healed so well. I knew if I made up my mind to heal well in my psyche, I'd heal well in my flesh and blood. Look at my scar. That's only a year old. Blacks have a tendency to keloid formation. Not me. My one failing is in the exercise department. I'm not pushing myself enough. I get in the car; I drive to work. If a shipment is wrong, I drive over to the warehouse. Every week, I say, 'Next week I'll do more physical labor for therapy.' I asked my cardiologist if I could do push-ups; he vetoed that. He wants me to walk, but that gets boring. I'm back to bowling once a week. Since my Bypass, my bowling average is down. I'd like to be in some kind of group exercise program, where I'd feel embarrassed if I didn't show up. In lieu of that, I'm going to start helping the men in the warehouse."

What did the Bypass do for you?

"Suddenly, I realized I was a very, very lucky person. That I was able to have Bypass, that somebody had devised such an operation, that people were skilled enough to do it, that I got through it without a mishap, that I could afford it, made me exceedingly grateful. My mother would have been happy to see how I thanked God. Bypass made me appreciate life more. It extended my life."

How long do you want to live?

"As long as I can be useful. I don't want to be a problem to myself or to anybody else. If I'm useful till I'm 125, that's fine. At all ages, people are able to contribute to society, as long as they're functional upstairs." Windsor leans back in his chair, smiles thoughtfully. "Scratch 125. I'll settle for ninety."

What else did Bypass do for you?

"I feel better. I don't get any pain. But I'm not as strong. It's a year. My strength should be back. I don't have any shortness of breath. Yet, *I'm not as strong.* That's a disappointment. Then, I have that numbness in my chest where they took the internal mammary. It's getting better. It's worth it, my doctor says, because the internal mammary stays open longer."

Has Bypass changed you in other ways?

"You want to ask me about sex? Is that what you're edging up to?"

No, I'll ask you about sex in a minute.

"I'm the same human being I always was. I'm more grateful, more conscious of being available to the world and its dwellers. My own personal philosophy is everyone should try to help somebody every day. If you don't reach out a hand to the next man, you'll have a lot of regrets. Your life won't count for much, when it's all over."

If the doctors said, "Mr. Windsor, you need another Bypass," would you have it?

"Absolutely."

Would you go to the same doctor and the same hospital?

"Yes. Only next time, I'll insist they put a stool solvent in with the painkiller. If they know pain medicine shuts up shop, they should anticipate the problem before it occurs. When a patient has to ask a nurse to break up the stool, it's bad for the patient, and it's not so much fun for the nurse."

*You said you waited six weeks to drive a car. How long did you wait
to climb stairs?*

"About two weeks. The first time I climbed stairs was real exertion."

How long did you wait to have sexual intercourse?

"Whatever the little booklet said." Windsor laughs.

Did the doctor talk to you about when you could resume sexual intercourse?

"No, only the booklet. White doctors don't like to talk about sex.
As black doctors move up the middle-class ladder, they're not so
willing to talk about sex either."

Were you afraid the first time?

"Since Bypass, I've not been as free sexually. I'd been conditioned
some about sex before Bypass. Sex, the exertion coming from plea-
surable sex, would set off the pain. Even if I'd go ahead, during
intercourse, I'd be anticipating pain. I wouldn't lose my desire, but
I'd be concerned. Since Bypass, I don't have any pain with intercourse, but a little man sits on my shoulder and says, 'I don't know.
I wonder if you'll have pain again.' "

Since Bypass, is your desire the same, greater, less?

"Right now"—Windsor sighs—"less. Even though I don't have chest
pain, it's less. For two reasons: number one, I've gone through a
period of being totally away from sex; and number two, the medications don't do your desire any good. I'm only on one Corgard a
day—and Tagamet for my ulcer. Both Tagamet and Corgard act
as sexual inhibitors."

*Does "inhibitor" mean they depressed your sexual drive or they de-
feated your ability to maintain an erection?*

Windsor's laugh is thin. "I don't know which comes first, the chicken
or the egg. But it's a loss."

Do you have intercourse now as frequently as you did before Bypass?

He shakes his head. "No."

How frequently is it?

"Only a couple of times a month. I had a girl friend I liked a lot. Before my Bypass, sometimes we'd have sex five times a week, sometimes only once a week. It depended on what was happening at home."

Do you have intercourse with your wife?

"No. Just with my girl friend."

Was your girl friend afraid the first time?

"That's another problem. Maybe you can help me on that one. My sex is not with my regular girl friend. It's with another friend. My regular girl, the one I spend most of my time with, has gone into a turnoff. She's having hot flashes, so she doesn't want to have intercourse. My cardiologist said, 'She'll work through it. Be patient. It's caused by the emotional problems attendant on change of life.' Meantime, I'm having intercourse with another woman. I don't like her half as well, so I don't have as much desire for her."

Did your first friend see a gynecologist? He might give her something for her flashes which would rekindle her desire.

"The flashes seem to be passing. As the flashes wane, her whole attitude gets a little warmer."

Fear for your well-being might affect her desire, even though she's unwilling to say it.

"It could have been. She's very fond of me. She was the last one to believe I had any kind of a heart problem. Maybe she didn't want to believe it. The night before the catheterization, she said, 'I *know* there's nothing wrong with your heart.' "

Nobody wants to believe someone she loves is sick.

"Maybe so. She's always been extremely attentive. This turnoff could have been fear. She didn't get like this until after my Bypass. We care about each other a great deal."

Did you ever think of divorcing your wife and marrying her?

"I feel responsible for my wife. After all these years, it's my job to be sure she's comfortable. The trouble is"—Windsor pauses—"I feel responsible for my friend, too. Not financially. Personally, as a companion, as a stay against loneliness."

Now that you're a Bypass veteran, what are your greatest fears?

"It's difficult to divorce the Bypass fears from the fears of growing old. I'm 61, you know. Since Bypass, I have fewer fears about my heart, but I dread the day when I can't do the things I love. I'm a physical man, I like hunting and fishing, I like the outdoors. I'm a sensual man." Windsor's face clouds. "I like my friend. I don't like using this other woman."

What are your greatest joys?

"Making people happy. Pleasing someone."

What's been your greatest disappointment?

"I'm dissatisfied with myself because I never could zero in on a single profession and say, 'This is what I want to do. This is what I want to be, whether it's engineering, medicine, law, to the exclusion of everything else.' I liked being a Renaissance man, but it catches you in the long run. Knowing a little about a lot of things, I've been happy with myself, but there have been times when I've regretted not knowing enough about one thing. If there was anything I would have changed in myself, it's the ability to hone in on a specific subject. Either way, you pay a price."

What explicit questions would you advise a prospective Bypasser to ask his internist, his cardiologist, and his surgeon, before and after surgery?

"Four months after Bypass, my doctor set up a reunion for all of us who'd been in the hospital at the same time. I went from work and got there early. I watched them all coming in, their wives driving them, helping them in. They looked sick, all bent over, walking all hunched and frail. These were whites, no black folks. I said to myself, 'Jesus! They look so sick! It's depressing to be with them.' Different people respond to heart surgery in different ways. My cardiologist says his toughest task is convincing people they can go back to work, even though medically they're sound as a dollar. Emotionally, they can't get themselves back to work. Some people get accustomed to being waited on and taken care of. The whole atmosphere of being an invalid feels good to them.

"Some people have difficulty going back to work because they've had so much heart trouble before the operation. If they were sick before, even after Bypass, they're afraid of every little extra effort. After I had that supposed heart damage in 1965, I never hunted by myself. Before '65, I'd go back in the woods for a week, just me and my dogs. After '65, I'd always have someone else, even though I felt it was foolish. If you're hunting five miles from anywhere and you have a heart spasm, what's *anybody* gonna do? Since Bypass, I go hunting alone again. That's better, because I can talk things out with myself."

How can Bypass, the hospital stay, the convalescence, and the present time be made better, easier, less traumatic?

"Before and after Bypass, a person has to work hard on his approach to the post-Bypass period. He has to think positively. If the Bypass is a failure, you don't need to be prepared. If you don't wake up, you won't know it. Before Bypass, you need to be sure you'll wake up, to be positive about the outcome. People need certainty that they'll get something out of every experience, even Bypass. Incidentally, I'd never been operated on." He laughs hollowly. "I was a little uneasy about what I'd say or do under anesthesia or coming out of it. I guess I didn't have to worry."

One last question: all of us have insecurities about things. What are your insecurities?

"One insecurity is whether or not I'll be able to perform sexually as I did before I was sick."

That's still a problem?

"No, not a problem, but I want to reach that peak of performance I enjoyed before. A mountaintop is different from a hilltop. Here again, I don't know how much is because of age, because of medicine, because of weakness after Bypass. Another insecurity is money. I don't have enough money for a comfortable retirement. In any event, I'd rather work as long as I can. I'm not looking forward to retirement. I hope I can work until I'm ninety."

Do you have any questions to ask me?

"I'm curious about the socioeconomic influences on Bypassers' reactions and postoperative responses. I think people are less affected by race and ethnic origin than by social and economic class. I'll bet the lower classes, white or black, have a higher death rate from heart attacks. They smoke more, drink more, eat more, sit around more, and see their doctors less."

You're right. Several studies show social-class variation as a significant risk factor. Another question is why there are so few black Bypassers. Blacks have a tendency to hypertension more than to coronary artery disease. As they move into the middle class, they retain their predisposition to hypertension; some acquire white people's affinity for coronary heart disease.

"Economics, no insurance, fear of job security, are all reasons, as I told you, why there are so few black Bypassers. But there's another reason. The blacks at the bottom of the socioeconomic totem pole, which means the mass of blacks, are harnessed to a rock-bottom fear of the unknown. These blacks have been fed on fire-and-brimstone religion, have been inculcated in a fear of the darkness, a fear of things not known, not understood. Many blacks, I strongly suspect, would choose to bypass a Bypass operation.

They'd be afraid to have anyone open their chests, touch their hearts. Blacks believe in ghosts and goblins. If you believe the old ghost stories, then you're afraid what might happen if you venture into the unknown."

Would blacks be more willing to go to a black cardiologist and a black surgeon than a white cardiologist and white surgeon?

"Ignorant blacks don't trust their own to be smart enough to do a good job. They think it's a mark of esteem to go to a white doctor— like a white lawyer or a white teacher. Yet they're caught: because they don't trust white doctors to take good care of them, they stay away from doctors altogether. If you want to judge doctors stereotypically, I had the best of both worlds. I had a black cardiologist-angiographer and a white surgeon. For my money, they could have been sky-blue-pink. All I wanted was for them to open those blocked arteries so my good red blood could flow through them again."

9. Abraham Stearin, M.D.
Psychiatrist
Age at Bypass: 53

Many doctors didn't want to discuss their own Bypasses. Many were doing business at the same old stand, working longer and harder than before surgery, competing even more aggressively with younger—and older—colleagues to demonstrate that they were better than ever. As though Bypass were some secret sin, many quizzed me closely as to how I learned about their surgery. One even asked how much I paid the interviewee. Yet Dr. Abraham Stearin, a psychiatrist and sexual therapist in Rockford, Illinois, was surprised that so many doctors refused to discuss their own experiences.

"I don't care who knows I've had Bypass. You can use my name.† I'm not ashamed. What the hell do those guys think we're in this game for, anyway, if not to help other people? And maybe, by helping them, to lend ourselves a hand?"

Tall, black-haired, gap-toothed, on this rainy Saturday Dr. Stearin is dressed in a navy sport shirt, open at the throat, a white Ralph Lauren sweater, and kelly-and-navy plaid trousers. Calling for me

† Nevertheless, Dr. Stearin's name is fictitious, as is his address.

at the Rockford train station in his fawn-colored Mercedes 450, he takes me to his small, dreary office not far away. He sits on a pale-green plastic-covered chair behind a large oak desk. The omnipresent couch, covered in grimy "coral" vinyl, matches my ballpoint-spattered chair. As we talk, Dr. Stearin alternately curls his long legs around the chair, puts them on the desk, raises his bushy brows, waves his hands, marks off his points on his long, thin fingers, chomps hard on his chewing gum, gets fresh gum. The rain beats remorselessly on the frosted windowpane, a lucky rain, because Dr. Stearin had tried to trade our appointment for a golf game.

What are the special problems of a doctor having Bypass surgery?

"Doctors' problems aren't any different from ordinary patients'— except in one area: *they know too much.* At least, some do—or think they do. They're aware of all the dangers, of the complications of Bypass. As a psychiatrist, I had an advantage. I didn't have so much information. I'm not exposed to cardiology, except when I get a neurotic constantly anticipating cardiac death, positive every *nudge* signifies heart disease. I've been an analyst for God knows how long—since 1963, which makes me an old chicken. I'm fifty-six years old. I'll bet you couldn't tell. I had my Bypass at fifty-three."

How does a doctor distinguish between neurotic fears of cardiac death and true heart pain? This questions bedevils patients as well as doctors.

"As a physician, I'm no expert in cardiology, but I do know medicine. When you get chest pain, you don't fuck[1] around. Many patients come in here with substernal pressure, sometimes with jaw or elbow pain. Before we can even talk about psychotherapy, I insist they see an internist. Occasionally, EKG changes turn up. Patients tend to deny symptoms, but sometimes they don't deny; they'll introject and make mountains out of molehills. As a psy-

[1] Inappropriate obscenity (as opposed to "appropriate obscenity") is characteristic of the Type-A personality, perhaps because the A considers all situations thwarting and stressful. Dr. Stearin's speech is a revealing amalgam of street argot, Yiddishisms, and psychiatric jargon.

chiatrist, I try to balance the deniers and the overemphasizers. I sort them out, but I don't take chances. It's too easy to guess wrong. Everyone gets tested; everyone with a heartache is referred to his internist. If the internist says, 'There's nothing wrong with you. Discuss this with Dr. Stearin,' then I feel a little easier, although nobody is a 100 percent *maven*[2] with heart disease, maybe not with psychiatric disease either.

"If my patient has EKG changes, then I assume a different medical role. I become the psychocardiologist, keeping in constant touch with the cardiologist. He and I should have a good working relationship, because we treat the same person. Many patients end up with Bypass, which I encourage. Some cardiologists, especially internists, have a tendency to treat patients medically for too long. I resent their stalling. They resent my urging Bypass, resent what they consider my butting in.

"Even I had trouble with the balancing act between denying the implications of my chest pain and saying to my wife, Dorothy, 'We'd better go to the Emergency Room.' Although I wasn't denying," he interjects quickly. "The pressure left. I said, 'Oh, well, probably it's a hiatus hernia.' I thought I was overreacting, the bugaboo of every psychiatrist. I'd already started dressing to go to the hospital when the feeling left. I said, 'Why am I acting like this? I'm behaving like a neurotic idiot.' I took off my pants, threw my shorts on the floor, and got into bed. As soon as I put out the light, the goddam pressure came back. I said to Dot, 'Kid, enough. Let's go. I won't be able to sleep. I want to know what's going on. If it's a hiatas hernia or good old-fashioned gas, let's find out.' I couldn't have been feeling too bad, because I drove.[3]

"As soon as we got to the Emergency Room, the pressure left. It came and went like a New Year's card from the *Malach Hamoves*, the Angel of Death. I was afraid they'd find something, but jackass that I was, I was afraid they wouldn't find anything; then, I'd look like a hypochondriac. As a doctor, you think certain ways; as a human being, sometimes you think different ways."

He shakes his head wryly. "So I wasn't such a neurotic. Wonderful. I'd had a coronary, or was well on my way to one. My face was saved, but my heart wasn't in such good shape."

---

[2] Expert.
[3] Unless they're very ill, Type A's do the driving. They need to control their environment.

To what did you attribute your coronary artery disease?

"Genetics was at the head of the list. After all, what am I a psychiatrist for if not to blame my parents? I am candidate A–number one for coronary artery disease. Both my mother and my father died young of infarctions. Villain number two was stress. There's the whole picture, nature and nurture. I was going through so much stress, I can't tell you how tough it was. My eldest son, Tom, is a physician who fell in love with a Puerto Rican girl. I'm Jewish. Even here, in America's heartland, I can't omit the Yiddishisms from my speech; maybe a part of me clings to them. In psychiatry, I'm orthodox-trained, analytically Freudian. As a child, I was Orthodox Jewish–trained. My grandfather would take me by the hand and we'd go to *shul*[4] every Saturday morning. Friday nights were big deals. We lived with my grandparents in the Bronx during the Depression. We'd lay *Tefillin*.[5] Do you know Jewish people? Did you ever hear any of these words? Do you know what I'm talking about?"

When I nod, Dr. Stearin rushes on, the words geysering.

"When my son was in college, I knew he was dating this girl. I understood. I had been to college. I'd fucked around. When he was accepted at medical school, I figured he'd leave her behind, he'd go on, meet other people. I wanted to give him a reward for being accepted. He'd worked hard. I also wanted him to get the message. I said, 'I'll buy you a new car; you'll need it for medical school. You won't be a college kid any more. You're a big boy now.' Fine. Carlotta came up that afternoon. She's a lovely girl, a bright girl, with her doctorate in economics. That's not the point. The point was, or so I thought, that she wasn't Jewish—which was dumb. Dottie would scream at me, 'Here you've been through analysis and you're nothing but a bigot. You're riddled with prejudices.' I said, 'I can't help it. It's been burned into my skull that my Jewish son should marry a Jewish princess. That's the way orderliness is perpetuated.'

"We went out and bought the car; we came home and were sitting and talking in front of the fireplace. He had to leave in a week for medical school, and he said, 'Carlotta's going with me.' I said, 'Is

[4] The House of Study, the synagogue.
[5] Phylacteries, small boxes holding four passages in Hebrew from Exodus and Deuteronomy, worn by adult men during morning prayer.

that necessary? If you go with baggage, how are you going to meet new people, make new friends?' He said, 'I'm in love with her. She's going to live with me. She's got a great job teaching economics at the university. We've been living together for two years.' Of course, I knew they were living together. That's what kids do today. I never took it seriously. Who in his right mind takes kids living together seriously? When he told me that he intended to marry her, I became furious. I was an absolute jackass. I stormed out of the living room and stalked downstairs to the family room. Some 'family room'! What kind of family was this? I started hollering at Dot: 'It's all your fault. You encouraged them. He'd never have lived with her if it weren't for you.' I had to blame somebody, but God forbid I should blame myself. Through this long tirade, Dot just sat there and went on painting. Dot's an artist, very gifted. Two months after we were married, she won a fellowship to study in Rome, but she was already pregnant with Tom, so she had to turn it down. Just as well. I didn't want my wife working.[6] Certainly, I couldn't tolerate a part-time marriage. Dottie knows how to handle me. She plays me like a violin. I'm not bad at playing her violin either. Finally, she said, 'You done, Abe? Now it's my turn. That's Tom's decision. He's a big boy now. You said it yourself, but you didn't mean it. Now, move a little to the left. You're standing in my light.' Eventually, I relented—sort of."

Did it bother you more because she was not Jewish or because she was Puerto Rican?

"Both. I said to Tom, 'Look, you'll have an interracial marriage. I know enough about society's attitudes towards interracial children. Your no-doubt dark children—because it's a dominant gene—will come home and see a white father and Hispanic mother. How will your children react? Will they have color discrimination? You're

[6] Most of the interviewees and the respondents had nonworking wives, perhaps a generational comment because many were over fifty, but more likely a Type-A comment. A's want to be depended upon. A's want to be boss, and money talks. Ironically, after they had had Bypass, the men whose wives worked were relieved to have their financial burdens shared. For a conflicting view, see the somewhat skewed results of Dr. Suzanne Haines's study in the *Journal of Epidemiology*. Dr. Haines finds a higher incidence of myocardial infarction in men with working wives, but bases her statistics on only 260 men of varied backgrounds and age groups.

not thinking ahead. You're taking on a great responsibility.' He said, 'All right,' which meant nothing, because Carlotta went with him just as they planned. I didn't say any more, but it was grinding away inside me. I reached the point that I was ashamed to visit my family. My brothers and sisters would ask, 'How's Tom doing in med school?' I never said a word about Carlotta. When he graduated, he told me that they'd set the date to get married; he wanted us to know. Further, he wanted to be married here, at my country club, which is mostly Jewish because the *goyim*[7] won't let us on their hallowed golf courses. The more irrationally I behaved, the more aggravated I got with myself.

"If I reacted like such a *meshugginer*,[8] how could I call myself a psychiatrist and help people with their *mishegass*?[9] I felt all alone. There was no one to talk to. I wanted to see my analyst, to call him, to pour it all out to him. But he was getting on in years, too. I kept debating, 'Should I call Kurt?' Ultimately, I called him up and said, 'I'm driving myself crazy with my relationship with my son. I adore my son; he adores me. I know that. I have to talk to you, get this settled in my head.' He said, 'I'm going away on vacation in two days. I'm booked solid. I can't see you.' He went away. And left me."

Dr. Stearin stretches his long legs, puts his feet up on the desk, and stares at the frosted blank window. "Seeing Kurt probably wouldn't have changed anything.

"The other stress was my relationship with this community. I had been taking a two-year course in sexual therapy. When I completed the course, I came to the chief of Psychiatry at my hospital and told him, 'I want to devote more time to the clinic, so patients can make use of my new knowledge.' He bit hard on that foul-smelling pipe of his and said, '*Absolutely not!*' Those were his words. 'This is a small conservative community. Discussing sexual matters is *not done*.' I said to myself, 'What the hell's wrong with society's attitudes?' Meanwhile, I had started treating a few sexual-therapy couples in my office. The OB-GYN Department invited me to lecture. Afterwards, but only after, I realized I'd committed a fatal error. I hadn't given them a chance to desensitize their previously

---

[7] Gentiles.
[8] Madman.
[9] Insanity, madness, fixation, an *idée fixe*.

chauvinistic approaches to women. Some OB-GYN men are terribly chauvinistic. They'll rip out your uterus; then they'll tell you
that you're the ball-breaker."

The stress prior to Bypass was your son's wanting to marry this girl?

"One of the stresses."

He married her?

"Yes. See this picture on my desk? See this blond-haired, blue-
eyed, little boy? He's my grandchild. His name is Abe Stearin, even
though Ashkenazic Jews don't name children for living people.
Which only goes to show you what *I* know about people and about
genetics."

*Besides your fraying relations with your son, your professional rela-
tions had worsened because of this course in sexual therapy?*

"They looked on me as an oddball: 'Why are you talking about sex
and showing films about massage techniques?' "

*Why did you take this course? What percent of your practice now is
in sexual therapy?*

"First question. In therapy, sexuality is important. You talk openly
about sexuality; at least, I hope you can. In my practice, I had
noticed if a young man comes to me because he is a premature
ejaculator, no amount of analytic work changed him. I couldn't
help a patient overcome her frigidity or her inability to achieve
orgasm. I couldn't help a patient with vaginismus.[10] Most sexual
dysfunctions did not respond to orthodox analytic psychotherapy.
When Masters and Johnson published their first book, I read it and
said to myself, 'Dammit, maybe this is the answer.' I enrolled in
this course for sex therapists. About 25 percent of my practice now
is sexual therapy. But when I got back from taking the course—
which was not long before Bypass, mind you—I ran into tremen-

[10] A painful contractional spasm of the vagina, usually preventing intercourse.

dous opposition. When I'd have a cup of coffee in the hospital cafeteria and bullshit with the fellows, they'd plunk themselves down at my table and say, 'Hey, Abe, when are you bringing in dirty pictures for grand rounds?' I'd get a *zetz*[11] in here." Dr. Stearin pounds his chest with his clenched fist. "I wanted to say, 'You dumb punks, you'll never understand this.'

"Because I'm so introspective, because of the analysis necessary to become a psychiatrist, I knew I'd gain nothing, that I'd antagonize them more because they're so sure they know all the answers. I'd lowered myself to respond to their idiotic 'humor.' I might make a fool out of myself. My insides would be churning. My ego was threatened by these *schmucks*.[12] I was *allowing* them to threaten me; my self-knowledge only exacerbated my stresses. I couldn't stop myself from this obsessive circling. Pretty soon, I was going to the hospital, taking care of my patients, no longer stopping for coffee in the cafeteria, no longer horsing around with the guys. I began to withdraw. Ours was an unspoken mutual isolation pact.

"After I finished my sexual training and supervision, I was invited to teach a course. I got along fine; I was with kindred spirits—physicians, social workers, nurses. All week, I'd look forward to those classes. But at this age, traveling down to St. Louis after a day's work, spending two hours in a class, and driving back the same night is a burden. I wasn't such a big-shot *shtarcker*.[13] Then again, Dottie and I are communicators. At night, it's a case of who'll shut up so we can get some sleep. I'd come home, puffed up about the classes. We'd talk till four in the morning, not only about my altered attitudes towards sexuality, but about my new ways of seeing. If you look carefully and you're open-minded, millions of little things reveal what's happening in a relationship. It was great. But I got tired out from traveling.

"My third contribution to heart disease was not being intelligent enough to say to myself, 'Stearin, you come from a stinking genetic background. For God's sake, why don't you start watching your diet, exercising a little? Before Bypass, I weighed thirty-five pounds more than I do today, not excessively overweight, but not so lean. All day long, I sit listening like a Buddha. Never mind your anti-

[11] Strong blow or punch.
[12] In this context, dopes, jerks, boobs.
[13] Strong man.

psychiatrist jokes about 'who listens?' My own stupidity made me look the other way about my elevated cholesterol and elevated triglycerides. As a rule, I'm never sick. I'm a healthy guy. I never get a cold. I don't go for annual physicals. Some people believe in them; some people don't. My analyst would say, 'The less I see a physician, the better I feel.' I agreed. I ignored tests. I'd say, 'I feel fine.' I'd eat steaks, hot croissants with whipped butter, chopped liver with chicken fat. If you feel well, you think you're immortal. You don't think, 'Pretty soon, I'm going to die, maybe sooner than later.' You don't think, 'The years are passing rapidly.' You think, 'Life will be like this forever.' You know life can't be good forever, or last forever; you know your parents died, yet you think, 'Not me, not now. I'm the golden boy.'

"Since my surgery, *my* surgery, not somebody else's *tsuris*,[14] my attitude's different. The stage was set: the genetic background, the stress of my youngster, the professional quarrels, the blind stupidity of not acknowledging the dangers of those test results." He stops. "If I'm confessing to my own self-destructiveness, I'll add one more *narishkeit*[15]: I was a two-pack-a-day smoker."

Do you still smoke?

He shifts uneasily, laughs. "Oh, once in a while, I'll have a cigarette; I'll puff on my pipe. Not like before. You sit here, you listen to patients. You light a cigarette, you put it out, you light another one. I've been smoking since I was sixteen. My father smoked. He introduced me to cigarettes. If it weren't for my father, I wouldn't have smoked. My son thinks anybody who'd inhale tobacco is an asshole."

What about pot?

"He smokes a little grass once in a while. I don't concern myself about his smoking a little pot; the amount must be minimal. If he were a pot-head, how could he function as a physician? How much can he smoke on weekends? He doesn't smoke during the week."

[14] Troubles, woe, worries, sufferings. Heartache. Dr. Stearin's Yiddish is quite explicit.
[15] Foolishness.

How did you decide to have Bypass?

"Deciding was easy: I had a left anterior descending. Knowing that the LAD is nicknamed the 'widow-maker,' I didn't have any questions about needing Bypass."

If you had had a less clear-cut indication for Bypass, would you have gone ahead?

"I can't answer that. I wasn't consulted. After the catheterization, my internist and my cardiologist put their heads together and looked at the films. Meanwhile, back in my room, I was trying to sweet-talk a nurse into giving me a cigarette. Shows you what kind of *schmuck* I was! They told Dot what they thought and asked her, 'What shall we tell Abe?' Dottie said, 'Tell him he has to have Bypass. Don't mince words.' I never had a chance to see the films. During the cath, I had seen this sturdy LAD shrivel into a thread, but I didn't grasp its significance. As I doused the cigarette in a glass of water under the table, they marched into my room with Dot and said, 'You absolutely must have Bypass—very fast.'

"If I go to a physician, and I hope patients feel the same way when they come here, I believe that I either trust my physician or I shouldn't go see him. Of course, sometimes I get so pissed off, I don't see anybody, but at that time I liked those guys, so I said, 'If you guys say I need Bypass, then I'll go have a Bypass.' Actually I had no idea what Bypass was, what it involved. I only knew that Zach, my best friend, had had Bypass and was not doing well. But I'm an optimist. I always felt that whatever will be, will be, and that I'll be fine. They started calling big-name thoracic surgeons, in New York, in Boston, in Milwaukee. All were booked solid. Zach had his operation in Los Angeles, so I had a little bit of *tziter*—a little fear—about going to L.A. I told them how I felt. 'Not that the doctors aren't good in Los Angeles, but Zach had pericarditis, he had postop bleeding, he had arrhythmias. Not that I'm superstitious, but . . .' They said, 'Look, they're the best[16] and you need this. L.A.'s trying to fit you into their schedule. We can't undo all

---

[16] Almost every Bypasser thought his or her surgical team was "the best." Dr. Meyer Friedman believes this attitude is consonant with the Type-A personality.

arrangements. We've made a million calls.' L.A. said, 'Dr. Stearin can come in Christmas Day; we'll operate a couple of days later.'

"*Tziter* and all, it was settled. For fifteen days, I sat around the house and waited to go. There I was, babying myself, and hating how I babied myself. I was extremely conscious, because I don't lie to myself, of how slowly I'd climb the stairs, one at a time, holding on to the rail. I used to take them two at a time. I said to myself, 'You're getting to be an old fart.' It didn't do any good. I pampered myself, carefully measured out my Inderal, my Isordil, my Valium, according to doctors' orders. Nobody could accuse *me* of patient-noncompliance! I hadn't had a symptom since the night I went to the Emergency Room, but the EKG and the cath said, 'Stearin's walking on eggshells.' "

You didn't have a stress test before the angio?

"Nope. I went from EKG to cath, from cath to surgery. 'Do not pass Go. Do not collect two hundred dollars.' That's me. I never even asked why. Christmas Day, Dot and I flew to California. The stage was set."

Did any of your sons go?

"No, I told Dot that I didn't want the boys to see me in the hospital."

Why?

"Another of my *mishegasses*. In case I died, which was a distinct possibility, although I did not believe it would happen, I didn't want my sons to have any lingering nightmares of the old man suffering, only the normal memories of horsing around with them, playing ball with them, going sailing with them. That was the psychiatrist talking. I didn't want them *ever* to see me in the hospital, hooked up to EKGs, tubes, and wires, being monitored, or to see me gasping for every breath, attached to oxygen. I told Dottie not to let them come to the hospital. Tom said, 'Look, in thirty minutes I can fly up there from med school.' Dot said, 'Don't come. Your father would be more distressed by your presence.' He never knew the reason: I didn't want him to have a memory of a debilitated, sickly father."

What about Dottie?

"That's different. I couldn't exist without her, I couldn't have had the operation without her. Every morning, she was there when I woke up. She was a bulwark for me. It was harder for her to go through than for me. I was doped up; she wasn't. She had to sit alone in the hotel, and wait for the liaison nurse to report how the operation was going. They kept her pretty well informed, but it's a long sit."

Would Dot have preferred to have your children out there or not?

"I suspect, although she wouldn't tell me this, she would have preferred the children around her to give her strength, but she accepted my reasoning. She respects me."

At Cleveland Clinic* and several other places in this country, they don't allow family members in to see the Bypasser for three days after the operation. How would you have felt about that?

"If she had not been there when I woke up, I couldn't have done it. Never."

After the surgery, did you review your life and its course, where you'd been and where you were going?

"Both before and after surgery, I looked long and hard at my life. Those three days before, tests or no tests, give you a lot of time to think, maybe more than you'd like. I thought about my mother and father and my relationship to them. They'd both died young of heart disease. They'd both worked hard all their days. I'm a first-generation American. They were both born in Poland. A stress that everybody looks away from is the stress of the marginal man with one foot in the old country and one foot in the new. Trying to achieve the standards of the old, to acquire the manners of the new. America was a new world for them, a world not kind, a world at best indifferent. My father is a very bright man. Or was.

"After I finished high school, I worked for a year. I told him, 'Pa,

* Not a fictitious name.

I'm unhappy every day going to work, being a clerk. I want to go to college.' He said, *'Far vos?'*[17] I said, 'I'm not sure. I'm a good science student. Who knows? Maybe I'll be a doctor, maybe I'll be a sculptor. I want to go to college and taste a few things. What I like, I'll eat.' That's all I told him, but he said, 'All right. We'll scrape together a few dollars and send.' But he added, 'If you go to college, you should not live home, you should not go to college in Chicago.' I was stunned. 'Why?' He said, 'You're still wet behind the ears. You've been no place. I want you to go to a new area of the United States, meet new people with different attitudes. You'll meet people who never even met a Jew, who think a Jew is somebody with horns.' I grew up in the Chicago ghetto, the *Jewish* ghetto, and I thought everybody knew about Jews. Oh, I'd been subjected to anti-Semitism. What Jew hasn't? But when you're young, who thinks the mainstream will look at him as a freak, just because of what he *is*, not because of anything he does?' I went to Nebraska. Sure enough, there were only a handful of Jews there. After Bypass, I lay in bed and remembered my old man taking me up to the bus station. I couldn't afford a train even. *He* was carrying my bag—'It's too heavy for you, Sonny.' My father was not a demonstrative man, but he put his arms around me and hugged me hard in the Chicago bus station. 'Study hard and write once in a while, so your mother shouldn't worry.'

"It changed my life. After my second year, the dean called me in and told me to start thinking about medical school. 'You're a good student. Your math stinks, but you could study over the summer and take the math exam again. You should go to medical school.' I owe that dean. I owe my old man. In the hospital, I kept going over my relationships to the important people in my life."

What about your other sons? You don't talk about them.

"One's a lawyer. The other's also a doctor, taking a year off in Europe now. He's a different kind of a son. He's Dot's boy. Tom is my boy. Matt loves music, plays the oboe, paints. Like Dottie, he's much more artistically inclined. Jeff, the lawyer, goes his own way."

[17] For what?

In the three years since the operation, do you think you value human relationships more?

"Yes and no. I'm much more selfish. Much more. Before Bypass, people would say, 'Come on over for cocktails and dinner.' We'd go. How could you refuse an intimate invitation to be with fifty of your 'closest friends'? No more. I don't go to parties. At the last gathering, twelve of us were together *Yom Kippur*[18] night to break the fast. Maybe it was a party. We were celebrating that we were still here, hoping we'd been 'inscribed in the Book of Life for another year.' But no cocktail parties with small talk to the same people about the same things, balancing a plate on my knee from the same 'new' cateress, drinking, messing around. Since Bypass, I have no patience with wasting a minute of my life. I'm protective of my time, even with patients. After the second or third session, if I'm bored with the patient, if I know I don't want this patient, I say, 'I think we should review these few sessions. Perhaps you would be better off with another analyst. Don't think I'm rejecting you, but for us to continue wouldn't be fair to you. I lack what you need.' I always put the onus on myself. I'm not wealthy. I can't afford to throw patients away, but it's too late for me to go through the motions. Maybe if more psychiatrists operated this way, they'd have a better success rate. I don't know. Surely, they'd be more honest."

After Bypass, did you become more irritable?

"I'm much more impatient with stupidity. I don't hesitate to show my irritability; I don't hold it in."

Since Bypass, has your practice declined?

"I used to work five or six days a week; now I work three days a week. Don't tell other doctors that. They'll think I'm retired. Now I pick and choose my patients. People still want to see me, although . . . well, I have openings on my calendar that I never had before. I like it that way. If I work from nine to twelve, I take an hour for myself. I don't eat lunch, just a cup of bouillon, a couple of saltines,

[18] The Jewish Day of Atonement, a day of fasting.

and some fruit, washed down by a Tab. I used to go out to eat, but I stopped."

You don't restrict salt?

"Of course, not! I'm not hypertensive."[19]

Why don't you go out to eat?

"Because I'd be tempted to sit down and have a corned-beef sandwich, that's why. I'm weak-minded when it comes to corned beef or hot pastrami, which even for me is too much salt.[20] And cholesterol. Besides, it's easier not to go out. I sit in my office; I listen to Beethoven or Brahms. I always have tons of reading; I'm never caught up with the professional literature."

Since the Bypass, are you more aware of things you wish you'd done with your life?

"My God, yes. Anyone who tells you he would do it the same way all over again is a *schmuck*. Boy, would I have done things differently!"

What would you have changed?

"Number one: I would not have become a physician. I would have become a sculptor, maybe a writer, like you. I keep a journal, I always have, except for the terrible period after surgery when I was in such deep depression. Even though my mother would not have liked having a sculptor or a writer for a son, I wouldn't have become a physician. As the years flew by, I have found them to be flat, one-dimensional types who can talk only one subject: medicine. If you count money, two subjects. I'm being unfair, because occasionally, you'll meet doctors interested in more than the beast and the buck. I shouldn't indict the entire medical profession, but the majority of physicians *I* know are plastic façades with nothing

[19] The villainous properties of salt, particularly for anyone with cardiovascular disease, rarely are appreciated by either Bypassers or non-Bypassers, unless they have vigorously antisodium physicians.
[20] Bouillon, Tab, saltines, are as forbidden as a corned-beef sandwich.

beneath. They wear their little white coats and run from cubicle to cubicle. At the end of the day, they count up their cash, and their successes are determined by their bank accounts. Money has never been a problem for me, thank God, as long as I have enough for my needs. My goal is not to pile up a couple million dollars. What am I going to do with it? Have them throw it in my coffin beside me? Leave Dottie a rich widow? I made enough to support the boys and put them through school. They never had the pressures of taking out student loans and having to pay them back, of starting out with a bushel of debts, as I did. I didn't want my sons to go through what I went through."

You're sorry you became a physician, yet two of your sons became doctors.

"They chose it. Not me. Don't blame me for that."

Your children are grown. You had Bypass. What's to keep you from chucking your practice now?

"I'm doing it. Slowly. I fixed up a studio. I've thrown out some carvings. I decided they weren't any good. It's part of the process of learning a craft, but it made me feel rotten. I wonder how many more I'll do."

Did the operation make you feel old?

"I went through a severe depression for two months. Thirty to 40 percent of Bypassers have post-Bypass depression. It's so easy to treat, so easy for me to treat. I pull up my shirt and say, 'Look at my scar. How's your scar coming along?' We'll talk about how it was for me, how I got through it. I don't treat Bypassers the way I treat other patients. Ordinarily, a psychiatrist doesn't tell a patient about himself. He's distant, aloof. With Bypassers, I'm much more involved. The treatment is short, because they come out of the depression."

A doctor whom I interviewed said it would have helped him enor-
mously if he had only known that the depression was temporary. And
yet he thought it not 'cost-effective' for a psychiatrist to be a member
of the team.

"He's wrong. If he was depressed, he should know better. He must
have been a surgeon. There *always* should be a psychiatrist who
sees the patient regularly before and after surgery and after he goes
home. Preferably, that psychiatrist should have had Bypass, because I don't care what anyone says, people who have been through
it are the best ones to help you out. The one person who helped
me *in the hospital* was the respiratory therapist. He'd had Bypass
and he showed me his scar. He told me about himself. A young
fellow, an uneducated Catholic boy, he'd had Bypass at thirty-five.
Originally, he'd been bitterly depressed because he thought he
'caught' an old man's disease. When he came in to see me, he made
my day. I felt great because I could say to myself, 'See how nicely
he's doing. I have more brains, more money, more years, than he
has, so I should be able to pull myself out of the morass.' But it's
not easy to do by yourself."

What professional help did you have for your depression?

"Nobody knew I was depressed except Dorothy. The wives are the
unsung heroines of Bypass. Your next book belongs to them."

Why didn't you tell anybody but your wife?

"As a psychiatrist, you're supposed to be able to cope with all
problems. You think people will say, 'Look at that poor psychia-
trist-*schmuck*. He can't even handle Bypass surgery. And he's trying
to advise us about our lives.' I knew I was being an idiot. I'd lie
awake at night and ask myself, 'What makes you think you're so
damned omnipotent?' One day, about three days after the operation, when Dot came in, I was weeping. Literally sobbing my heart
out; I couldn't stop. Terribly upset, she said, 'I'd better call your
surgeon.' I said, 'Don't you dare. You do and I'll punch you out. I
don't know what's going on with me. I've never been depressed in

my life, but for the first time, I sure know how it feels. If I'd known what I was going to have to go through, I'm not sure I'd have had it.' I knew it was ridiculous; I had to have Bypass to live. She tried to calm me down. 'Don't placate me,' I bellowed. 'You know I hate to be placated. You're just doing that to aggravate me more.' I ventilated all this depression, heaped it all on Dorothy. Later, I could interpret my depressions as internalized anger: *Why me? Why me?* I was wild with rage at my ancestors. Why couldn't I live to be 103 like my grandmother? Why did I have to have my father's and mother's genes? A completely infantile response which I had to ventilate.

"The worst was that one awful day in the hospital. After that, the depression was different because then you are dealing with *yourself*. You're having to face facts: you're not the same bundle of energy as before. Constantly, you're reminded you have no stamina, you've had a big operation, you're healing so slowly. Over and over, you ask yourself, 'Is the operation a failure? If it's successful, how long will it last? How will I know?' It's a true endogenous depressive neurosis,[21] which lasts a few months. I vacillated between thinking mine was a neurotic response or a normal reaction to a massive somatic[22] and psychic assault. While I was getting stronger, I could accept or reject my physical debilities, be patient with myself or angry with the world, angry with my body because it had let me down, angry with myself because I'd let all this get to me."

When you returned from California, did you call your analyst?

"No, I had written him before I went. I'd told him what had happened. He never answered. Besides, what could he do? He couldn't possibly understand because he didn't have Bypass and wouldn't know what I was going through. How could he know what I meant when I said, 'When the weather changes, my chest hurts.' Then I agonize: 'Is the pain from the weather, or are my vessels closing off?' My mind runs a review course of all the terrible postsurgical complications."

[21] Despondency, despair originating from within, as opposed to *exogenous* depression derived or developed from external causes.
[22] Of or pertaining to the body, as distinguished from the mind, the emotions, or from external environment.

Is it better for patients to know about complications or not to know?

"How could you ask that? Of course it's better to know. Most of the complications are transitory, are commonly experienced. If you know that lots of other people are suffering what you're suffering, it's a different ball game entirely."

Do you prescribe antidepressants for Bypassers? Did you take any yourself?

"No, because I was analyzing myself. I stopped taking the hospital's Valium because it made me flaky—and it's a depressant. I need to have a clear mind. I'd take Ativan—one or two milligrams—to calm me down. I work out my own problems."

Don't some antidepressants trigger arrhythmias?

"It depends on the antidepressant. Psychiatrists have to be careful. I usually put a patient on Sinequan or Desyrel. I won't keep a patient on a drug for more than two weeks. I don't want them crutching their way through life and *kvetching*[23] in here. Some psychiatrists use Desyrel much longer. I don't like saying, 'Look, you're depressed; this medication will help you.' I want patients to know that medication will help temporarily, while we work together. I tell them beforehand, 'You'll only take this for two weeks. It'll help you open up to me, so we can do some therapy.' "

Before the surgery, did you have any preoperative fantasies or nightmares?

"The night before surgery, I dreamt I was talking to God."

What did He have to say?

"God was dressed like Kurt Lundberg, my analyst, with a little mixture of my grandfather because He had a beard and Kurt does not; He rumpled my hair and Kurt is not affectionate. But the speech pattern was Kurt's. I was *kvetching* at God. I told God, 'You

[23] Complaining.

really know how to make a guy suffer. Who do You think You are, anyway?' I never told anybody about the dream. I didn't even tell Dottie until months later. The dream may have been provoked by medication or God knows what."

Do you have nightmares now?

"No. Well, once in a while. When Carlotta was in labor, Tom called us. I said, 'Mother and I will drive up to keep you company.' He said, 'Stay home.' I did it to him with my Bypass; now he was making me stay away. But mine was sickness. His was new life. I fell asleep and had the worst kind of nightmare. Everything went wrong. Everything ended in death. The phone rang, thank God, and awoke me. It was Tom: 'We have a little boy. Everything is fine. Go back to sleep.' I wanted to be with them so much; they kept me away."

Did your surgeon talk at any length to you before the Bypass?

"That's why I loved him, although I'm not sure if he explained it well because I'm a physician. I'm sure he didn't talk to lay people; I have two patients in town whom he never talked to.

"When we arrived on Christmas Day, I was pissed. 'Why doesn't he come to visit his nice Jewish patient who's come all this way for Bypass?' I realized he had a family, that it was a holiday, but I couldn't restrain my antagonism. How could such a serious operation be treated so cavalierly by the doctor? By the next noon, I was biting my fingernails to the elbows; I still hadn't seen him. He was operating that morning.

"Late that afternoon, he came in. He's handsome, young, quiet-mannered, witty. He got to me. Here am I, sitting with my pipe in my mouth, my tobacco pouch on the nightstand, and in he walks. He gave me such a look and picked up the pipe: 'If I had known you smoke, I wouldn't have taken you as a patient.' I was ready to kill him. Here I'd come all this way and he was lecturing me about smoking. Of course, he was right, but I couldn't admit it. 'I'm going to assume this belongs to someone else,' he said. He broke the pipe with his bare hands, and threw it in the wastebasket. A $150 Meerschaum! Next, he threw the tobacco in the basket. He turned to Dorothy and asked, 'Why do you let him smoke?' I said, 'See here, don't put the onus on Dottie. Yell at me.' He asked me about my background and history. He never sat down. He stood, and his liaison nurse stood beside him."

Did you mind that he didn't sit down, that he didn't talk to you alone?

"Not at all. They're busy, they don't have time. Well, maybe I would've liked to talk to him by himself. I might've asked different questions. But he did something very nice. After that, he could've done anything, it would've been okay with me. He said, 'I haven't seen your films. Have you? Would you like to go with me to see the films? Let's look at them together.' I had two reactions. Simultaneously. 'Yes, I want to see the films. No, the less I know about it, the less I have to worry about what could go wrong.'

"As I was debating, Dorothy stood up and said, 'That's very sweet. Seeing the films would be helpful for Abe—and for me too.' How could I say, 'I'm petrified, I don't want to see the damn things. Look at the trouble they got me into'? All four of us went to the screening room and looked at the cath films. I could've *plotzed.*[24] That LAD looked like Coney Island on a Sunday, a strip of beach at each end, with the middle clogged so with people, or with fatty plaque, that you can see neither sand nor sea.

"He said, 'It looks like I'll only have to fix one. But when I go in, if I find another vessel like that one, I might have to do more. When you wake up, don't ask me, "How come you did three or four?" When the nurse brings in your release, just sign on the dotted line. As a doctor, you should understand why we do business that way.' It's the same as my attitude with my patients: 'If you don't trust me, you shouldn't be here.' I said, 'Fine.' "

Now do you think much about your Bypass?

"I don't think much about my operation, but I'm obsessed by my mortality. Even as I talk to you, I'm saying to myself, 'How many more years? How many more years?' That question never lets go of me."

---

[24] *Plotz*—to split, to burst, to explode, to be infuriated, aggravated beyond enduring. Dr. Stearin's subconscious uses a Yiddish slang verb appropriate for his LAD.

What do you think Bypass did for you?

"Bypass gave me a chance to live longer, but I can't tell how long. I'd like to believe that I'll outlive at least 50 percent of the male population because I had more coronary arteries repaired."

How long do you want to live?"

"Forever. I worry that I won't dance at my grandson's wedding. Just after my Bypass, Matt, my baby, came home to inform us that he's a homosexual, which didn't help those arteries of mine. I keep thinking, 'Where did I go wrong?' All that crap. I know. These things happen, nobody understands why. People become gay—such a nice word to have its meaning so warped! Strong mother, strong father, nobody really knows what causes it. Harry Stack Sullivan said that something occurs sexually at an early age which fixates sexuality. It's been tough to take. With all my street language, sometimes I think I'm as old-fashioned as my grandfather. Matt has great difficulty in getting along with me, because he knows I have great difficulty in getting along with him. He knows I've accepted his life; surely I don't make snide remarks about it, although I feel so raw when he and Dot talk, because he's very open with her. He'll go into certain details of his love life. As an artist, she finds homosexuality old hat. If I'm there, I'll interrupt: 'Matt, please spare me the particulars,' because Matt'll be telling her, 'Oh, he had biceps like this. He has such lovely, soft hair and dark eyes.' You picked this up, because you said I talked about Tom and not about Matt or Jeff, so I decided to tell you, to lay it all out in the open.

"Because Matt told us, he now comes home frequently, and our relationship is much better. In time, perhaps he'll forgive me; maybe I'll forgive myself. Right now, I don't forgive myself. Now I hate myself for my own stupidity and my lack of patience with him. For God's sake, I'm a psychiatrist! I see these people, homosexuals, every day. How can I help them if I can't help myself, if I can't help my son? Like a jackass, I keep worrying, 'What if somebody found out he's gay?' Then I realize, fuck 'em. Like Tom said about Carlotta, 'If they don't like it, tough shit.' Matt and I are working to develop mutual respect each for the other. I keep thinking, 'It's easy for him to respect me, but how can I respect him?'

Then I become so enraged at myself because I have such blinders on. I'll never forget the New Year's Eve when he told us. What a way to begin the year! For him, too. I worry about the difficulties he must experience, about the life he's cursed with. How many relationships must he go through before he finds someone who has some significance for him? Will he pick up some terrible physical illness, herpes or even, God forbid, AIDS?"

Since Bypass, how's your marriage?

"The same, the same. Maybe I'm more irascible and selfish. I guess I take advantage of her."

As a sexual therapist, you must know the old cardiological dictum: after a heart attack or a Bypass, you can have intercourse, but only with a woman to whom you've been married for at least twenty years.

"If a married man has had a good sexual life with his wife, it'll be good after Bypass. If he's had a bad sexual life, or an unhappy marriage, after Bypass he'll have a poor sexual life. Surgery won't change it. If a male patient says, 'After surgery, I had my first affair, and I really feel good. I finally got laid and overcame my anxiety about it,' I'll reply, 'Why with her? Why not with your wife? How was it with your wife before surgery?' If he says, 'It stunk,' then I make no comment. But if he says, 'It was good. I enjoyed it and she enjoyed it. We had a good sexual relationship until the operation,' then I'll investigate it because he's trying to prove certain macho shit. He's stressing himself by trying to prove something dangerous to himself—and to his marriage: he's capable of screwing anybody he chooses. He's attempting to prove a neurotic premise, no better in sex than it is in geometry; but in sexual relationships, there's no such thing as a perfect triangle. He'll be much more comfortable with his familiar wife than running around with some young chick, who might be adorable and a great piece of ass, but who also might push him into a performance of which he is not psychologically, or even physically, capable."

Should the first sexual experience after Bypass be initiated by the patient?

"Absolutely. For the woman to initiate puts pressure on the male. If the woman has had Bypass and the man initiates, it puts pressure on her. While a woman can fake orgasm, as a man cannot, this is a poor way to begin their new life after Bypass. If Bypass patients themselves initiate the first time, then they have no pressure to perform because the sexual act has been requested or even alluded to in veiled hints by the other person."

Many Bypassers have virtually no information about when they can resume intercourse. Either they are afraid to ask their doctors, or the doctor says, 'When you feel up to it,' which, they object, tells them nothing. Many Bypassers waited four to six months. They were afraid of what intercourse might do to their newly Bypassed hearts.

"More time than that even. I did not wait, thank God. It was a little more than three weeks. When I had the courage to trust myself, I could turn to Dorothy. Nobody should wait months for intercourse; that's the doctor's fault for not talking about sexual matters to the patient. The longer the waiting time, the greater the fear. Anxiety builds up, patients are less likely to be successful. Many male Bypassers masturbate after the operation as a kind of trial run. It's hard for them to tell me. Very often, they'll say, 'I'm crazy, a man of my age,' and I'll ask, 'What do you mean?' They'll hesitate and say something like, 'One day when I was still home, my wife went shopping and I was horny. I started to play with myself. When the feeling was so good, I continued to ejaculation.' Sexually, we're still living in the Dark Ages, because they look so shamefaced when they tell me. I ask, 'What did you feel? Were you frightened about it? Did you experience any physical discomfort, any chest symptoms?' They say, 'Oh, sure I was frightened. I remember the things my folks told me, but I knew I was going to ejaculate; I didn't know what it would do to me.' You pass a point of inevitability and you can't stop. You just can't stop in the middle of an orgasm. After it was over, they saw that they might be breathing a little heavily but everything was fine. Masturbating felt so good to them that it gave them the courage to go to their wives the next time they felt sexual desire, and they were able to perform."

An internist just published an article stating that masturbation imposes greater stress than does sexual intercourse. Do you agree?

"It depends. That kind of sexual *non sequitur* is senseless. So much depends on the individual's attitudes towards masturbation and intercourse. Many people think masturbation is a sin, it's not good for you. God will punish you. I've seen women patients who say, 'My goodness, I wouldn't touch myself in a million years.' I feel like saying, 'You're missing a lot,' but I refrain and try to explain to them. Psychologically, if a man is unsure of his performance and masturbates to ejaculation, if he finds he's had no untoward physical symptoms, if he's received pleasure, which is the driving force behind sexual congress, he'll have intercourse and won't be so worried. The first time, the wife is more anxious by far than is the patient."

Was Dottie afraid the first time?

"Afterwards, I asked her. I'm a sex therapist, we communicate well, or as well as can be expected after all these years. Yet I couldn't bring myself to ask her before. That first time, my chest muscles were far from healed. Despite all the fancy improvements, I like the missionary position. I like to feel her tits against me, pressing into me, but I couldn't . . . it hurt too much. So I used the rear-entry position. When you live with someone long enough, you know certain responses; there's no doubt in my mind that, for her, some were missing. She was tense. When I did ejaculate, and I am a loud ejaculator, I whooped and she heard me. Many women are not aware of the ejaculate entering them, sometimes they are and sometimes they aren't. That time, apparently, she wasn't so sure. Later she told me, 'I was afraid to move, and the next thing I knew, you had fallen asleep. You were holding me, I was grateful life was beginning again for us, but I put my hand very lightly on your chest to make sure that your chest was going up and down. All night I kept waking up and putting my hand on your chest just to check.' The anxiety for the spouse is as great if not greater than for the Bypass patient."

Do you think a sexual therapist should be a member of the Bypass team, to instruct the Bypasser and his spouse?

"Absolutely. The first consulation with the sex therapist should be before the patient leaves the hospital, so that the Bypasser knows he's coming back to life, that nobody thinks of him as a cardiac cripple.

"A cardiac surgeon should do several things. Number one, he should insist that the patient find a psychiatrist with whom he can develop a rapport. Preferably, of course, that psychiatrist should be a member of the Bypass team, but many patients go out of town for surgery so the follow-up isn't there, although patients should at least begin with a psychiatrist at the hospital. If the psychiatrist himself has had Bypass, then he's perfect; if he hasn't, he still can be competent, can have the compassion and understanding to help the patient through the dark tunnel of depression to the light at the end. No matter how much he denies it, every patient has to slog through depression; Bypass constantly confronts him with his own mortality. He's forever asking himself, 'Am I going to keel over this minute or the next?'

"Second, a patient needs a psychiatrist or a sex therapist to educate him about sexuality, because 90 percent of our population is unsophisticated sexually and censorious about sexual knowledge and pleasure. So few people realize that there's more than one position and more than one way to achieve climax. It's essential these be gone through with husband and wife. If the patient is single, he still should be taught, perhaps all the more so because he feels so ineluctably alone.

"Third, patients need to know that their exercise program is far more important than they realize. Because they feel lousy early on, they tend to goof off. Later, because they feel well, they lose interest in exercise. Taking a little walk will do more for a patient than taking any kind of pill or tranquilizer, because he is helping himself physiologically. That's where the cardiologist fails. He fails in not helping the patient discuss his fears, he fails in not encouraging, not demanding, exercise be performed. I have patients not told to walk, not told to do anything except what they wanted to do. That kind of laissez-faire cardiologist is a *putz*;[25] he's reneging

[25] A tool. Also the Yiddish word for the male organ.

on his responsibilities. Doctors should demand that patients exercise, demand that they follow their diet almost compulsively.

"Fourth, surgeons and cardiologists should encourage patients not to hestitate to call about any kind of symptom, even if they need another EKG, or another ten EKGs. When I compare what I did with what other Bypassers could do, I feel sorry for them. If I had chest pain and it made me anxious, I'd get on the phone and call the doctor's office. I'd see him; he'd have the nurse do an EKG, ask me what I was feeling. He'd say, 'It's probably the wires knitting, just the healing process.' I'd be reassured—until the next time. But doctors encourage patients to be passive, not to insist on their rights; they intimidate patients because they don't want intrusions on their days. I have a yearly stress test and semiannual blood tests, but never did my doctor check my HDL. That's my baby, my HDL; I order my HDL when I get to the labs. I never thought about HDL before. Never have I been called in by my internist. Never did he say, 'Hey, Abe, come in and see me.' That's probably because he has to give me professional courtesy. People think doctors get better care because they're doctors. Don't count on it. Doctors get worse care because, supposedly, other doctors observe the Hippocratic Oath,[26] although that's a thing of the past. Doctors get worse care, too, because their own doctors think that the doctor-patients know more than they do about their own illness. Heart surgery is almost as foreign to a psychiatrist or a pediatrician as it is to a bricklayer. Doctors also get worse care because their physicians think that the doctor-patients are looking over the doctor-doctors' shoulders and criticizing. I'm not happy with my doctor. I remember leaving his office the last time and saying to myself, 'I don't like him. He doesn't like me. He wants to be rid of me.' Our relationship, which had been so close—*before I was ever sick*—has changed. I don't know why, I don't care, and I won't waste a minute analyzing it."

Why do you remain with this internist?

"I don't. I got a new internist in another town. I told this one not to mention it to the old one. Funny, how doctors feel that patients are their property.

[26] "The Physician's Oath," sworn by graduating medical students since about 400 B.C., in which physicians "swear by Apollo the Physician, by Health, by Panacea" to certain ethical creeds, among them the promise never to charge other physicians and their families for medical services.

"I don't know how to help patients be less intimidated and less suspicious, which is the other side of the intimidation coin. I told you before, 'If you don't trust your doctor, get a new one.' I had trusted him at the time of the operation. Fine. Now I don't, and that's not so fine. It's hard getting used to somebody new. Like breaking up with a lover, you hang in there too long because you're afraid of the outside world. When you start with a new lover, you keep comparing her or him with the other one and wondering if you'd acted too rashly."

Has having had Bypass affected your relations with other physicians? Do you think they look at you differently, treat you differently?

"Not now. Oh, after the operation, my colleagues were very solicitous, but as I got stronger and sassier, as I became my old self, our relations became even more fractious. For a year after Bypass, I covered my share of night calls, but getting up in the middle of the night wore me out. Even now, my fatigue is a bone-tiredness, much altered from the way I was before the operation. Usually I'm in bed at ten, read till ten-thirty, get up at six. Once I'm asleep, it's tough for me to have my sleep disrupted. When I was on duty and the phone would ring, if I had to go into the hospital, I'd get stressful for a day or so afterwards.

"After my surgery, I'd promised myself, 'No more!' I went into my chief, a horse's ass, and I said, 'I need a sabbatical.' He said, 'What for? You're doing fine. You're jogging and golfing.' I said, 'Screw you, that's different. I don't like getting awakened in the middle of the night. I don't have any stamina for getting up in the night, driving to the hospital, seeing the patient for an hour or two, driving home, trying to get to sleep, and then starting all over again the next morning. I've paid my dues in duty call to this hospital. If I can't take a sabbatical from my hospital responsibilities, then I resign. That's that.' With much reluctance, he gave me the sabbatical."

What about with other colleagues? Some people have said that their colleagues have tended to write them off, to treat them with much more reserve.

"I'm the writer-offer. I'm more aloof, I don't tolerate the social crap, and I don't socialize with physicians. I have two dear friends.

Having one dear friend has its limitations. All friendships impose certain limitations; you can let your hair down just so much; you can discuss one problem confidentially with one kind of friend and something else with the other friend. I needed these fellows for different reasons. They're a good balance for me. Actually, I have a lot of friends because we belong to the country club."

How do you define 'friend'?

"A friend is someone you can trust, someone who keeps his counsel when you talk to him and doesn't tell the whole town, someone who gives the best counsel he can, someone who just listens, someone who can come to your house without calling you, someone whose house is open to you, where you can go without prior notice and know that you'll always be welcome. There is freedom to impose on each other. He can impose on me, and I can bitch about it *to him*, not to anybody else; I can impose on him, and he can bitch to me."

You have this kind of friendship with the members of your country club?

"Look, *I* don't ask *you*, 'How many friends have *you* got?' "

Usually, I don't make people count either. This is special. Do you believe in God?

"My God! What else?" He laughs. "I've been searching for a relationship to this word, 'God.' There must be a plan, but God only knows what it is, and how much we're lousing it up or fixing it up. If someone asked me, 'Do you think all this happened by accident or has been in existence forever?' I'd have to say, 'I don't know.' Things are not for forever, that I'm sure of. Except that the idea of God is forever. Am I making any sense?"

Do you think He was in the operating room with you?

"He? How do you know It was not a She? But no, I don't believe such a thing. That's silly. What I do believe, and this'll sound kooky to you, is that what happens in our lives can be controlled by our minds." He taps his forehead. "In there is a remarkable organ, never to be duplicated by any machine, perhaps never to be understood completely either. If you have the ability to use this brain, if the brain cells doled out to you are sufficient, then you're fortunate. But I'm too scientific to say that God had something to do with what's in our skulls."

When you awakened, after the Bypass, what was your first thought?

"When I opened my eyes and felt this lousy endotracheal tube, I didn't say to myself, 'God, how lucky I am that I'm alive. Thank you, God.' None of that bullshit. Being introspective—yes, and selfish—my first thought was, 'Take this fucking tube out because it bothers the hell out of me.' Nothing was worse than that tube."

Is there any way to make the tube easier to tolerate? Or is it a necessary evil?

"There are ways to help. I was lucky because I had a marvelous male nurse, who deserves a raise and who saw me thrashing and trying to pull out the tube. He spoke very quietly to me, held my hands down, and said, 'Doctor, that tube is breathing for you. It's an endotracheal tube, and you know why it's there.' 'That doesn't mean I like it,' I thought, and fell asleep. Once in a while, he'd come over and reassure me. He wouldn't wait for me to start thrashing because, of course, I couldn't talk. I couldn't say anything. You have no idea how important it is for the Intensive Care nurse to hearten the patient's flagging spirit, even though the patient himself may not remember the touch, the word. Because he was so comforting, I said to myself, 'Look, *schmuck*, you're a doctor. You know you need the endotracheal tube. Shut up, it won't kill you. They're watching you, you don't want to look like an asshole, so go to sleep.'

"Every patient should be told about the tube by the anesthesiologist, the night before surgery."

You weren't told about the tube?

"Not a word. Today, every surgical procedure has an endotracheal tube; perhaps they thought I'd know enough to expect it. But it's the responsibility of the anesthesiologist to sit down and tell the patient all about it. You're going to think I'm some kind of half-assed doctor, but I never once thought of the tube before the operation. I never thought of the tube in connection with me. Magicians though they may be, it's their duty to explain everything in detail. In some places, not only do they tell you all about the tube, but they give you a little code to use when you can't talk. That way, you can answer when they say, 'How do you feel?' 'Are you awake?' 'Where do you hurt?' 'Do you want more pain medication?' With such a code, *you* can ask *them* questions. Another thing, along these lines, is that patients are undermedicated. Studies have shown that doctors underprescribe, ordering inadequate dosages at inflexible intervals, and for a majority of surgical patients, nurses don't dispense maximum narcotic orders. Pain is stress, which can trigger a coronary. The risk of addiction is rare. Patients usually are too intimidated, once they stop being intubated and can speak, to ask for pain medication. Doctors don't appreciate that their patients are at the mercy of the house staff and the nursing staff."

You said that every surgeon should recommend that his patients be followed by a psychiatrist. Should there be a psychiatrist who sees you regularly while you're in the hospital?

"In the beginning, the psychiatrist should stay out of the picture until about the fourth day, when many patients have that terrible melancholia. Then, if all seems to be well, the psychiatrist should talk to the patient before he goes home, because sometimes people live in communities miles away from any psychiatric help, one of those little places with a name ending in v-i-l-l-e. Someone besides the surgeon should answer questions and encourage the verbalization of anxieties, because surgeons aren't good at answering questions. Maybe that's why they become surgeons."

If you had the operation to do all over again, would you have had it?

"Absolutely. Even if I didn't have a left anterior descending, I would have the operation. If the main blockages were on the right side and I had severe angina, it would restrict my activities so much that my life would not feel like a life to me, that I would not feel like me—whatever it is that I feel like. And whatever *that* is, it's not a Bypass 'patient' or 'veteran' or whatever you call it, because I don't think of myself in those terms. I know that I'm the same person I've always been except for certain modifications. I know I had surgery. I know I came through successfully, I was lucky, that much I know. I give it no more thought."

What do you want to do with the rest of your life? What do you fear? What do you wish for?

"Even without Bypass, I'd fear that I wouldn't live long enough to do everything I want to do with my life."

A lot of people don't know what they want to do with their lives. They only know that, at this stage of the game, they don't like what they've got.

"I want to dance at my grandson's wedding. I want to be a sculptor, to pursue this long-neglected dream of mine. I'd like to give up practicing, but for financial reasons I can't. I'd like to create figures from stone that would touch people's minds and hearts. As an analyst, I've done that already; I know I have. But now I'd like to do this in a more abstract way, to touch someone's heart, someone whom I don't know, yet whom I know in the most intimate way. I want to leave a piece of me, a piece of me for posterity, not for anybody else, but for the generation that comes from my loins. After all, my name is Abraham. I want my children, my grand-children, my great-grandchildren, and the generations after oc-casionally to talk about me. Selfish, isn't it? I don't know, it's so personal, but, yes, I want to have a piece of me carried on through the ages. I don't like the thought that whatever years I've had and will have on earth will come to an ending, a conclusion, and be nothingness after I'm in the earth. I don't know if that's my ego or my superego talking, but I'd bet on my ego."

Dr. Stearin's face darkens, he bites the edges of his lip, plays with a smelly unlit pipe. "The outside world will remember me better than any fruit of my loins. Tommy had a vasectomy after the baby was born, Jeff doesn't want children, and Matty's hom-osexual. Some Abraham I turned out to be! I told Matty that if he could find a relationship that is good and significant, then he and his . . . friend should consider adopting a child. He should give the benefit of his knowledge and experience and education to another human being, the closest thing you can do short of fathering a child yourself. Sometimes, he thinks about marrying and fathering a child. A lot of homosexuals do this. It's good cover for them; it's a comfort as well. A part of me wishes he would, but the better part knows that would be disastrous. He'd be having homosexual affairs, and then what would happen?"

After Bypass, is there a greater desire for an extramarital affair?

"For whom?"

For the patient, not the spouse.

"Sure."

How?

He shakes his head, leaps up for a fresh pack of gum.

Did you lust for an affair?

"Absolutely."

What is it that makes you want an affair after Bypass?

"You misinterpreted. I said, 'Yes, I thought about it.' I'm not saying what I did, or *that* I did. But what I felt after surgery is no different from what I felt before Bypass. As a sex therapist, I'm convinced that if your sexual life is one way before surgery, it'll be the same after the operation, unless there are physical complications."

But there are two exceptions to the rule. One, some people yearn for an affair, in the abstract, or yearn for somebody else specifically, but don't have the affair until after major surgery, because now they want to extract all life's sweetness. And two, most married people's sex lives are a lot of ways—not just 'one way,' good, bad, indifferent, exciting, comforting—which may be the appeal of the affair.

"I understand what you're saying, or trying to say, but you're not getting at it very well. Let me reword it for you," offers Dr. Stearin.

"What you want to ask me is, 'What happens to a Bypasser who says to me: "I've never been happy with my wife. She's my major stress. If I ever loved her, I don't now. I've hung around for my kids, who now are older, yet I feel a responsibility, indoctrinated into me since I was a child. My mother always said, 'You're responsible. Be a man and accept your responsibilities.' " My approach is: 'You're a fool to continue this marriage. You're digging your grave faster by maintaining a stressful relationship in which you don't love this albatross around your neck. I hope you find somebody whom you can love, and maybe you already have.' If they have, they usually tell me. Frequently they already have before they tell me and are looking for my approval. Then I say, 'It's up to you whether you marry her or live with her, but you've got to decide how to conduct your life. You can't control other people. You must try to control yourself and your own life, which is much harder.' "

In all our discussions, you've talked almost exclusively about male patients."

"Depending on whose statistics you read, 80 to 85 percent of Bypass patients are male. I've had women Bypass patients."

If a woman in her forties, or in her fifties, has had Bypass, is unhappy with her husband, and if she breaks off her marriage, she has much less chance—

"Yes. She has much less chance of building a new life than a man does. That's the nature of the world, of society."

Do you encourage such a woman, as you encourage such a man, to build a new—

"Absolutely not. Good advice in my office and good advice for that Arctic Circle outside don't always connect. Life has to be adjusted to society's rules."

That's easier for men to say than for women.

"I'm aware of that. I can tell a man this afternoon, 'You should get rid of this stressful marriage.' In two weeks or a month, he'll be happily ensconced someplace else. I can't do that with a woman. Part of the reason is financial. How many women can earn good livings in today's world? How many women have marketable skills? Part of the reason is supply and demand—a good part of the reason, I guess." He chews the corner of his mouth. "A woman Bypasser might be considered damaged goods; some people might say that a woman got what she deserved for trying to enter a man's world. A male Bypasser would be deemed a macho price-payer, worthy of sympathy for all he suffered to be successful."

Don't you have any patients with marriages both comfortable and comforting? Is that the wrong question to ask a psychiatrist?

"Some Bypassers tell me they like their wives, they don't want to break their marriages, but they find it necessary, or think they find it necessary, to have an affair. For all the good it does, I tell them that these desires are psychosocial aberrations. They're content— or so they say; their partnership is significant to them. Why do they need anything? What are they proving? What reasons do they have?"

What do they reply?

"They have no answers. I tell them they'll produce more heart-damaging anxiety to go fooling around in somebody else's bed than to stay home and 'lust in their hearts.' They're sure they won't feel guilty; they're sure they won't get caught. Maybe they're right. The female Bypassers are another story. If they have longings for someone else, they're afraid they'll get caught or the would-be lover will be revolted by the scar. While women don't have the same performance anxieties as men—every woman's a bedroom Bernhardt, at some time or other, unless the man is terrific or the woman is unique—women fear social sanctions and sanctimony. Ironically, a lot of men feel their worth has been validated by the need for Bypass; a lot of women feel their worth has been invalidated by Bypass."

Your own real rock seems to be your marriage.

"My marriage helps. My real rocks have been my relationship to my parents, especially to my mother. I never wanted to resolve my

Oedipal conflict. I loved it, I love it now, even though she's gone. She was a remarkable woman, talented, smart, persistent, but she could not pursue her talents for lack of education and because my father always held her back, always wanted her home, even though *he* was never home. The other significant force was my good fortune in being psychoanalyzed by Kurt Lundberg, who contributed to my philosophy of life."

Did your wife ever have psychoanalysis?

"No."

Did she ever want to?

"One time, she said she'd like to see somebody, so I told her, 'Go see whomever you want.' That was the last I heard of it. Later, I asked her if she was going to see someone, and she replied, 'No, I'll get along without it.' I asked, 'Is it something serious?' Immediately, I take the blame on myself: 'Did I do something wrong? What's the reason?' She said, 'It's personal and none of your business.' I said, 'Okay,' because that's the way it should be, but I don't think she ever went because she didn't want to spend the money. Most psychiatrists are like cardiac surgeons: they don't give professional courtesy to doctors and their families."

Do you give professional courtesy?

"I did until I had Bypass. When the surgeon billed me two grand in addition to what Blue Shield allowed, I quit."

In what particular ways could doctors treat Bypass patients better—besides omitting the $2,000 surcharge?

"You're dealing with a multitude of personalities. Each patient is unique, each doctor is different. None of us is the same. You can group patients together as you're doing, by occupation, by sex, by color, by income, by God knows what, but no two are the same. No two should be treated the same. Everyone in a family is a special combination of nature and nurture, of heredity and environment."

Are you close to your brothers and sisters?

"We see each other often enough for my tastes."

That doesn't sound like a close family relationship.

"Some families spend every weekend and every holiday together. That's not intimacy. That's loneliness. They don't have anybody else to spend time with."

The theme of most of these crucial conversations has been that arteries may be Bypassed, but loneliness is endemic and epidemic in America. Most of the middle-aged Bypassers I meet feel as though they don't have any friends, as though their families, especially their children, are grown and gone far away; even if their children are all they wanted them to be, they're still far away and no longer attached to them.

"Some people can't function as well as they could or should."

He stops, looks searchingly at my face, waits.

The operation is billed as improving the quality of life, which is why having a psychiatrist around is important. What about you? Is life sweeter to you since Bypass?

Tired and annoyed, Dr. Stearin's voice gets louder, harsher: "I told you . . . How many times do I have to tell you? I'm the same person. When people make statements about making the quality of life better, they're talking about physical conditions: you won't have the angina, you won't have the shortness of breath, your chest won't hurt, you'll be able to get around more. But psychologically, you'll be the same; never forget that."

Sometimes people aren't the same. Sometimes they appreciate life more. Sometimes they have severe psychological problems which may have been contained before but now are running rampant.

"Even with psychiatric help, most people will be unhappy."

The Angel of Death has hovered close, yet you say people don't change and you didn't change.

"My only difference is that I don't bottle things up as I used to. I say what's on my mind. I'm not concerned, as I was when I was younger, with what other people think of me."

Were you so concerned about people's opinions because you're Jewish?

"Nah, it's my nature. If I were Italian, I'd worry what the Mafia was doing to the Italian image. Maybe that's why I went into psychiatry; by helping other people cope with their anxieties, I'd release my own fears, so that the patients I'd help would be helping me. There's a magnetic pull between occupation and occupier . . . I think I did a good job, I know I'm doing a good job with Bypassers. And they're doing a pretty good job with me."

10. Ben Rand, M.D.
Internist
Age at Bypass: 46

A sea wall is an unlikely place for an interview, but having consented to talk, albeit only "by the pool," Dr. Ben Rand seems little
concerned with Acapulco's surf and sunshine.

Ben Rand is a cube of a man, his skin soft and white, his hairless
belly drooping over the waistband of his gray athletic shorts, each
of his white legs streaked with an angry red ropey scar. Rubbing
his gray wispy beard—"I grew it to hid my weak chin"—Ben Rand
concentrates on the details of his Bypass, while a steel band plays
"Yellow Bird," that staple guaranteeing banana trees and tropical
paradise.

"I practice medicine in Lafayette, Indiana. I was born in Chelsea,
but wanted to escape the 'Big City.' I'm still on my first marriage,
thank God. I've got two children: a son, twenty-one; a son, nineteen;
the usual statistics. I'm a pretty good doctor. I'll be fifty next
Wednesday. To be accurate, 49 and 51/52," he corrects himself.
"My family history isn't bad—considering. My father died of a
stroke at seventy-two. My mother's still alive. My brother's thirty-
eight, a dermatologist—less work and more money than an internist. A real exercise freak. He's got a nice resting bradycardia,

but his normal EKG shows a right bundle branch block. When his group switched insurance carriers, they rated him.[1] He runs six miles a day; he doesn't have angina—and he's rated. That kind of stuff gets my goat. I had a patient who's a professional tennis player, not the best, but second-best. They wouldn't sell him insurance because he had an abnormal EKG which reverts to normal when he exercises. He even had a normal stress test. Still, they rated him. Insurance companies are one of my peeves. I have too many peeves to single out any one as a 'pet.' "

[This extra information is the usual stalling device of doctors until they decide how much they want to say. They'd rather do the asking than the answering.]

Tell me about you and how you came to Bypass.

"I don't know where to begin, because— Well, my Bypass was on April Fool's Day, 1980. How's that for a good Bypass day? I was forty-six years old, but Bypass was no surprise. I'd had an MI ten years before, at thirty-six. My family history looks better on paper than it is. Even though my father didn't die of his stroke until he was seventy-two, he'd had an MI at fifty. I can never remember my father not sick. One of his brothers had died young of heart disease and diabetes. My father was diabetic. Both his parents died young, in an accident in Europe, so I don't know what would've happened to them if they had lived. The Nazis probably would've gotten them; they got the rest of my grandfather's family. Funny, my mother's family lives forever. Her parents and grandparents died in their nineties, probably because the machine just gave out. Why are defective genes so dominant?"

But you had a coronary at thirty-six, much younger than your father. Did you smoke?

"Not then. But I had smoked from the time I was a young kid, fooling around in Chelsea, until I was twenty-nine, when my son was born. I stopped smoking because I was a father. I felt a responsibility to set a good example for my child—and to live for my child, because, by then, *my* father was dead. It's ironic that I

[1] The insurance company forced him to pay a higher premium rate.

stopped smoking for my son, because he was picked up for selling dope and snorting coke at least three or four times in high school and again in college. He's such a smart kid, too. He used to write term papers and sell them to pay for his drugs. He's clean now. I think. But I worry about him, where he's going, what he's going to do with his life. What can you do with a communications major? He hasn't communicated with me in years."

Dr. Rand squints into the sun at a parachutist floating down to the water.

"Just think of the waste. Fifteen dollars, or whatever it is in pesos, for a two-minute ride. Why do people need all those thrills? Like my son with his drugs.

"There was another reason I stopped smoking. When I was a resident, I'd had an episode of paroxysmal atrial fibrillation, for whatever that's worth in my history. They used to say that PAF came only to young, healthy hearts, but I figured that the smoking couldn't be doing me any good. Besides, they didn't pay residents the way they do today. Smoking costs money, children cost money. So I stopped."

If you had a coronary at thirty-six, how did you come to Bypass at forty-six?

"I did just fine for those ten years. Funny, how clearly I remember that first infarct; afterwards it seemed to me that I had never thought about my heart. I had my infarct on a Saturday while making rounds in the hospital. I know just when it happened. I was on 5-M. In those days, the EKG Department was one floor down. I had some discomfort in my chest. I got sweaty, I went downstairs and had the technician take an EKG. It didn't show any changes, no diagnostic changes. Then I went and got a chest x-ray just to make sure I didn't have—well, *you know*.

"I must have looked pretty lousy because a resident saw me and put me in a wheelchair. Of course, the chest x-ray didn't show anything. I got an SGOT because, in those days, we didn't do much more than that. I felt a little better. Mostly, it was shoulder and jaw pain, nothing you could call chest pain. My partner took the rest of the day for me, and I went home. My friend was visiting that weekend. That night we went out to dinner. I got a call, climbed two flights of stairs to see a lady whose pacemaker wasn't working.

I didn't have any pain or shortness of breath. On Monday, I said, 'I'd better get another cardiogram.' That one showed I'd had an inferior MI. The worst of it was that my friend who was visiting, a classmate from high school and college and medical school, died suddenly the next day. He'd left on Sunday morning. Tuesday, his wife called; in bed that morning, she'd found him dead. A very dear friend of mine, the one real friend I ever had. And now he's gone."

For a minute, Dr. Rand doesn't seem to see me, then continues matter-of-factly: "Anyway, that was when I was thirty-six. I did well from then on, until one night about ten years later, I was reading cardiograms in the EKG Department and I felt a worm in my chest, sort of twisting around my sternum. I said, *'Uh-oh.'* Probably, I had known something was going on because I had been getting discomfort while exercising, not that I exercise so much. If I walked the hills in my neighborhood in cold weather, I'd have a twinge. Then I'd been getting slight discomfort on rounds in the hospital, so I'd slowed my walking pace. But now, sitting there in the EKG Department, I got rest pain. *Talk about* déjà vu! *Both MIs while I was reading EKGs in the hospital!* I walked over to where they keep the nitroglycerin on the stress machine and took a nitro from the treadmill. The nitro didn't help. I took another one and called to the nurses around the corner at the CCU: 'Come and get me. I'm not well.' They brought me to the CCU. I told them to call my friend Mark, the cardiologist, because I thought he was in the hospital. Another friend, an ENT[2] man, walked by and I asked him to call my wife. Ten years before, when I had had my infarct, she'd come running in and bumped into this same ENT man. To tell the truth, these guys aren't friends; they're colleagues. Whenever Jack, the ENT man, hears anything about a heart attack, the first thing he does is run to get a cardiogram on himself. A nice guy, bright, although ENT men don't have to do much to stay caught up with the literature. A hypochondriac.

"Mark wasn't in the hospital, and I was beginning to feel pretty funny because I needed morphine. I told them to give me morphine, but it didn't help. I needed more, so I told them to give me more. I hate to order something like morphine for myself, but you can't

[2] Ear-nose-throat specialist (otolaryngologist).

become addicted from taking morphine just once or twice. I told the girls to put a nitro patch on me."

You were giving all the directions?

"Well, Mark, the cardiologist, was on his way in. The only doctor in the house was Jack, this ENT man. He was sitting on a chair, calling for the nurses and gasping. He was sure he was going to have a heart attack. I felt funny giving all my own orders, but there wasn't much choice. The morphine gave me no relief. The nitro was no help. The next morning the pain subsided all by itself."

Did the pain keep you up all night?

"Just drifting pleasantly. Morphine makes me sleepy. They took a series of cardiograms and other tests, but there was no acute MI, just *unstable angina*. Obviously, without an MI, something had to be done medically or surgically. Mark ordered Inderal. The pulse slowed appropraitely, the rest pain went away, but I was having exertional pain on minor exertion, like walking to the bathroom. The choices were surgery or—I don't know what.

"Meanwhile, on the very day that I got sick, my partner had left for a vacation in Italy. He didn't know I was sick; he had to turn around and come back. That was bad."

Who made the decision for you to have surgery?

"Plainly, I needed catheterization, at least to define the anatomy, to see what could be done, and how urgently it needed doing. Mark, the cardiologist, and my wife were busy fighting about a dozen different things. Mostly, she was right, but I'd get aggravated and yell at her. I couldn't yell at Mark. The problem was that we do catheterizations at our hospital. A delicate position. Here I am, a physician, working at this hospital. Mark did not do, even now rarely does, unstable anginal patients. He'd be stupid to do them. If he got into trouble, we don't have the backup. What a setup for a malpractice suit! Nevertheless, I'm a physician at this hospital and I'm going somewhere else to be cathed. How does *he* look? Patients have come to me since, and I've advised, 'You need a catheterization. I'll call the cardiologist and see if he agrees with me, and if he does, we can—' They say, 'Well, where did you go? You didn't have it here.' When I reply, 'Well, no, I didn't,' the explanations ensue: 'I had unstable angina; if you were unstable—, 'Forget it. *You* didn't have it done here.' It's a tough problem, the special problem of the doctor who is a patient.

"I knew all this must be going through Mark's mind. I wasn't privy to his arguments with Myra, but I'd hear bits and pieces from the hallway. He was uncertain. He was thinking, 'If I don't do the angio on Ben, what's it going to do to my reputation as an angiographer in this town?' Myra kept after him to call Cleveland for me. I had sent patients to Cleveland* for fourteen years, including one of their first Bypassers, because I had heard some of their talks, had seen Sones's[3] early x-rays. Mark called, and they told him, 'We can do him in three weeks, maybe four.' "

How did you feel when Cleveland put you off?

"Not surprised. Not even betrayed."

Don't you think that doctors are owed some courtesy, some special care and handling?

"Sure, it would've been nice, but that kind of kid gloves is gone. Maybe courtesy went out when they started letting ordinary guys like me into the profession. I don't know. They've got a schedule, too. These delays are built into the system. I've gone through them time and again with my own patients. But—I had sent Cleveland a lot of work. Anyway, a local medical center about fifty miles away could catheterize me the following week. So I transferred there."

By ambulance?

"Yes, and that caused a fight, too. I didn't think I needed an ambulance. I would just as soon have gone by car, but Mark insisted, maybe to show other people how sick I was. My wife said, 'Fine, if I can go in the ambulance with him.' Another fight, about the

---

* The Cleveland Clinic.
[3] Dr. Mason Sones, pioneer in angiography.

insurance: who would be responsible for her? Finally, she stormed: 'Look, I'm goddam well going in that ambulance with Ben.' She had to sign a release. If there was an accident, the insurer wasn't responsible. They tried to keep all these altercations from me. I knew. Of course, this fighting stressed me. The whole thing was stupid. It was stupid to have to go in an ambulance. As it turned out, the ambulance broke down five miles from the hospital. We went about five miles an hour for the last five miles. But the medical center was all right. Having dealt with those people on the phone and at meetings, I felt comfortable going there. Compared with Cleveland, where the neighborhood is terrible, this place was better. My wife was able to stay across the street and not be afraid of going out in the dark, even in a car."

At your medical center, could your family see you right away after the operation?

"Absolutely. I'll go into that in a minute. Infection rates are higher when families show up.

"They catheterized me on Thursday. The next day, the cardiologist invited me to go with him to look at the films. I was ashamed to tell him that, running after him in the corridors, I was getting angina. He walked too fast for me. I used to be such a fast walker. I couldn't say anything. He was busy. He was anxious to get to the next patient, so he was running ahead of me. I was trying to keep up, getting pain in my chest as I chugged along.

"The films were not very exciting. The old occlusion was a distal branch vessel with just minor damage. There was another occlusion in a distal in the right anterior descending. That was it. At this point, Bypass was purely elective. If that vessel had occluded completely, odds are that I wouldn't have died. *But I couldn't function.* I couldn't walk from here to there. So I said, 'I'll take surgery. When can they do it?' He said, 'We have two cardiac surgeons, Dr. Lash and Dr. MacDonald.' I knew MacDonald, I had sent patients to him, they'd done okay. I didn't know Lash from Adam. He's on the Cardiac Council, does research on artificial hearts, but I'd never laid eyes on him. The cardiologist said, 'MacDonald is better at valves. Both are good at Bypass. That's not tough surgery. There's nothing so picky about Bypass. Lash could do you Friday. MacDonald could do you Monday. It's up to you.' I said, 'Friday. Who needs to wait over the weekend? I'm doing this because I want to function as a normal, healthy human being, and I can't wait.' "

Friends came from Vermont to keep Myra Rand company. "We told the hospital that she was Myra's sister. Nobody cared. They go through the same rigamarole that a lot of places do. Preoperatively they take families and patients through the Recovery Room, show them the I.V.'s, the tubes, the aches and pains. That way, they'll know what to expect when they visit Intensive Care after their special person's surgery. The preoperative trip probably is a good idea, but I wonder how patients feel at being displayed in their misery: wouldn't films make patients feel less uneasy? Some patients complain about hospital dehumanization. Others object that seeing films isn't realistic enough preparation. They're both right.

"My family was pretty well prepared with booklets and pep talks. *I* didn't get much instruction. Because I'm a doctor they assumed I knew the ropes; I would've welcomed more instruction. A few things could've, should've, been improved upon. During all this time, in two hospitals, nobody did a rectal on me. Okay, for sure, I wouldn't tell them to do a rectal, but I didn't like the idea that they omitted it. An intern came in to draw blood and couldn't find my vein. It hurt like hell. Myra went and found an oncologist-friend, who came in and drew my blood. Another intern said, 'You know, this is the first time I've ever had a doctor for a patient. I don't know what I'm supposed to do. How am I supposed to handle you?' I said, 'Handle me no differently from anyone else. Ask the same questions. Don't assume that I'm going to volunteer any information that you don't ask. Don't assume that some questions are too personal. Don't skip any questions in your history or your physical exam. Remember that a good exam is 95 percent history and that doctors are notoriously poor historians. Don't try to be kind to me. Don't assume that I have any more knowledge than any other patient—or any greater support system here or at home. Treat me as you would any other patient.' He stood there with his mouth open, but that's the best piece of advice he'll get in medical school or in training."

Dr. Rand laughs. "But *he* didn't do a rectal either. There's nothing there, I guess, just hemorrhoids, but that's not the point. They're still treating the doctor differently—not looking up his ass. Maybe they don't do rectals on any of their cardiac patients. If so, it's wrong. Here I am, forty-six years old. The last time I had a rectal was when I bought insurance, in my thirties. Now they could give me ten rectals, and they wouldn't sell me insurance."

You're a shoemaker's child. You should be going yearly to an internist who gives you an inside-out exam.

"I have a flexible sigmoidoscope[4] that I use in the office."

On yourself?

Dr. Rand laughs because I fell for his joke: "It's not quite long enough. Maybe I'll be able to get a plumber's snake. My Garden of Eden is already despoiled." The smile vanishes and the parentheses about his mouth, half-hidden by his wispy gray mustache, deepen.

When you made up your mind to have Bypass, what helped you?

"Going over the films with the cardiologist—once I caught up to him. Talking over the pros and cons was all I needed. He told me—without being asked—exactly how he rated their surgeons, what was their mortality rate, their complication rate, even, *mirabile dictu*, their success rate and how long I could expect to go on one operation. I didn't need any more than that. I'd been recommending Bypass since 1968, which in the history of Bypass is a long time, practically the age of dinosaurs."

[Dr. Rand had come to Indiana, an outsider from Boston. Within five years, he'd begun sending patients for what seemed a crazy, risky operation.]

Do you think you are more open to new ideas and new procedures than most internists? We hear so much about conservative versus aggressive treatment.

"I can't compare myself with other people. Yes, I guess I'm receptive to new ideas. I'm probably getting more rigid now. I worry so

---

[4] An instrument used in a complete physical examination to visualize the lower bowel and to check for rectal polyps or lower-rectal cancer.

that I've left some stone unturned, although sometimes it's better not to disturb the stones."

Your patients must have had a lot of confidence in you, and you had to have confidence in yourself.

"I'm supposed to have confidence, or I'm in the wrong business. When I went for my own Bypass, I wasn't afraid I'd die. That's too easy. I was scared that the operation wouldn't be successful, that I'd still have that goddam angina."

You were sure you were going to live?

"I didn't say that!" Dr. Rand's voice is angry. "No, I wasn't sure I was going to live. I wasn't sure at all. But I knew what the odds of dying were. Believe me, dying would've been preferable to living like that. If I died, nothing. If I lived with angina, I'd be worse than nothing. I *need* to be doing things."

Did Bypass make you more aware of your own mortality?

"I didn't need Bypass for that. I've been well aware since that MI at thirty-six."

A doctor from Boise who also had a coronary at thirty-six, and then did well for twenty-five years, said that the first MI didn't affect him.

"He lied."

He said that the drama of the surgery traumatized him.

"Sounds like a psychiatrist. 'The drama of the surgery.' I don't know if it's so all-fired dramatic. I'll tell you what I was afraid of, what I'm always afraid of when I go into hospitals. This'll sound crazy to you, but I'm afraid of making a fool of myself; I don't like being dependent on people. I hate being dependent on anybody. In a hospital, you can't do much for yourself. They force you to be dependent on them, then they get sore when you press the call button. I don't like to *bother* people. I want to take care of myself.

I don't want to be a pain in the ass to people. I don't want them to have to do for me."

If people are sick, how do you feel about having to do for them?

"Doctors don't do for patients like nurses do. It's a big difference."

After the surgery, did you become irritable?

"You'll have to ask my wife. I'm usually irritable," he replies with an apparently cheerful laugh.

"My kids say I'm forgetful, more so since the operation. They don't understand. I'm no more forgetful than before. *I have things on my mind.* My only memory loss was the day of the operation. They prepped me the night before, awoke me at five so I could shave myself. I wasn't going to let some technician shave me. After they gave me preop medication, my surgery was postponed because the OR had an emergency. Because they couldn't do me for several hours, they warehoused me someplace. I don't remember any of it. My brother was there with me, until they threw him out. The operation was performed on Passover. I was hallucinating bread. My brother asked, 'Do you want bread just because it's Passover?' I said, 'No, I'm hungry!' After that, all I remember was awakening and trying to yank out my endotracheal tube. That's one of my big fears: choking to death. I knew I didn't want that endotracheal tube in my mouth. I pulled hard on the end of it. I don't know what happened next."

Did anybody talk to you about how you'd feel with the tube?

"*They* wouldn't know. *I* knew how I would feel. An N-G tube[5] bothered the hell out of me. I'd had minor dental surgery once with the N-G tube, and I pulled that out immediately. Before I went into the OR, I *knew* I'd feel miserably uncomfortable. My brother was there then. The nurse said, 'Oh, look, he's so alert, he's waving to you.' My brother retorted, 'No, he isn't. He's pulling out the endotracheal tube.' He was right."

Dr. Rand places his hands around his own throat, sticks his

[5] Nasogastric tube.

tongue out, and presses on his windpipe. "Aaaagh! Like that! I remember the surgeon and his gofer, the research fellow, standing over me and discussing how low my blood pressure was, as though I didn't have any ears. I wanted to tell them that I needed blood. I couldn't speak and I wished they knew. Finally, the fellow said, 'Maybe I'll give him a couple units of blood.' I thought, 'Thank God, he's so smart,' and went back to sleep.

"I suppose I could have communicated in some way with them, but because I felt so rotten, I was so scared. It's all mixed up with the morphine, but I knew I needed blood before he said it. Even if I could have talked, I was sure they wouldn't have listened to me, because they'd figured, 'What does *he* know about Bypass?' "

Did you have any postoperative depression?

"Oh, no! For the first time in ages, I didn't have any pain. I was weak, sure, but without pain. It was terrific."

What about any severe pain from the operation itself?

"It's different, completely different."

Some patients panic because they're fearful that they're having heart pain.

"No way! Anyone could distinguish between the two! I hurt but I didn't have angina. I was ecstatic. The surgery had worked! Every time I got on a scale, I'd lost another kilogram, even though, every day, I ate a chocolate-almond bar, my favorite. Eating chocolate-almond Hershey bars and losing weight, isn't that heaven? That particular paradise only lasted two weeks, but by that time, I'd made up my mind to lose more weight. I dieted. I lost twenty pounds. And I've gained it all back—with interest. After the operation, I watched what I ate, I exercised every day, I jogged. The last six months, I've eaten the legs from under the table, and I quit jogging. Just laziness, lack of discipline, boredom. Jogging is unadulterated boredom. I have a stationary bicycle, which I use sometimes, when I watch the 7:00 A.M. news, but an exercycle is not so good as running. It's better than nothing, I suppose."

You seem to work hard, to take the practice of medicine seriously. Did Bypass encourage you to alter your work pattern?

"I guess I don't go out so much at night. I try to handle things on the phone, to stall till morning. I don't like doing that. What if someone has a coronary and I'm too tired to see him, to pick it up? Mine is a two-man practice, that's all. Right after my Bypass, my partner took sick. Five weeks postop, I went back into the office half-days—and my partner became acutely depressed. So by six weeks postop, I was back in harness full-time. I was by myself in the practice for two months. He's back now. I still feel responsible for his depression. When I had the MI, he had to return from Italy to take over. One hand washes the other."

Bypass or not, you work as much as anybody else in this world— maybe more.

"That's what the Bypass was supposed to let me do. When calls come in the night, I may depend a little more on the Emergency Department doctor than I had in the past, I may not rush in so quickly. *But that's wrong.* The operation did make me regret how little time I'd spent with my kids when they were growing up. As for any other regrets, I'm not so unhappy with what I've done with my life, although I've not succeeded as much as my twenty-year-old self had hoped. My marriage is about the same, perhaps, no— My wife was very important during the operation; she battled for me when I couldn't fight. It was worse for her than for me. Chelsea kids learn to fight early, but the street scene doesn't tell you what the prices will be. Bypass isn't that bad for the patient. It's rough on the family."

After the operation, did the surgeon explain much to you?

"No. Surgeons have a cavalier attitude. By the Thursday before the operation, I'd still not met the surgeon, so I said, 'Hey, I'm not going to the OR until I know what this guy looks like.' The nurse told me, 'He's tied up.' 'By whom?' I wondered. Finally, he showed up.

"The surgeon never sat down. He stood with one hand on the door. Minor things, but they bothered me. After the operation, I had a few problems which he was exceedingly un-upset about; an internist would've been upset. Every evening, I got shaking chills. With those terrible chills, naturally, I was afraid of endocardititis. One day when I was in the bathroom, a huge hematoma[6] broke in my thigh. They'd done a lousy job suturing my leg. It must have been done by a first-year resident.

"That leg gave me such problems. Like a lot of patients, I guess, the leg is more of a pain than the chest, but this busted hematoma was worse than most patients' leg mess-ups. The blood was all over the place. It sprayed the whole bathroom. I tried cleaning it up, but I was very weak, because I still had night chills and fevers. I kept trying to sop up the blood in the bathroom, but I couldn't. I went back to my room and fell into the chair, which got a little bloodied, too. Finally, I crawled into bed. That bed looked nine feet high. The whole time I was there, they never cleaned the blood out of the bathroom. Whatever blood was on the wall, remained. Naturally. An intern came in. I asked him to clean up the chair. This is a bug of mine. The hospital was filthy. If they don't have to, nobody sweeps under the beds. Dust balls as big as your fist accumulate there. It's terrible. Nobody ever comes in to check if the place is clean. Sometimes, they check with the cleaning people, but they never look to see if the job's been done.

"Anyway, the fevers went away, but nobody seemed too concerned. The surgeon stuck his head in the door almost every day, but just looked at the chart, never examined me. One day, they inspected the incision and decided to pull the wires. I have Raynaud's.[7] My hands were getting blue, so you can see I have Raynaud's. With these chills, I don't know why, I would get tremendous spasms. One hand was getting white and blue. The anesthesiologist was the one guy who came by every day. *He* was scared about these chills, and my mother— No, not my mother. Jesus, that's Freudian. *My wife* said, 'Isn't that nice? He's coming here every day.' I said, 'He's coming down because he's scared stiff. He thinks I may lose my hand.' It bothered me that nobody examined me after the operation, any more than they had before. . . . For six grand,[8] the

---

[6] Caused by broken blood vessels swollen under the skin, it is commonly called a black-and-blue mark.
[7] Vascular disorder of capillaries, usually of fingers and toes, and marked by pallor, blueness, redness (in that order) on exposure to cold.
[8] Fees vary around the country.

least they could do is the kind of insurance physical I do for thirty bucks. But look, I don't want you to think this is all complaints. I felt so great when I awakened. 'Great' isn't the word; it's 'relieved.' I was alive. I knew I needed blood. I was afraid they'd let me slip away. Once I got the blood, I knew I'd be all right, I knew I was going to make it. It was dark outside when I waked. Thank God, the CCU had a window. CCUs ought to have clocks, too, but I'll tell you something: it wouldn't have mattered to me; without glasses, I can't see two feet in front of me.

"Even though I woke up during the night, on Saturday morning, I woke up for real. The nurse asked if I wanted breakfast. I still had the tubes in, the arterial line and the venous line in my arm, but I said, 'Oh, yes, I'd love it.'

"They brought a tray in to me and left it on the table. Suddenly, I realized, 'Either I'm feeding myself or I'm not getting anything to eat.' So I fed myself a liquid breakfast. I guess it was part of the therapy, dropping a tray on the table and walking away. I don't know. Then the surgeon came by with his fellows. They took the tubes out, they took out the chest tubes, and off I went to the general floor that day, that morning. That afternoon, I walked. Only three days in Intensive Care, how's that for speed? A nurse came by and showed me how to cough—two days later. They should have shown me before the operation and again, just after removing the tubes. She gave me a good coughing lesson, but she was a little late. They didn't do any pulmonary function tests, because they don't have a pulmonary department there. They're not much interested in breathing and coughing. They claim there's no room there for a pulmonologist. Pulmonary function's not one of their priorities."

The worst part of Dr. Rand's convalescence was postcardiotomy syndrome. "Nobody's quite sure what causes postcardiotomy syndrome. Some doctors think it's an inflammatory reaction of the pericardium (the membrane encasing the heart) to surgical invasion. Other doctors think that an autoimmune response may manifest itself as the heart, the body itself, heals. While I'm sure that anginal pain and postcardiotomy pain are easily differentiated, some patients confuse the two; they worry. Anginal pain commonly is pressing, sometimes crushing, usually can be relieved by nitroglycerin, while postoperative soreness, whether from postcardiotomy syndrome or not, is more persistent, more likely to be helped by aspirin, Indocin, or cortisone. With chest pain, it's better to be safe than sorry, better always to call the doctor, even if you've just called him the day before or the morning before." He laughs. "End of lecture."

Dr. Rand prescribed aspirin, eight to ten every day, for himself, ruefully adding, "Sure, I know the doctor who treats himself has a fool for a patient, but I used to read George Herbert a lot in college. Do you know him? The seventeenth-century poet? Anyway, Herbert, that lovely man, said, 'Go not for every grief to the physician.' I'll stick with Herbert. I'd had enough with doctors. I'm beginning to sound like the patients.

"Maybe the worst wasn't the fever and aching of postcardiotomy. Maybe the worst was that damned leg. It was bad. For six or eight weeks, every time I stepped down, it hurt."

Dr. Rand had gone back to work, was standing on his feet all day. "It wasn't just the pain. It was this mess here." He lifts his leg onto the sea wall to show his scars. "I have lousy veins, so the incision is huge; it goes from here to there. Nobody checked the leg or the postcardiotomy for six weeks after discharge. By that time, I was better, and I didn't have time to wait in *their* offices. I had my own office to run. But my pantleg used to stick to my skin from all the wound-oozing."

You didn't have a left main. You had a tough time postoperatively. What do you think the operation did for you?

"First, it enabled me to function, which I couldn't have done otherwise. It gave me some ten years of comfortable life—I hope. Three, so far. We shall see what we shall see. Last night, when you asked me if now I smell the flowers, I told you, 'Nothing has changed.' Yet Bypass is one reason I'm down here in Acapulco. Not that I need the rest, but ordinarily, I would've said, 'I can't take off that much time.' Now I'm not afraid to take off a little more time."

He stops, looks out across the water. "I've got no strong attachment to *my* hospital or *my* doctor. It doesn't matter. I hold no brief for him or for anybody else. It's whoever is capable at a competent hospital fulfilling the *New England Journal of Medicine*'s minimum daily requirements. Sounds like vitamins, doesn't it? Surgeons will argue, but they're all alike, with the exception of a few superstars, and I'm not sure about them either. For all you know, you might get a resident running the show. Surgeons do their thing. They're interested in technical aspects: whether it works or not. They cut and run. Internists pick up the pieces. But internists won't cut. We internists are guys who can't stand the sight of blood."

The first three weeks postoperatively, Dr. Rand paced himself, slowly but surely speeding up. "I drove a car in about three weeks. They let me drive early because I live in high, steep hills. I had to drive to flat ground to walk. I couldn't wait for someone to drive me down. That's silly. I waited about two weeks to climb stairs. We moved our bed into the family room."

How long did you wait to have sexual intercourse?

"About a month."

Did the doctor talk to you about sexual matters?

"Of course not. They gave me a booklet. No living human being talked. Talking is for internists and psychiatrists. They had their own pass-out booklet, about when you can do this and when that."

That first time, were you afraid?

"No."

Was your wife?

"You'll have to ask her."

Is your sexual desire the same, better, worse?

"The same. The same." Flatly. "The same. I'm not on any medication. No antihypertensives, no nitrates, no Inderal. My greatest fears are that I'll get angina again."

If the angina started again, what would you do?

"If medical means were completely unsuccessful—a lot's been accomplished in three years—then first I might give angioplasty a whirl. I don't send my patients directly to surgery. Unless they're high-risk or LADs."

What are your greatest joys?

"Being alive. Being able to function. I'm happy. I really am happy. Look, I had an infarct at thirty-six. I'm happy just to be alive. Oh, I know all the statistics that say there's long-term survival, that the prognosis isn't as bad as it used to be, but I still have patients with inferior MIs, they're not supposed to die, but they die anyway. They get arrhythmias and they go out."

What's been your greatest disappointment?

"Not my children. No, not my children. It's myself, I'm disappointed in myself. I haven't been able to keep my weight down, to keep exercising. I wish I were stronger, but I know myself, and I know it's hard for me. I'll get my weight down. You'll see. When I'm motivated again, I'll lose the weight."

What did the operation cost?

"Well, Major Medical covered it. Total fees for hospital were, oh, about $12,000 and the doctor was another $6,000. I don't remember the numbers."

If you'd had to pay for the operation yourself, out of your pocket, would you have had it?

"No."

No?

"No."

Why?

"Because I wouldn't have, that's why. Well, maybe I would have, I don't know, maybe Myra would've nagged me. But it would have involved borrowing. I don't have that much savings. I hate to be in debt, just hate it. I have a good practice, a busy practice, yet over the years, our income was never what it should have been. For a variety of reasons. I made money, but not a lot. Part of it was Blue Shield reimbursement, which we've given up. We don't accept assignment. I won't go into that, period. Part was sloppiness in pursuing bad checks. My wife comes in part-time. Since she's in the office, we don't work any harder, maybe less hard, and our income has gone up considerably, especially because we banned Blue Shield, which says, with its infinite wisdom, 'This much.' What they do is pay you for your office, your help, your overhead. Your part, the doctor's knowledge and skill, is the part they won't pay for. This country respects doing, not thinking; hardware, not software. That's why I never have any cash, surely not enough cash for a big operation."

What explicit questions would you advise people to ask their internist, their cardiologist, their surgeon, before and after CABS?

"It surprises me when sometimes people don't want to know; sometimes they say, 'The less I know, the happier I am.' But most people want to know, need to know, deserve to know. When I refer my patients to a major medical center, I tell them to ask, loud and clear, 'What is this center's experience of mortality and morbidity?' I tell them to ask, and to discuss specifically with that particular hospital, 'How long is recovery time?' How much time are they going to be spending in Intensive Care? Whether or not their families can visit them right away, because Cleveland Clinic and some other hospitals don't allow family visits for three days.

"A friend of mine went to New York University Hospital* for Bypass, and theirs was a distinctive setup. They use a motel for out-of-town patients' recovery, so they don't hustle them from the hospital cocoon to an airport's barbarism in the dead of winter—or the heat of summer. It's time medicine started being more civilized, having some manners, using some common sense. I tell my patients to ask the questions which they gave me the booklet for: 'When can I drive? When can I climb stairs? When will I be able to do what I want?' "

* Not fictitious.

Do the patients whom you recommend for Bypass find that your having had Bypass helps them?

"In a small town like ours, and Lafayette is a relatively small town, believe me, all my patients are aware that I had Bypass. For instance, a woman patient had a situation similar to mine: single-vessel disease with unstable angina, maybe not so severe as mine. I tried to make it clear that her Bypass was elective, that she could get along without it, that she might be able to be handled medically, but she was miserable. She couldn't function at the level she liked. After my little speech, she asked, 'What do you think I should do?' I said again, 'It's an elective procedure.' She went ahead and had Bypass, because, as she said, 'You'd already given me your answer: you had the operation.' "

Don't patients find that comforting?

"I don't know. My Bypass turns some patients off, the idea that their physician was sick. Some people don't like that. It's not just in my mind, not that I'm projecting my concerns onto them. I don't know how to put it, but some patients are disturbed that I had coronary artery disease, that I'm trying to tell them what to do when I had it myself. They look at me. I'm still fat, I'm still soft. I can see what they're thinking."

How does that make you feel?

"Depends. Sometimes, I think, maybe they're right, that I should have taken better care of myself. Sometimes I feel it's none of their business. Sometimes I resent their making me feel like this about myself."

One reason you'd don't take such good care of yourself is that you're out there taking care of them.

"Maybe. Doctors don't have to run every minute. It's a good excuse not to confront ourselves. But to go back to your question about questions to ask doctors. Some people want to put blind faith in physicians. Too frequently, doctors playing God encourage such trust. Most of my patients ask penetrating questions. I encourage them to know. The mechanics of the surgery are questions people ask after the operation. Preop, patients ask—rightly—'Do I really need this Bypass? What can Bypass do for me that benign neglect would not do?' Postoperatively, they need to know, 'When can I do certain things? Why do I still have pain? How can I differentiate surgical pain from heart pain? I've been through this operation to make me well; why don't I feel great?' Some operations aren't successful. That's why patients don't feel well."

Spelling out the details varies with the attitudes of the surgeon and the medical center, says Dr. Rand. His objection to the hospital's booklet was its vagueness about how, when, and what can be done: "Such books should say, and the doctor should reinforce in a predischarge discussion as well as in postop visits, when you can drive, when you can have sexual intercourse, when you can go back to work. This booklet said, 'If you are a secretary, you can go back in five to six weeks.' But people feel, 'This is what I do; when can I go back? I'm a living human being. I'm special. Treat me as though I'm unique.' "

Tell me about your uniqueness. Describe yourself. First, physically.

"I'm overweight and uncomfortable, because my clothing is getting tight. I'm five-seven and I weigh 180 pounds.

"I'm not a good athlete. I play some racquetball, but I'm lousy. If I'm not good at something, then I don't do it. Nothing in between. So I don't do much athletics. I feel well. My limitations are not from my heart, but from my inabilities. I'm not a great mountain climber, a great golfer, a great tennis player, but I wish I were better. I don't pursue anything as deeply or as long as I should. I suppose you could call me a dilettante. I admire people who single-mindedly commit themselves to becoming expert in a field. Even more I respect those people, like Lewis Thomas, who can be so articulate, can know so much about philosophy, zoology, and history. It's not just because he studies—he remembers. I'm not able to synthesize information as I'd like to. I'm a good physician, but I'm not the best, because the best can put things together."

At the half-century mark, with a Bypass behind you, are you glad or sorry you moved to Lafayette?

"Oh, glad. It's a nice community, even though Bostonians look down their noses at such places. In Lafayette, I can do much more than I could have in Boston. In big cities, everybody is pigeon-holed. For seven years, I was a nephrologist.[9] I started the Dialysis[10] Unit there. We sent the nurses away for training. We had a manual, we read the book, all self-taught. Somebody once showed me how to put in a catheter, so we put in catheters, did acutes, ran the machines, did kidney biopsies. Hell, I never could have done that in Boston. I've got lots of interests. In Lafayette, I can do oncology[11] and hematology,[12] whatever I want. In Lafayette, I get a lot of respect, a lot more, I guess, than I would in a larger place where doctors are a dime a dozen, although we're approaching that ratio back home, too. In the last five years, the number of physicians has increased dramatically. I worry about that."

Describe yourself psychically, philosophically.

"I get misty-eyed easily. The cup—that standard question—may be half-full, may be half-empty, depending on how well things have gone that day, depending on my mood. I'm a perfectionist. How could a physician be anything else?"

Some physicians aren't perfectionists.

"They're not good doctors. That's one of my problems. I'm a perfectionist, but I can't achieve perfection. Some physicians come much closer to perfection than I. You've got people's lives depending on you. How can you do anything half-assed? For me, the salt hasn't lost its savor. I like taking care of patients even more now than ever. The trouble is, you get to know people, to like them, then it hurts when somebody dies. When something goes wrong, you say, 'What did I do that I shouldn't have? What didn't I do

[9] A specialist in kidney disease.
[10] Mechanical elimination of impurities from the blood during kidney failure.
[11] The branch of medicine dealing with tumors.
[12] The study and treatment of blood and its diseases.

that I could have?' You can always find things. Well, not always, but sometimes. I have a short fuse. Mostly, I blame myself a lot when there's trouble in the hospital. The nurses know I don't take any nonsense. I can understand their making mistakes, but not sloppy, stupid errors."

What about at home?

"What can you do? Probably I pour catacholamines from irritability at home and in the hospital all day long. At least, in the hospital, they respect me."

What about the Type-A characteristics? How do you rate?

"God, I'm one of the two fastest eaters in the world. My partner's the fastest. I won't wait in lines. I like to do at least two things at once. I don't make lists, but I feel guilty that I'm not organized enough to make lists."

Do you feel guilty about a lot of things?

"Oh, yes, sure. Is that normal?"

I don't know normal from abnormal. I just ask questions.

He laughs. "Okay, you win. I'm always on time. I mutter in traffic, but not as much as my wife. Now there's a Type A for you! I don't honk if I'm behind someone and the light changes. That's the New York Olympics: how fast can you blow the horn? Years ago, Russell Baker wrote an article about horn-blowing New Yorkers. 'Course, if they're preoccupied with doing something else, like putting on lipstick, and if I know it's a short light, I might wake 'em up gently. I listen to someone with half an ear and think about other things, but not with my wife. She's the boss. I wanna keep some peace in the house. But I won't go shopping with her. She knows that. Shopping is boring, number one; and two, in large department stores, I get disoriented, even vertiginous; and three, shopping is a big, fat waste of time."

All of us have insecurities. What are yours?

"Living, just living. If I'll live, how I'll live, how long I'll live. The other is my ability as a physician. I worry: 'Am I good? Am I keeping my abilities? Will they deteriorate? What don't I know that I should?' I worry a lot about that. I try to keep up, I read, but I'm unsure what kind of doctor I am. That's my most important insecurity. Being an internist is connected to being insecure. There's so much to know; it's impossible to master everything new." Ben Rand stops, takes off his photogray sunglasses, wipes them on a corner of his terry beach jacket. "You're caught in a Catch-22: you can't know everything, but you have to. If you don't know everything, you're no good."

11. Jason Master, M.D.
Chief of Gynecology
Ages at Bypass: 49, 55

Dr. Jason Master lives in a white house high on a wooded hill overlooking his hometown of York, Maine. In his knotty-pine study, politely he offers me a chair, then eases his gangling body into a worn leather rocking chair, which squeaks in protest every time he shifts his large frame. His eyes pale-blue and watery behind bifocals, his once sandy hair the color of shorn winter wheat, his face gray, his voice weary and halting, he seems much older than his fifty-five years. He'd had his first Bypass in 1975, his second one, six months ago, he notes matter-of-factly. His older brother, like Dr. Master, their father, and grandfather before them, is also a surgeon. His brother had offered to give blood for him in 1975, but had been so anemic that the Blood Bank had refused him. "Then," Dr. Master adds carefully, "he had a GI series which turned up a CA;[1] that was successfully resected. *He's* had no recurrences. Unlike me, he's been fine since."

Dr. Master had never smoked, had lived a clean old-fashioned life. "I drank moderately. My weight hasn't changed much over

[1] Cancer.

the years. In the past ten years, I've deliberately lost about ten pounds. I've always tried to keep in shape, to keep my heart in good condition. I jogged, I skied, I swam, I enjoyed sports," Master confesses. "My wife and children had enjoyed sports, but mostly I was careful to keep my body in good tone because I thought exercise would help me avoid heart trouble. Somehow, I knew I'd come to Bypass. Yet I didn't figure on having it twice.

"My father had his first heart attack at thirty-five, although he lived to eighty-one, a ripe old age. He didn't marry until he was forty-two, and he never participated in sports. I figured I'd be on the heart-trouble list. My wife thinks I'm a little obsessed, because I'm always making contingency arrangements. Statistically, Bypass always threatened me. All that exercise helped me avoid a life-threatening infarction. Initially, I just had angina, appearing out of nowhere. It took me a while even to realize what it was. All I had was a pain in my throat after a large meal. The pain wasn't much; it would disappear after a few minutes.

"I almost forgot. The month before the throat pain began, I'd almost blacked out at a meeting I chaired out of town. I didn't know what in the world was happening. Instead of going on, I turned the meeting over to someone else and came home. In four days, I felt better and went back to work. It was another month, the beginning of April, before I noticed this throat pain and recognized—finally—that the pain must be angina. It kept getting worse. On May fifth, I went to Galveston. One week later, May twelfth, I had the Bypass. I was forty-nine—almost fifty. I thought I was a pretty young forty-nine. That's the average age for Bypass at many places. It wasn't so surprising.

"I went to Galveston to get away from my friends. I didn't want my colleagues to feel responsible for my surgery if anything went wrong. My new chairman had trained there; he said that it was one of the best places in the country. I don't like New York City; I didn't want my wife all alone there. The second time, I didn't go back to Galveston—it was too hard on my wife. It's miserable to be the patient's family there. You stay in this one motel. My wife was afraid to be out at night. She was pretty unhappy there. Besides, the hospital restricted my wife from seeing me for the first three days after the operation. I was surprised that they were so harsh about families. It didn't make much difference for me because I was so sick both times. I was almost unable to respond.

Seeing her, that second time when she could come in right away, was difficult. I wanted her near me, but it was distressing. It was really hard on me, but I guess it was better to see her, at least briefly."

Dr. Master claims that he never asked, "Why me?" because, "I kind of expected it. I'd accomplished a reasonable amount of what I set out to do in my life. The idea of having to plateau out didn't overwhelm me. Even if I were quite disabled, I knew I could continue to work, to contribute to society, so I didn't feel so cut off from the world. There'd be opportunities for me. In some measure, I'm grateful. Heart disease is better than multiple sclerosis, which my brother-in-law has. That's absolutely devastating.

"Before and after both operations, I looked back at my life and tried to decide what I could do. Depending on varying degrees of disability, I figured out contingency plans. My nature is to be orderly. I need to have thought through what avenues are open for me. I don't like being forced to take action before I've charted my course.

"Before and after the second operation, I was a lot sicker than the first time. The second procedure took more out of me, but, then it took a lot longer: five hours instead of three, four Bypass grafts instead of just one. The emotional debilitation after the second operation appalled me. My wife says that I was just as depressed the first time, but I felt much more wretched the second time. I'm not depressed now—at least, I don't think so. My mentation is better than at any time since the first Bypass. A year after the first operation, I gave up private practice and went into academic medicine. I became professor of OB-GYN, which I had always wanted to do. Since this second operation, I fatigue less readily, but since the first surgery, I've gone to bed at eleven, and I've made it a point to take a nap every afternoon. One thing about being a surgeon: you learn to sleep anywhere, anytime. I'd lie down for that nap. I'd drop off to sleep in about one minute."

Asked whether he was disappointed about the need for a second operation, Dr. Master doesn't answer directly: "A year before the second one, I had a small MI. In the hospital, they advised surgery, but I didn't think I was bad enough—yet. I told the cardiologist I wanted to go home. He wasn't too happy. I went home anyway. I went back to work. I felt pretty good right through Christmas. By March, I was a lot worse; I knew something had to be done. I let them catheterize me; all three vessels were involved, so I knew I couldn't put it off much longer. In the hospital, with nitroglycerin and Nitrobid and I forget what else, I still was having unstable angina.

"The worst was that I changed from a healthy middle-aged young man to an old man, older than my father ever seemed to me, older than I ever thought I'd be—at this or any other age. I was no longer vigorous. I couldn't do sports or the heavy work I'd always liked to do, puttering on cars, working on the house. I had to give up some of my aspirations. I wanted political jobs in medical organizations. I wanted to work for the abortion clinic. If I hadn't gotten sick in '75, I would have been chairman of the Federal Advisory Group on Contraceptive Research. That job would have led into other national jobs. I was supposed to be president of the state medical society. I may say yes to them next year; I haven't decided. My wife's always glad when I give up something. But I'm not glad. She worries that I'll do too much: I should be sensible, she says. But being sensible, as they call it, makes me feel old. When you're young and full of beans, you don't have to 'be sensible.' Her concern and, I guess, my own fears generate a stress of their own. Not that it's avoidable.

"It's funny. I didn't worry about having the operation. Bypass doesn't hurt that much. The postop period's not like the pain of orthopedic or abdominal surgery. The depression bothered me, but you forget it. You don't remember depression that well, which is a blessing. At one point, after the second one, I was suicidal. That scared me. Because I was so weak and sick, because I was stuck in the hospital, I could do nothing. Fortunately, my gun was home. I didn't have access to a syringe or to pills which I could have self-administered in fatal doses. I wasn't strong enough to get to a window; I'm not sure that the Coronary Care Unit should be on the tenth floor, because if I could have, I would have ended my life then and there. What was the use of going on? Not enough is done with Bypassers and depression. It's not good enough for someone to pop his head in the door and say, 'Cheer up. You'll feel better soon. Stop giving in to yourself.' And then to go flying out the door again. The fifth postop day is the worst. That day, my suicidal fantasies were acute. All I wanted was to say, 'Enough! Game called because of rain.' After that, the depression began lifting. I'd lapse back, but nothing like that fifth day. Once I got home, I had times when I'd get down, but not that much. One time, I looked for my gun. Betsy must have hidden it; it wasn't in its usual drawer in my desk.

"At home, convalescing, I hated not knowing how strong I'd be, how much I could do. I couldn't plan for the future. I didn't know whether to retire or to look forward to going back to work. The best thing was that after six weeks, I started going into the office. Ben Frank flew here from California and we wrote a paper together. Working on the paper was exciting. It did a lot to turn my convalescence around. It made me realize that I'd be able to get back on my feet—at least for a while. Ben's a good man. He says he would've come here to work with me anyhow; I'm sure he came across the country to get me going again. And he did."

Dr. Master complains that, although the second operation was six months ago, he still gets tired. "I should have been over the effects of surgery after two months. I went back to swimming a mile every day. I could do a mile right away, the first time in. I jog a mile around our hill here. I'm not the athlete I wanted to be when I was young, but I enjoy the well-being of athletics, which helped me recuperate better both times." He stops, looks out the window at the sun, its hectic edge just visible above a copse of blue spruce.

"The hardest thing was, when I awakened, the business of the intubation. Especially, the second time, not being able to talk and wanting to. Those idiots—not the doctors, the nurses—were asking me questions. I had the tube in and I couldn't talk."

Some places have a pad and pencil nearby.

"What good would a pencil and paper have done? I couldn't write, because I had an arterial catheter in one wrist; I've forgotten what was going into the other arm. They kept asking me questions. There was no way to reply. They should know better, should have a better means of dealing with the acutely ill, alert, intubated patient."

As chief of Obstetrics and Gynecology at the hospital, didn't you comment to the staff about ways of alleviating these problems?

"Last time, a year ago when I was in with the MI, I wrote a letter containing what I thought were a few constructive comments. As

I look back on it, maybe they were just petty things, perhaps the administration thought my complaints only minor. I wanted personnel to wear their nametags so I could read their names; if they wore their tags at all, usually they had them on upside down. I've a poor memory. I like to see people and know who they are. I like to call them by name and I like them to call me by name—not my first name! What a demeaner that is! Knowing people's names helps me orient myself. I feel more human, more as though I'm connecting with other people, if I know their names. Then, the food knocked me for a loop because it had too much salt in it. I was on a regular 'house' diet, but I didn't want all that salt. Soup, meatloaf, fish, it was all loaded with salt—and cold.

"I wrote them about it and I never got a reply. They don't welcome criticism. I don't like to do things unless I think they will be acted upon. I think the hospital rejected my suggestions because they didn't want to hear them; they didn't want to be forced to make changes."

You're the chief there. If they don't listen to somebody like you, how would they listen to an ordinary patient?

"They believe that doctors tend to be overreactive, hypercritical, which some of us are. I try to be a reasonable patient, but I do see every little thing."

Is it more difficult for the doctor to be a patient?

"It's a lot easier because I know my way around the 'system.' If I want something done, I know how to get it done. When I decided that I wanted to go home, they weren't ready to let me go. I got the resident and the nurse to warn the cardiologist. By the time he had gotten to me in his rounds, he knew I wanted to go, and that I'd go home whether he let me or not. So he had adjusted his own thinking to my way and he let me go. If he hadn't let me go . . . Well, I was just fed up with the place. I'd been there too long. The food was dreadful, it tasted dreadful, it was repetitious, boring—and salty. I couldn't eat much. I was getting a tachycardia from eating. I had postcardiotomy syndrome both times, after each surgery, which was bothersome. The second time, they had me on Indocin, which helped. I still have to eat carefully. If I could just go home, I knew I'd be more interested in food, that Betsy would fix me things I like.

"Both times, they were pretty good about spotting the postcardiotomy syndrome. Galveston had had a lot of Bypass experience. They put me on aspirin and digitalis. Trouble was, they didn't get the dig. dose up high enough. My own internist finally pushed it up to a therapeutic level—at home. Aspirin always irritated my stomach. I tolerated the Indocin a lot better. Even so, I had to take food with it. Each time, it lasted about a month, maybe. I was always afraid it would come back."

Some people have said that postcardiotomy syndrome was worse than the operation, worse even than unstable angina.

"It was bad, yes. I couldn't talk from it, especially this time. I didn't feel like seeing people—friends, or even family—because I couldn't talk to them. I wanted to talk, but my voice wouldn't work. Even today, people say my voice is faint and apathetic.

"My voice always has been weak. That's why I'm a surgeon, I guess. It's pretty good now. Years ago, when talking to patients, I tried an amplifying system, because my voice would get so tired. Some days I talk all day. You see thirty or forty patients, you run out of steam. You get a deaf patient with a prolapse, it's hard to communicate. After the second operation, I kept a log, so I'd know when things would slump and when they'd get better. I kept it because my cardiologist wanted it. Before the operation, I was on nifedipine (Procardia), which then was an experimental drug. I'm not on any drugs now. I don't like drugs. Even so, when my cardiologist wanted me to have this second go-round, I didn't want it. I wanted to try the medication. I'm glad I waited. I got at least another year out of the first operation. I tell you, I don't want to have another Bypass. Because I waited, I figure my chances of going on longer might be better. Who knows? Nobody can be explicit about how much you can do. You're told, 'Do what you can tolerate.' That's not good enough. You like to know exactly what you can and cannot do, what they think you can tolerate. My greatest disappointment now is my lack of stamina, my lack of energy. My lost responsiveness."

Responsiveness?

"Oh, you know. Somebody makes a request; I'd like to be able to respond, to do what they want. I'd like to be able to work on a car and take the front wheels off, do a brake job. I've got a car down cellar needs a brake job. Normally, I'd do that. Ten years ago, I'd have done it in a day. Now, it'd take me a week, even a month. I couldn't do it. I can only work now if I feel good. If I'm tired, there are times that I can't do anything, and *it burns me.* I'm afraid I might default on some medical job. That's why I don't do any more emergency surgery. I can't go back into the hospital at night. Some nights, I'm just too bone-tired. The only surgery I do is on an elective basis. If I do a hysterectomy, that's all I do that day. My secretary doesn't schedule anything else. I used to see patients in the office, operate, go out to dinner, go to a play or a concert, work on a paper after I got home. I can't do that any more. If I'm entertaining a visiting professor, I get very tired, I can't stay with him all the time, I can't take him round to all the people he should meet, places he should see. I have to go off by myself. Since the first Bypass, I've had this energy crisis."

What did the two Bypasses do for you?

"Oh, they relieved my angina. People don't realize about the severity of angina pain. It's intractable. Like cancer pain. I had it in my arms, my chest, my back. That's all gone now. I still get a little in my throat, but that's the old angina. It goes way back to before the first Bypass. That first operation never relieved the throat angina, but it's not bad. It's fleeting, maybe it lasts a few hours at most. It's not enough to demand medication. If I swim, it'll go away. If I eat, it goes away instead of getting worse, the way it used to. My cardiologist doesn't think it's angina, but I'm sure it is. *I know.*"

He leans back in his chair. "The second Bypass made my sex life better. It's made quite a difference. Since the first operation, I couldn't sustain a *reliable* erection. It's not what it was, it's considerably reduced, the ability to *perform*, but the past few months, it's better.

"I tolerate cold better. Here in York, the winters are pretty bad. People ask me whether Bypass prolonged my life. I think so. I'm not sure. My dad got along without it. He protected himself; he regulated his activities even more than I do. See that shingle? That's my dad's shingle up on the wall. That's his clock from his waiting room. That clock used to be in my grandfather's waiting room. It still runs, it doesn't miss a minute—without Bypass.

"I wonder if I'll live as long as that grandfather's clock. Sometimes I wonder if I want to. If I can perceive, can communicate with people, can contribute to society, then, gosh, I'll go on to ninety. If I lose the ability to read, to hear, to talk, then it'd be ridiculous to keep me alive. I've pretty well decided that I'm going to do more because it feels good to me and I enjoy it. If there's a little risk, well, so be it. I can't be superprotective of myself; that's not living. I'd rather feel myself alive."

Are surgeons more or less aware than internists are of their own mortality? What role did the operation play in that awareness?

"The first operation made me aware that my life span was shorter than the Brooklyn Bridge and not so secure. Now I know that mortality is just around the corner. I knew something would happen to me before it happened to other people—and it did."

After that first surgery, did you change your work pattern?

"I withdrew from my old partnership. When I left, the partnership fell apart. We had six gynecologists; we were the biggest office in town—and the best. I was the group's president. I kept peace among them, and gave them direction. Doctors are prima donnas. I was sick of playing Rudolf Bing to their opera company. After the Bypass, I didn't have the energy. With the schism between town and gown, I got sick of being an LMD,[2] as the residents refer to us, of being a townie, being just a referring physician. I decided to get some of the privileges of being a gownie, to be a full-time medical academician. In that respect, that first operation did me a favor; it brought me up short. I'm not so sure about the second one."

---

[2] Local medical doctor.

Was your depression anger turned inward at being sick?

"It's hard for me to believe I was that angry about being disabled. I was disappointed. I know when I get angry. I wasn't enraged about my disability in the same way. Either time. I get angry about other things—like drivers. I love to drive. It bothers me to be behind a slow driver, not to be able to drive as fast as I want to. I'm learning to accommodate. I realize I'm getting old, too; I'm also going to be inept and fearful on the road. In years past, I'd honk at a Creepin' Jesus, then blast by 'em, but now I don't get so worked up. If I'm feeling irritable, I'll take off and pass them, but I don't honk."

In such mild tones, you talk about anger. Are you more irritable now than before the operations?

"Absolutely not. I'm under a lot less strain. Very few people recognize the stresses of obstetrics. When you're carrying a full practice, you may get home for a meal because your wife and kids are after you, but there'll be six people waiting in the Emergency Department. They're all angry because they had to wait in the hospital; the hospital is angry because you went home to eat instead of coming directly into ED. That kind of stress, day in and day out, makes you irritable. You get calls from patients, they want this or that. You go to bed and they wake you up. You go in early to make rounds before office hours or operating, which means you're lucky to sleep four or five hours a night. It doesn't matter how big the office is; each man ends up with a work load like that if he's successful and doing good work. If he's not, you don't want him."

Given the nature of the beast, why do doctors clone doctors?

"If you like it, your children see that it's satisfying and rewarding. I've always liked being a doctor—most of the time. I didn't like having so much of it, but you can't put a lid on. I hate to say no if it's something I like or want to do. That's what gets me in trouble."

Is that your nature or the nature of medicine?

"Some of it is my training. The way we train our residents, we dump things on them, so that only the most gifted and the most motivated prevail and excel. Sometimes they burn themselves out. I've seen this happen. Who knows? Maybe I burned myself out. I always wanted to be an engineer, I wonder what my life would have been if I'd stuck with engineering. I was accepted at MIT, but World War II came along. I thought I'd be drafted right away, so I went to the University of Maine in premed because my dad thought it'd keep me out of service. He was right, too, at least till the Korean War. The dean of the medical school was dad's friend; he took an interest in me. He was on the draft board; until he retired, I was never inducted.

"My father never kissed me. Our family doesn't express emotions easily. I have trouble communicating with the children in that respect. Yet I've always felt a little tearful at weddings, funerals, in church, for reasons I don't fully understand. After each heart episode, the two Bypasses and the MI, I'd have periods of increased lability. I'd cry a little easier. Now that I'm doing better, I don't get misty-eyed so much. I'm not depressed the way I was on the Inderal. The nifedipine depressed me, but the Inderal really got to me. Funny, those are billed as nonemotionally reactive drugs."

The doorbell chimes. Mrs. Master effusively greets visitors. Restless, Dr. Master looks at his watch, then checks it with his grandfather's clock.

"I don't choose my friends. I take the ones who are friendly to me," he notes, tapping a pencil on the desk. "Some people I used to think I'd like as friends, but they didn't cotton to me. That bothered me. I've always wondered why. Lately, I've decided that kind of friendship isn't important. You gravitate to people who appreciate you. I guess I've never felt close to people. It's funny. Implicitly, I guess I trust people. I'd do anything for them that they wanted; but to exchange confidences about how one feels about all kinds of things, no. I don't mind being alone. I'm happy to read, to be entertained by my own thoughts, to travel alone. Usually, I take a paper along that I'm writing. I enjoy writing."

He looks at the clock again.

What would you advise someone who's been told to have Bypass?

"Go ahead and have it. I went once locally and once far away. Other things being equal, I'd stay local. If the mortality rate is the same, I'd stay with the local group. It's a lot easier on the family. Goin' away is pretty harsh for families. Talk to my wife about that."

Should there be a member of the team who is psychologically trained and who sees you regularly?

His no is flat and final as he adds, "It's a waste of time and money. The physiological responses produce depression. It's pretty common; probably there's some chemical cause that we don't know. No psychological reinforcement would make any difference. What you need is support—lots of support—from family, staff, clergy, the church, other people who've had Bypass."

You seem involved with your church.

"I'm a lousy churchgoer. I go four times a year, but I give them money. I don't have time. My wife represents me at church."

Do you believe that there's a design to the universe?

"Yes—well, maybe to some extent; nevertheless, I can affect what happens to me. Oh, I believe in God. Sure. He was in the operating room. When I'm operating and I'm not sure what to do surgically, I ask God to tell me. It's worked out quite well. Sort of a *quid pro quo*.

"What bothers me is that Bypass changed the way people treat me. They don't respect me so much. They're less likely to disagree and argue. I depend on discussion, maybe even on argumentation, to find answers. Mine is a committee style. I get my ideas there. If you have a lot of gray hair, if you've had a couple of Bypasses, if you're a professional, a chairman of a department, it's hard to get young people to express their ideas—students particularly. That's what I have to overcome. I don't like being dogmatic, shutting off someone's intellectual ferment before we can talk things over."

The gray hair was there before the operation.

"It's gettin' grayer steadily. People shelter me too much. I s'pose I should be grateful. I'm not afraid for me so much as they're afraid. What I fear is gettin' the angina back, having my coronaries shut down on me."

Would you have the surgery again?

"I don't know. Maybe. Maybe if they showed me an angiogram which, based on my own knowledge, made sense to go through all that again. It's the first time I've said this: I don't relish another trip through Bypass.

"The postop period was rough. But I suppose"—he stops, looks up at his grandfather's clock ticking loudly, surely, on the wall—"I suppose if I could continue to work, to be with my wife, to watch the family grow and flourish, if I could continue to teach and to be around the students, I'd consider it. Doctors need to tell you the score, need to level with you better. Oh, I know all the arguments doctors propound against too much information. In some ways, no matter how many T's are crossed, how many I's are dotted, informed consent is a myth. Still . . .

"I wish they'd told me that depression was in the cards, that the second time around was tougher than the first. If they'd warned me ahead of time, I'd have accepted depression. Surely, I'd have expected it to disappear instead of thinking that depression was mine forever; knowing would've made those black days more bearable. All I knew came from a neighbor who'd been through the same thing. He'd been through the same thing, and said, 'Just remember, the fifth day is the nadir, but *you get better, you climb out of the pit.* The depression doesn't last forever; even when it comes back, each time it's not so bad as the time before.'

"Fortunately, every time I seemed to hit bottom, I'd remember his words. But if the doctors had warned me in advance, had recognized the depression, it'd have helped. When I know what's happening, what's going to happen, usually I can accommodate. The unforeseen unsettles me."

12. Kurt Ranter, M.D.
Family physician
Age at Bypass: 62

Kurt Ranter is a short, muscular man, with deep-set, piercing blue eyes, thorny charcoal brows divided only by the fierce furrows over his hawklike nose. His rare smile briefly lightens his constant glowering. Having consented to talk only because his wife, also a Bypasser, had persuaded him, his impatience repeatedly and sometimes deliberately breaks the tenuous connections between us. He dials his answering service, riffles through his mail, looks at his watch, angrily erupts at my remarking how many Bypassers are refugees from other countries.

"We're not refugees! What kind of refugees are you talking about? I've been longer in this country than you've been alive. Are you a refugee, answer me that? Talk about refugees does not apply to Milena and me, number one. And number two, if stress has a lot to do with heart disease, and it does, genetics is the single most important factor. So you should not talk about refugees, because you are proceeding under a false premise. Now"—Dr. Ranter points his finger at me—"what do you want to know? But make it short."

How old are you?

"I'm seventy, but I'm a young man yet. Chronological age doesn't mean anything. What means is what you've done with your life. I was always active in sports. In my youth, I coached two hundred youngsters while I was going to school in Vienna."

What year did you leave?

"Nineteen thirty-eight. Milena got me out—she was always smart, always beautiful. She got me into Italy, and then to England. In 1940, I came here. Here in Norfolk, I started complete new graduate training." He stops. "If you don't need this information, cut me short," he barks.

You said heart disease is genetically based. What's your family history?

"In my case, there's no heart disease in the family. In Milena's family, yes. For me, no genetic origin at all. But this doesn't mean genetics doesn't play a primary role."

When did you find out that you had heart trouble?

"When I couldn't play a full afternoon of racquetball. After the first game, I started to get short of breath. The only trouble before was once, in 1974, sitting in the family room, I'd had sudden arrhythmias. I signed myself into the medical center. Everything was negative. A resting cardiogram, what does it prove? I insisted to have a stress test, had it done; it showed some changes. So we cut out skiing, and proceeded our lives as usual. Milena was already sick from skiing; it was no loss. Nothing more until I visited my son in Montreal two years later, and again arrhythmias, but this time, shortness of breath. My son and his wife were having trouble. This was the first we know that things were not so good between them. Later, they divorced. The new wife is not well. Again, I signed myself into the hospital. The first time, I had a fast pulse, a tachycardia, regular, but unpleasant. In Montreal, I was unusually tired, walking around, big dinners, theatre. In Montreal is so much to do, it's a little like Europe. I think I got carried away. Funny expression, in English, that 'carried away.' At the theatre, I had a spell, a little perspiration, a little fast heartbeat. I left the theatre and walked back to the hotel. That same night, I woke up with arrhythmic beats. I told Milena, 'We go to the hospital.' I didn't take my pulse, but *I knew*. It was irregular. By the time I got to the hospital, the pulse was all right. The EKG showed only a left bundle branch block, which covers up everything; you can't tell what's going on. I continued my investigation at home. The same as in Montreal: nothing. The thallium test was negative. Still, I insisted to go further. Something was seriously wrong. An angiogram showed obstruction. They dillydallied. I didn't like that. I got a second opinion from another cardiology group, who agreed I had obstruction of the left anterior descending and the circumflex. The right coronary, they felt, was a spastic reaction to inserting the catheter. Then what? The two groups got together. In two days, I was on a plane for Colorado and had four bypasses grafted."

Who made these decisions? Who decided on the angio?

"I pushed for the angio. They couldn't make up their minds. I couldn't wait for them to invent the wheel."

Did stresses or your responses to stresses accelerate in the year prior to this?

"Not really."

What's 'not really'? Do you think of yourself as a stressful man?

"Of course. I consider myself Type A, but I didn't need any Meyer Friedman to tell me. Before I heard about Type A or Type B, I knew the problem. When you are in stress, you accelerate your pulse and your blood flow. This factor should be obvious to any layman. You do not have to be a scholar and give alphabetical letters to personality traits."

Did you ever try to modify your behavior?

"Behavior type is in your genes. I have a different opinion about psychiatry from Americans. I was brought up with Freud and Adler and Jung, the whole group in Vienna. When I was fifteen, it was like we have here rock-and-roll; there we had psychoanalytic discussions. We were brought up, so to speak, on the mother's milk of psychiatry."

You don't believe in behavior modification?

"Yes, I do believe. But it is very difficult. There is the teleological outlook and the causative outlook. The teleological philosophy says everything is predetermined. The causative, the more scientific, believes everything has its reason. If we don't know the reason, we are just not up to it yet. Going to the moon, cardiac surgery, extracorporeal circulation, all things we never dreamt would be possible, are due to advances in technology and medicine. Psychiatry today is scratching the surface. They will find out reasons for behavior in the cell or in the electronic data of our brains. If we get to it, then all psychotic situations may be treatable. I don't know if it's in our time or not. For now, you can only modify behavior externally. Internally, character can never be modified because that's the way it's been made. Our characters are stigmatized by genetics."

You accepted the decision to have Bypass? You wanted it?

"I did not *want* it. I *had* to do it. As a physician, I had sent a dozen cases for surgery before I myself went. What's good for my patients is good for me. A decision like that is tough. Going for Bypass, a garbage collector is better off than a physician, who knows exactly what will happen, all the dangers. Although the mortality is low, down to 1.5 or 2 percent, for the one or two they lose, it's 100 percent. Being active all my life, I couldn't live the way I had to without Bypass. I am happy I did it.

"I am back to full-time work; I work more than I used to. Lately, I get a little tired towards the end of the day. I think I am getting a little older. I am not thirty-eight anymore. I am starting to be thirty-nine. As a doctor, going for this surgery, the fear is greater, but the rewards are greater. You understand what feats have been accomplished medically."

Your wife had Bypass. Is it harder to be the patient or the husband?

"Aach, harder to be the husband. No question about it."

Why?

"You know what's going to happen, you know all the dangers. It's harder to watch someone I love go through such an ordeal than to go through it myself. After the anesthesia, you are out. The next thing you know, you are fighting for air and that's about it."

After Bypass, did you value human relationships more? Did you change in any way?

"After Bypass, you are euphoric. Even with the tube in, you feel exultant—well, not with the tubes in, that's exaggeration, but after the first couple of days. When the tubes are in, you have no thoughts about being euphoric or not euphoric. You fight for breath, more or less. My worst experiences were immediately afterwards; I was operated on with a chest cold. I told them to wait, not to operate. They went ahead. They don't listen to anybody; the schedule must go on. I had slightly complicated postoperative course."

Which was what?

"I had pneumonia. My lungs were not so clear. But after the first couple of days, everything went well. You're euphoric, you're glad to be alive; you came through, you're beginning again! You have the idea, from now on, your life will be on a different level. Your life expectancy is up. After a while, you get rebound: you're depressed because you don't see yourself getting better fast enough. After all, it is a major procedure. They open the chest. They cut the bone. With any motion, you feel the crepitation of the sternum. Your recovery takes longer than you think it should. After three months, I went to play golf. I put on a smiling face. I told everybody how wonderful it is. I don't like being pitied. But it takes a good year before you're yourself again. Even then, you have certain times when you might have chest pain. If you are a physician, you wonder, 'Is it chest-wall pain or is it cardiac pain?' I suppose the nonphysician is troubled by the same questions, but Milena never said anything, my son-in-law never said anything. In my case, I still had arrhythmias. I was on Pronestyl and Quinidine. Naturally"— he grimaces—"I had to develop Quinidine fever. All these little things eat at you."

Do you still have arrhythmias?

"No. I took myself off completely from all medication. The arrhythmias disappeared just like that. After a while, drugs themselves can take over and cause arrhythmias. About a year ago, I got fed up. I took a chance, I stopped everything, and I am fine. I don't like for my patients to do things like that, but I know better."

How long were you depressed?

"Not 'depressed,' but not euphoric any more. I never had deep depression. That's for women."

After Bypass, did you become irritable?

"I would not say so." (Milena Ranter, also a Bypasser, had complained about her husband's irascibility.) "But I am an explosive person. I kept my fuse. Age may mellow me, but not yet. My values have changed. I never was interested in material things; I sacrificed a lot for my medical studies and development. While others went out and made money, I spent ten years working in hospitals. Fortunately, I earned a good living, not fancy, but comfortable. After Bypass, any interest in material values faded completely."

Do you value human relationships more?

"I always valued, always."

Are you more willing to go on a vacation with your wife?

"Why go on vacation? Who needs it? This summer, to please Milena, we'll go to Vienna for the first time in forty-five years. Why she wants me to go so much, I don't know." His face darkens. "You should not go back, you can't go back. Other than Vienna, my *modus* of life hasn't changed, I haven't changed. Medicine is still my life. It will be until I die."

Did Bypass make you feel old?

"Old? Never! You were surprised that I am seventy. I do not feel seventy. Nothing is changed. Since Bypass, I may be less active in sports, but I have taken on a greater work load."

Did Bypass make you feel as though you had a new lease on life?

"In the beginning, for a very short time. Maybe a year, not now. The arrhythmias disturbed me."

Did you ever feel angry at the universe? Did you ask, 'Why me?'

"Never. No physician could do that. He knows what's happening. He knows how his heart disease developed. I could never understand how anybody familiar with heart disease could be angry. In me, there's no Jonah syndrome. Not Job either."

You treated yourself very aggressively.

"Let's just say I was helpful to my physician."

Did the operation make you aware of things you wish you'd done or not done with your life?

"No. I would wish everything the same, except"—Dr. Ranter averts his face—"I don't know if I would have come to this city. The doctors here are jealous. They don't like 'foreigners.' I don't know about Norfolk."

Since Bypass, is your marriage the same, better, worse?

"Always it was good. This has nothing to do with Milena and me, but when you hear people say, 'They are the ideal couple. They never argue,' that marriage is the most endangered species, because most of them get divorced. Communication is the most important thing. Even if you are temperamental and blow up, you have reestablished your relationship. Milena and I are as young as we were when we got married. We have the same attitudes towards each other." (Milena Ranter had said her husband brooked no disagreement on the smallest matters, that with each year, he became more demanding and rigid.)

Did you like your surgeon?

"No."

Did he talk much to you before the operation?

"I am an outspoken man. When I came to this medical center, I said I would like to see this surgeon who is operating on me. I never heard of him. I had never seen him. I had been sent here thousands of miles from home. I wanted to look in his face. When he came in, the first thing he did was to deliver a fifteen-minute tirade against physicians as patients: 'They are the worst patients,' he said. I said, 'Listen, if you would be in my place, you would be much worse.' He didn't know me. He didn't know if I would be a good patient or a bad patient. What's 'good' or 'bad'? How much you bother the doctor. I just asked to see him. When he delivered his monologue, I put him in his place, in a nice way, by telling him he wouldn't be as good as the doctor-patient I was. Then I told him, 'If you want to know whether I'm scared, yes, I'm scared. Only a fool would not be scared. Those heroes in war are as scared as anybody, but the job has to be done; so they do it. You think over the operation logically, but it does not take away your fears.' After that, he calmed down.

"As a matter of fact, he never sees patients postoperatively, but I insisted to see him before I left. One night, in the hospital, when I woke up with sweat and fibrillations, I wanted to see him; no doctor is on duty there at night. Only physicians' assistants. Better than nurses: yes. Not so good as doctors—or as doctors with physicians' assistants helping them. That's a shortcoming. Those surgeons make enough money to hire a resident physician to be on duty twenty-four hours a day. I told him so. But he didn't come until the following day. He never came while I was fibrillating."

There are no resident physicians on duty at night?

"No resident physicians. Just physicians' assistants, well trained, but not doctors—not enough protection for seriously ill patients. This is what I criticized about the institution—and I still do. The next day, the surgeon came, he sat down, he took my hand, which I withdrew. If anything would be serious, he told me, he would be there. All that malarkey, he told me. I listened. I didn't feel like putting up an argument. What could I do? Not having a well-trained medical staff on twenty-four-hour duty is a great short-coming, a serious flaw in a setup."

Did Milena go to him or to another surgeon?

"She wouldn't go near him, she hated him. Yet for her, it was the same problem. Different doctor, different hospital, same setup: only physicians' assistants at night. Godfrey, my son-in-law, had Bypass at thirty-eight, at yet a third place, famous, where everybody tiptoes when the surgeon walks by, and still no house staff at night. The private institutions rely too heavily on physicians' assistants. That's my objection to all three places; it's a big objection. They say physicians' assistants are better-trained than house officers. With that kind of reasoning, why do we need doctors at all?"

How long was the tube in?

"About eighteen hours. It was terrible, terrible not to be able to talk."

Did they instruct you beforehand in any sign language?

"Nothing."

Breathing exercises?

"Nothing, nothing. They assumed I knew everything, which I did and did not. These seem like simple matters to them, but so many little things could make life easier for the patient. I objected tremendously because they did not have a sheet of paper and pencil for me to communicate. The worst thing is not to be able to communicate with the outside world. I took the nurse's forearm and scratched a word with one fingernail, so she would know what I wanted. With pencil and paper, I could have written, not been so cut off. They hover over you, they don't leave you for a minute by yourself, but you can't tell them what you want or need. You can't see a clock. I would have liked a clock. I wasn't going anywhere, but I wanted to know if time was passing, or if I was passing."

What was the worst aspect of convalescence for you?

"I don't know. What I expected, I got. I expected I would have problems to move fast or to go back into my usual routine. I was right. The time of the year was nice. It was May. In three months, I started to play golf, to go out."

How long did you stay out of work?

"About three months. I did not go to the hospital . . . I went to the office full-time. I drove myself. I don't like to wait for people."

How long did you wait to have intercourse?

"I don't recall, but soon, very soon. Milena is always lovely for me. She says I waited longer after my Bypass than after hers. The hospital said, 'Go ahead whenever you feel like it.' They didn't give instructions; I didn't need instructions. Milena says I rushed her, but I was careful with her. You have to modify your activities a little in the beginning. You can't do the chest any harm. Sex is better for the chest than driving a car."

Since Bypass, is your desire the same, more, less?

"I don't think this has to do with surgery. You are on certain drugs. Inderal, for instance, deters—deteriorates . . ." He laughs harshly. "I was on Inderal, but no more."

You're on no drugs now?

"Nothing. Only an aspirin a day, and to avoid possible arrhythmias, I'm on what's virtually a placebo, Lanoxin, 125 milligrams daily. Just because it is already a tradition: 'You are doing well with it, so leave it.' Lanoxin is a nice old drug. With all the fancy new ones, it has the fewest side effects. Of course, it doesn't always work."

After you and your wife had Bypass, your son-in-law also had Bypass?

"About eighteen months later. He just fooled himself by not admitting the problem. He was only thirty-eight; accidentally, he found out. We had the whole gang to our cabin in the Berkshires for a big birthday celebration. When your children are grown and live far away, you don't see them much. It was Milena's birthday; we paid everybody's way. What did somebody say? 'When your children are small and have birthdays, you buy them gifts to make them love you. When your children are big and you have a birthday, you buy them trips to see you, so you can tell yourself they love you.'

"Carrying some wood into the fireplace, Godfrey hit his head on the door, and had a severe headache. We drove him into the hospital. In that little place, they did a routine EKG, and would not let him out any more. He had a stress test; they did not see anybody with a worse stress test than his. It was hard for him. He thought Bypass was an old man's operation. He should be all right." Dr. Ranter raps the desk with his knuckles. "He has Janey and five children to take care of. The children are young yet. Janey never knew how to be a breadwinner. Doctors' daughters don't know how to support a family."

What was the worst part of the operation? Is there any way it could have been made easier?

"First of all, I had amnesia. All I remember is telling Milena, 'It's all my decision, this Bypass. You don't have anything to do with it. Whatever happens, you should not blame yourself.' That helped her, she said, because she was in favor of Bypass, too, but she worried if it was right. The next thing I knew, I woke up. I don't recall the preparation or anything. It's very common, this partial amnesia. I was all right afterwards. I have had patients who worried about the amnesia, who thought they'd had brain damage or a stroke. I tell them, 'It's okay. I'm the same tough guy I always was. It didn't weaken me; it's a blessing not to remember!' "

If you had to have it over again, if you had to have a second Bypass, would you have it here in Norfolk?

"I would not have a second one."

Why?

"Because it is too much to go through. No doubt about it. The first one, I would always go ahead. The second one is too much. I have seen patients who have Bypass a third and a fourth time. . . . Apparently, they think it's an appendectomy."

All of us have insecurities about certain things. What are yours?

"What do you mean, 'insecurities'?"

We are uneasy, we are unsure, about our lives and the directions in which we've gone, about the roads not taken.

"I have no regrets. In any field. I am now happy, uniformly happy with what's going on. How long it will go, who knows? Whether life will be shortened or not . . ." He clears his throat. "Right now, I have the impression, probably a foolishness, that by having had the surgery, I will have my normal end of life. I am definitely convinced that Bypass surgery, the revascularization of the heart, does prolong life. For how long, we don't know. You don't have to have statistics, but if you think logically, you have new circulation there. The coronary heart disease is not cured—far from it—and is not being treated—except for preventive measures. Bypass is a preventive measure. It will take another period of years to obstruct these vessels again. You cannot tell how long it takes. Each individual is different.

"My conception of heart disease, and you may assume I know it quite well as a physician and a patient, is you should not ignore minor symptoms. If, like Milena, you're fortunate enough to discover obstruction beginning or progressed, with only minimal symptoms, you should follow this lead. With Milena, it was optional. The main obstruction was in the left descending—85 percent. The only thing I told her was, 'Milena, if I would be you, I would go for it. But it is your decision.' This is tough. As a prophylactic measure, it's a tremendous operation, tremendously invasive, but I felt it was worthwhile. In my practice, anyone past thirty-five wanting to engage in vigorous exercise must first go through a stress test. A routine EKG is for the birds. Because the resting EKG was normal, there have been many deaths. First, the regular stress test, then, if necessary, a thallium stress test. Any question: do the angiogram."

Since Bypass, have you had an angiogram?

"I had the thallium stress test."

Every year?

"Once is enough. I don't have symptoms. I know, I know, I contradict myself. What doctor doesn't? The body is not a computer. My Milena had minimal symptoms, just a little something when she played tennis, nothing more. I would not suggest angiogram, but deep down here in my heart, I knew it would come to that. Her cardiologists are conservative, yet both opinion number one and opinion number two favored her having the Bypass. If it would have been my patient, she would have had the angiogram already, a half-year before, but I waited for them to make their decisions."

After Bypass, didn't your wife have to go back to the operating room? She told me she bled.

"Yes. From the destruction of the platelet cells. One out of four goes back from bleeding. You never can tell whether it's from oozing or if those sutures blew."

Which was tougher on you, the first part or the second part?

"Both. I was there like a hawk. They hated me. I said, 'It's my wife.' I said, 'I'm the physician. I'm the referring physician, and this is my wife. *You are not going to lose her.*' They had some ideas about waiting until she lost 260 cc. of blood. I said, 'Listen, losing 60 cc. was fine. Now it is up to 180 cc. I would not wait until 260 cc. Get it now, right away. . . .' They are reluctant to call a doctor. If they had a resident there, the nurses would not be so reluctant.

"Nurses are intimidated by doctors. They had orders to call him when it was 260 cc., not before. I said, 'You call him right now.' They had a tough time getting him, they couldn't get him by beeper. I said, '*Get him right now.*' I did not know that they did not have a resident staff.

"All over this country, the heart surgeons make fortunes. It's unbelievable. They get bad marks on how they treat their patients, yet they get millions of dollars. You know what they want? They want to get in and get out of the sternum—one, two, three—to make their millions of dollars. Bypass surgery should be reorganized and resupervised. The whole thing. No institution doing Bypass should by permitted to exist without resident surgeons there who know their business.

"They can afford to pay postresidency surgical fellows even $100,000 per year, but they don't want to part with a nickel. And the doctor should see you every day. My doctor had an associate who saw me every day. But Milena's doctor—nothing—nobody, just physicians' assistants. Milena told them, 'Afterwards, I want to see my doctor every day.' A couple of times, he came in the afternoon; but a couple of times is nothing. The guy has one case at seven in the morning, one in the afternoon, then comes an emergency, and pretty soon, he's not slept for twenty-four hours. I don't like a surgeon to operate on me when he has not slept for twenty-four hours. That's when slip-ups come. That's why I worried so about Milena being the second case. That's why I kept my nose in all the time.

"I said, 'If you do not have a resident, I will be the resident!' but they kept pushing me out."

Did you have any chest pain while she was in the operating room or in the hospital?

"No, but it was stressful. I slept very little. Aach! so stressful. Doctors should not be allowed to do more than one case a day. They make enough money with the one case. Then, they could do proper postoperative care."

Do you think that the fee for Bypass should be lowered?

"Sure. Medicare pays them if you're over sixty-five. But most Bypasses are on people under sixty-five. Whatever the insurance plan says, Blue Shield, Red Heart, Green Chance, surgeons and anesthesiologists should not be allowed to charge more than the insurance pays. Even that's too much. Bypass is not so hard for the surgeon. Here in this town, they are the worst. A bunch of— I think it's terrible. Surgery should be more regulated. All these FDA regulations for testing drugs, and what mechanisms for controlling surgery? Did you see the Bypass on TV? It was a performance, a beautiful performance. He could operate on me any time. I don't want to see his face, I just want him to do the anastomosis. He anastomoses quarter-inch vessels, big vessels, and *that's all he does.* Then, he walks away and the other fellow closes up. Someone else opens, and someone else closes. Pretty nice. Another team prepares the vein for the graft, which is very important."

You talked about genetics. Are you concerned about your children's heredity?

"Two of my children smoke. One daughter smokes dope! 'Only on weekends, Daddy,' she says. My son Howard is thirty-six; he's never had a stress test, except for his marriage." Dr. Ranter barks a dissonant laugh. "Tell me: do your children listen to you? They only know what they want, what they need, what did you do for me today? Only Janey, Godfrey's wife, my eldest, listens, and she's up to here with a hotshot husband who's had Bypass at thirty-eight, who's out to prove he's stronger than everybody else.

"When Milena was out from Bypass only six weeks, Howard's wife, that's the new wife, took very sick. She'd had cancer before he married her, had been told never to have children. After five years in remission, she had a baby. The cancer kicked up. Her mother 'wasn't up to taking the baby,' so Howard brought the baby to Milena. She loves that baby. She called her 'my therapy,' but nine weeks with a new infant is not easy, even when you're feeling 100 percent."

Dr. Ranter's sigh hisses through the summer air. "All right. You bothered me, you made me talk to you, then you have to take care of what goes in your book.

"You *must* write this in your book: as skillful as the assistant may be, he or she must have the surgeon's okay on what to do. If he or she has to get somebody to come in from home, valuable time is lost. If the patient goes into ventricular fibrillation, a doctor must be right there. By the time they come in, it could be too late. I don't care if they have only one or two well-qualified resident surgeons or fellows on six-hour or eight-hour shifts, but somebody, a well-trained surgeon, must be *there* for twenty-four hours. If I would not be there, it would have been another hour before Milena would go up for the second surgery to stop the bleeding. I asked the nurse to call him, and she said, 'I couldn't reach him. Now she's lost 260 cc. of blood, so they should try again to find him.' I blew my stack. People don't know what's going on. That's why I kept my nose in when my son-in-law was there. If not for me, he wouldn't have made it, a young man, thirty-eight years old, with five children. They have to pay attention, not be casual. They come to the lunch table in the hospital and they talk about how much they worry about their patients. Talk is cheap. You have to be there." Abruptly, he stands up, "Okay. Enough. Was I helpful to you?"

Very helpful. You're a reflective man who, besides himself, has had a wife and a son-in-law with coronary Bypasses.

Suddenly, he sits down, shakes a bony forefinger at me: "How old is your husband? Did he ever have a stress test? Did he have a thallium stress test?"

He doesn't have symptoms.

"You should make him go. If not for me, Milena would not have had Bypass. I don't know how grateful she is to me, but it was the right thing. Remember what I told you to write in your book—and send your husband for tests. You have no right to go running around asking people about Bypass unless you have a heart for what's happening at home. Have your husband's heart checked, *then* write books."

13. Pierre Borget M.D.
Internist
Age at Bypass: 51

Dr. Pierre Borget is a short, stocky man. His long white lab coat droops over his beige glen-plaid trousers. A paisley silk tie tries nobly to light his weary gray face, but his sagging jowls, his gauntly hollowed eyes (it's called periorbital pigmentation), his sparse sandy hair spiking over his long-lobed, creased ears, overwhelm the tie. Sagging into a side chair in his massive wood-paneled office at Overbrook Hospital in Fall River, Massachusetts, Dr. Borget's tired face and body contrast with his high-pitched voice exploding in passionate torrents as his hands flutter their birdlike counterpoint. He shrewdly examines me. "Before we go any further, don't you want some cold data about me?" The chief of Cardiac Rehab at Overbrook had twisted Dr. Borget's arm to come and talk to me; I had no information. Quickly, Dr. Borget fills in the blank spaces, carefully spelling his name.

"You'll never guess how old I am. I'm sixty," he says triumphantly. "When I was nineteen, I looked twelve. I used to be so thin and rangy. Now I've caved in."

Are you married?

"No." He pauses, looks down at his hands spread out on his starched white lab coat, adds in a low voice, "Never married."

You're an internist. What's your title here?

"I'm director of Medical Education for Overbrook Hospital. My full-time job since 1969. I had my coronary on Election Day, 1968. The day Richard M. Nixon first was elected president."

Am I to adduce any kind of political—

"No, no, no. I just mention it. You might think, 'Why is he so obsessed with this, that he remembers the day?' I never went to vote that day. Now wait!" he chortles. "I think I was going to vote for Mr. Nixon. With my background, I would have liked to have voted for someone of a more liberal stripe, but I found Mr. Humphrey difficult to support."

What's your family history? Anybody—

"You mean vis-à-vis coronary artery disease? Nobody. Just nobody. I come from people who are all very long-lived. I had an old grandmother whom I knew so well because I grew up with her. She was a widow when I was born. My mother was the youngest of eleven children. My grandmother lived with us all my life. She had been a diabetic as long as I knew her. That's the only positive quadrant of my family history. She died of a coronary at seventy-five, which is not significant in looking at a family tree."

Was she a juvenile diabetic?

"I can't tell you. It's funny, the important things we don't know about our families. She was insulin-dependent, but her diabetes began in her middle age, before I knew her. What the nature of the disease was, I don't know. I have no other siblings, except my two unmarried sisters. My father's family had no arterial history; yet when he died, he had a cerebral hemorrhage. I refused to believe that this man had vascular disease. We did a postmortem—I insisted—and holy Moses, he had an occult carcinoma of the lung with metastases to the brain, into which he'd hemorrhaged. And his *arteries* . . . If I could have just put his arteries in a bottle! They were magnificent! He had the arteries of a boy, which had always been my . . . contention."

How old were your parents when they died?

"My mother's still alive at eighty-three. My father died at seventy-four. He'd had an accident and was quadriplegic. For ten years, we took care of him at home. His death had nothing to do with his accident. Our family's had a lot of illness in the last twenty years, which kind of absorbed all our energies. We have Mom at the end stage of senile depression. She took care of Pa for ten years in the most *incredible* way. When he died, all she had left was this great big vacuum."

Does she live with you?

"We live in her house, my two sisters and I. *We live with her, okay?*" [Other adult caretakers of elderly parents emphasize whose house it is.]

How did you come to Bypass?

Dr. Borget's voice rushes in torrents of recollection. "You asked about family risk factors. I was always a slim, trim normotensive[1] young man, who worked and worked—and worked some more. I was Dr. Friedman's Type A model to a T. In medicine, I was a Primary Care-ist. I went into medicine because I liked people. That challenge never diminished. I would put all my emotionally disturbed patients in at the end of the day. They'd come in; they'd want to talk. In the ordinary run of the office day, they couldn't talk as long as they wanted. I didn't have time. I'd have them come back at night. As often as not, four or five nights a week, I'd be in my office until midnight, just letting them ventilate and helping them as best I could.

"I'm from this area, I've always lived around here, I've always

[1] Having normal blood pressure.

known all these people, what they've gone through. I've been to their christenings and their wakes. We all had to go in service. We had nine months to train after medical school; I knew I didn't have time to become an internist. My rotating internship[2] prepared me me for my mental image of myself, the fantasizing of a young doctor, a healer on the front lines. The Army made me a psychiatrist!

"After the Army, I went into practice. By 1960, with this busy practice, I became volunteer director of Education at Overbrook Hospital. In those days, it was a small institution, nothing like it is now, more like a cottage industry. What an exciting time! Our group in internal medicine was interested in establishing rigorous programs. We'd always been a teaching hospital, but when I interned here, there were just interns, no residents. When I came back from the war, the young guys had put residencies in place. The sixties, in community hospitals like this one, were the time to connect with universities; we did academic things that were *thrilling*. I was part of that movement. I loved it, but I was doing two jobs. In terms of stress, what I demanded of myself in days, weeks, months, *hours*, was crazy—but I loved it. I was always thin, I was active, I never did much physical stuff, no tennis, no competitive sports, I never had the time. I was always on call. But about 1967, I began noticing that when I would make rounds in the hospital, I was getting tired in ways that I never measured exactly. Not until I had my coronary and had nothing to do but lie in bed did I realize my fatigue wasn't normal."

You were only in your forties then?

"I was born in 1924. This was '66 or '67, when I noticed that, although the hospital was not getting bigger, in walking the hospital corridors, carrying my bag to my car in the hospital garage, I'd feel heartburn." He stops, narrows his eyes, as if to measure the shock effect. "Something else. I smoked."

---

[2] Post–medical school training in several specialties—surgery, internal medicine, obstetrics, pediatrics—as opposed to a "straight" internship, which focuses on a single specialty.

How much did you smoke?

"Two packs a day. I never smoked until I went to medical school. When I went there—I'd never been away from home before—they had a beautiful new library. In front of each chair was a shiny, new pewter ashtray. You looked down the row; all the little girls and little boys were smoking. If you didn't smoke, you were a freak. As an intern, I was paid fifteen dollars a month. Cigarette money, they called it, so I used it for cigarettes. It wasn't good for much else."

You smoked two packs a day from medical school until—

"Not two packs. A pack a day. I'd bum another pack. Until? Until the day I was brought into the hospital with my coronary. I was remarkably good at getting patients to quit smoking. They'd look at me and say, 'Dr. Borget, when are *you* going to quit?' I'd say, 'The day I have the time to apply my mind to it.' If they came into the hospital for a gallbladder operation or even a hernia, they couldn't smoke. When they left, I'd say, 'Hey, you've done it! Now don't start in again! I brainwashed myself into saying, 'If ever I have my gallbladder out, when I leave the hospital, I won't be smoking. But I've got time. Look at the good family history I've got.' Funny, I was revolted by the habit. My chest felt raw, just awful. My mouth tasted rotten in the morning. Okay, heartburn.

"I've had osteoarthritis of the hands since my forties. When I wrote a prescription, my hands would hurt. By taking a couple of aspirin, I'd get relief. In four to six hours, my hands would get stiff again; I'd take a couple more aspirin. Long before my coronary, I was eating aspirin like popcorn. I also carried antacid tablets in my pocket; if I'd just taken a couple of aspirin, my gut might feel irritated. My pockets looked like the corner drugstore."

Come to your coronary.

"I'd have this heartburn; I'd take antacid for the heartburn. Then, one day, the great American doctor made the brilliant association that the minute he got to his car and rested, the heartburn went away. The antacid didn't put it away, resting did. I began to correlate cause and effect." He bangs his fist on the highly polished mahogany desk. *"Effort brought heartburn. Heartburn wasn't heartburn. Heartburn was angina.* Literally, my heart was burning away. I didn't tell anyone. My associate is a cardiologist, but he was tired, too. I didn't want to burden him. I did have him give me a complete physical. He found *nothing.* It's no wonder insurance companies won't permit doctor-prospects to be examined by doctors in their own offices. You don't see the forest for the trees. You're in great shape, quote, unquote."

You didn't tell him that you thought you had angina? Don't internists say that a good physical is 90 percent history and 10 percent examination?

"I didn't see any point in listing my symptoms. He didn't do a stress test. Remember, this was back in '65."

You didn't say, "I'd like to have a Master's Two-Step"?[3]

"No, nothing. Within months, this heartburn of mine became more and more, provoked by less and less. Finally, it came out of the closet and became pain."

Were you crescendoing?[4]

"Within a year, I was crescendoing like Beethoven's Ninth. So I knew where I was. It was April, I remember. In Freshman English, I read a poet who said, 'April is the cruelest month.' I always wanted to read more of him, but never had time. Now that I've got time, I can't concentrate. Anyway, it was April; Jim, my associate, was going to Europe. I wanted him to take that holiday.

[3] The ancestor of the contemporary computerized treadmill test was conceived by Dr. Arthur Master and consisted of two wooden stairs, of measured height and depth. Patients made prescribed numbers of trips up and down the stairs, with an EKG done before and after as a means of objectively assessing functional cardiac status. Some doctors still use the Two-Step in their offices.
[4] Sometimes called preinfarction angina, crescendo angina is characterized by persistent unrelieved pain lasting more than half an hour, not responding to nitroglycerin, and accompanied by EKG changes. Frequently, such patients are hospitalized in the hope of controlling their angina and avoiding an infarction.

"I said to myself, 'What the *hell* am I going to do? If I tell people I have angina, and my cardiogram is normal, my heart size is normal, my blood tests are fine, I look well, and I'm young, *young*, what will they think of me? It's going to get everybody in a tizzy.' I had to keep our practice together, I had to run the education program here, so I said, 'We've got to wait for the tiger to come out of the bush. There's no point in stalking a tiger you can't smoke out.' Know why?" Not answering his own question, Dr. Borget rushes on: "I wasn't terrified. What was there to be terrified about? I kept it to myself. In fact, I signed up to go to Warsaw for an international medical meeting in September of that year. Now, remember, I was to have my coronary on Election Day. When I saw myself in Dubrovnik and such places with their paltry little hospitals, I thought, 'You are such a damn fool! Suppose anything happened.' Till the day I got on the plane, going was a Las Vegas flip of the coin. But I went.

"On that trip, I felt angina more and more. Incidentally, I never did get to Warsaw or Prague, which was the reason I took the trip. I had some residents who came from Prague and had to go back. Communists, but delightful young men, and I was dying to see them again. At the rate I was going, I was dying to see them. The Russians marched into Czechoslovakia. Like the Russians, the coronary was marching on, the arteries were shrinking up." He claps his hands in rhythm to the Coronary's March. "I was threatening to have a major coronary. I didn't tell anyone."

Why wouldn't you tell anybody?

"Well . . . *denial*, you know. I knew I would have a coronary. *I* knew I was a setup. I've forgotten some details. My father was crippled and downstairs. My mother was exhausted taking care of him. I was the third member of that little trio. My sister Violet was doing graduate work at Rutgers. My other sister has always had all she could do to take care of her own problems. Well, *why should I have told anybody? Tell me, why should I? What* should I have done? Gone to bed and rested? You know, we didn't Bypass then, darling. Remember, our *attitude* toward this disease, this heart disease, had been *total*. There was *nothing* you could do. You could lie there, that's it. Everybody would have wrung his hands over me, sent me flowers which I loathed, and fruit which I couldn't eat. It made abundant sense to me to keep quiet about it.

"Finally, one night, I remember, I went to an executive meeting which went on until *midnight*. At three o'clock in the morning— good morning!—there it was, the pain, full-blown, incredibly painful. That was all right. It was about time. I called my associate to come see me. Suddenly, I realized he couldn't get into the house. I didn't want to wake my mother and father. I crept down, opened the door, and crept back up, but I couldn't lie down. I was in such pain. I was better if I moved around until he came. Then, boom, boom, chop, chop, into the hospital, and that was it."

That was in 1968? Fifteen years ago. Then what? How did you come to Bypass?

"Then I rested. What else could I do? Oh, there's a bloody, psychologically relevant part of the story that follows. This is '68. Bypass is '74."

We should talk about Bypass.

"I never really blew. I never had a big coronary then; I kept threatening to. I had T-wave changes, but I never lost much heart muscle. Fortunately. Because I remained Bypass-eligible. But I kept having all this pain over and over again. They put me into CCU, out of CCU, until all I could think was 'God! Why doesn't this heart attack just happen?' In despair, I went home. My angina, then, was in spades. It was very limiting. But remember, darling, in '68 and '69, surgery wasn't even an option. Oh, it was beginning to be done in some places, but the Ivy League places sneered loudly at Bypass; they acted as though it was one more gimmick.

"Every year, I'd go to a medical-education meeting in Chicago in February. The surgeons go to Hawaii for their winter meetings. Only the internists can figure out Chicago in the winter. With thirty-nine inches of snow, the wind would whip around the corner. That November, I thought, 'By February, I'll be up to going to the annual meeting; it'll be my stress test. If I can't swing Chicago comfortably, then I won't be able to practice.' That decision just made itself. Obviously, I wasn't going to be able to lead the life I'd carved out for myself. I knew myself well enough to know that I could *never* practice, given my own nature, except the way I like to, the way my patients expected me to. I could never practice by leaving the door only *that* far open. If I had to leave it *that* far open, it would be over, it had to be over.

"So I went to Chicago, and I'll never forget it. We were in the Palmer House. Have you ever been to the Palmer House? Lines for everything. You can't get the switchboard because it's overburdened with calls. This meeting went on for three days; you never got out of the Palmer House. There was too damned much snow and winter outside. I couldn't walk without getting angina. I couldn't go to Brentano's across the street without angina. I sat down in my room, right in the Palmer House, and on Palmer House stationery, I wrote my patients a letter and said, 'I'm awfully sorry this happened to me. I can't practice medicine any more. I can't be your doctor any more. I can be your friend, but that's it.' It was the hardest letter I ever wrote.

"I came back from Chicago, and my associate, I think, was prepared for my leave-taking. He already had lined up somebody else. Funny, how easily we are replaced, we the irreplaceable.

"Fortunately, my volunteer job had grown enormously. They'd been pressing me to do it full-time, irrespective of my health. If I hadn't said yes to them, they'd have hired someone else. I just slid over into this nice, cushy job, with this big fancy office, much nicer than my private-practice office, where I sit behind a desk and talk on the phone. But I had such angina, I couldn't talk on the phone. If I hadn't had Bypass, I could no more have given you an interview, have sat and talked like this. I'd have had to stop every little while and say, 'Nancy, do you mind if I come back in fifteen minutes?' I had angina that woke me from sleep. I had angina postprandially.[5] I was very limited. And I missed my patients so." His face is wistful. "I miss them now. Even now."

Didn't you read about Bypass in those days? Didn't you think of seeking out an opinion about—

"In '68 and '69, Nancy, it wasn't an option. In '70, I went looking. I went to New York. With Violet ensconced in her new career, it was easy not to upset the old folks: I was just going to visit my

[5] After eating.

sister Violet. I checked into the hospital. I won't go into the gory details of the most miserable medical experience. It was *dreadful*."

Why was it so bad? Why was it any worse than any hospitalization?

"In every way. The way they handled me psychologically was not to be believed. They admitted me on the service of a very famous cardiologist who shall be nameless and whom I ended up never seeing. He was off giving lectures, adding luster to his fame."

Just because you belong to the doctors' guild, he doesn't have to be nameless.

"Well, I would rather not say. I was in the hands of the house staff, not even house staff, but medical students. They kept me busy. Occupational therapy. I went in on a Sunday for a GI series, which I didn't need, then a gallbladder x-ray. They had to do something, so they did the angiogram, performed dreadfully by these two kids who got lost in a maze of arteries. I got a clot which they had to flush out. Just a nightmare.

"Come Friday, no one had talked to me, no one had told me what he or anyone else had found. Suddenly, it occurred to me at four o'clock on Friday afternoon, that if I didn't speak up, these sons of guns were going to keep me till Monday. I guess they were waiting for Dr. XYZ to come back from wherever he was wowing them. I said, 'Hey, I'm leaving—if necessary against advice—if you don't give me information. I insist upon seeing a physician, *a real live doctor*.' They sent me a surgeon. I'll never forget the crudeness of this man. He came in and said, 'You must know you've got dreadful disease.' Apparently, I had congenitally small arteries. Practically no right coronary. I'd been going all my life on my left, which was diseased all over the place. He said, 'You should know there's nothing we can do. You probably knew before you came here. Some people are fooling around with Bypass surgery, but we've been through all that. We've gone through the Beck procedure[6] and

---

[6] Claude S. Beck, a Cleveland surgeon, was a CABS pioneer who wrote a paper, in 1935, on "The Development of a New Blood Supply to the Heart by Operation." In 1951 Dr. Beck first recommended prophylactic Bypass in asymptomatic but susceptible patients to prevent progression of heart disease and to prolong life.

the Vineberg operation.[7] It's all a crock of crap. Don't let anybody put you on.' He was so insensitive. He never sat down. He delivered this ultimatum with his hand on the doorknob: 'At this institution, we have nothing to do with arterial surgery. You had better go home and take it easy. You know what the prognosis is. I don't have to tell you.' I just looked at him; I didn't know what to say to the man. He turned on his heel, and walked out without another word. To this day, I get an annual request for funds from their development office."

And your Bypass?

"Okay, that was '70. My Bypass was '74. I went home. I sat under my rock; I was pretty depressed. I lived with it, but there was no living—even though, Nancy, I worked. I came to this office every day and I worked. Working saved my sanity. Just don't tell me about the *Protestant* work ethic. We first-generation French-Americans outwork those laid-back WASPs every time! Even with plugged-up hearts. But I kept waiting for something to happen. Finally, I went to an American College of Physicians meeting in New York, one of those deals at the Hilton and the Americana. You walked a block between the two hotels for different sessions, but *I* couldn't walk that block. I couldn't even walk across the lobby of the Hilton without getting belted by pain. I made it up to the room. I had taken so much nitro that my head was blowing off. I fell into a chair and said, 'Borget, what in *hell* are you doing at these meetings? Get thee home.'

"At this point Cleveland* was being heard. Even here, our cardiocath team was catheterizing people, and even doing some Bypass, although not enough, not as they are today. I said, 'Let's get this show on the road.' Nobody was winning, me least of all. I was prepared to die, Nancy. This is crucial to my attitude towards what was an amazingly successful Bypass. I'm a triumph!"

[7] A. M. Vineberg, a Canadian, in 1950 pioneered the techniques of implanting an internal mammary artery into the myocardium, by making a tunnel through the myocardium. Vineberg's operation solidified the concept and technique of arterial anastomosis (joining) to the heart.
* The Cleveland Clinic.

That's wonderful!

"I had my ninth post-Bypass anniversary last Sunday."

That's great.

Dr. Borget turns his face away, replying weakly, unconvinced, "It's all right.

"Anyway"—he shifts gears—"I came home from those meetings in New York. I called my associate and said, 'Let's get this done.' Our cath team here checked me in that afternoon. I was done the next morning. The New York angio was terrible. With that information, they could never have operated on me. Our cath showed that I had diffuse coronary atherosclerosis, but surprisingly good muscle. By all criteria, then and now, I was a good candidate. I lay there wondering, 'What now? Where do I go?'

"Into my room waltzed a little gentleman, smaller than you, Nancy, a nephrologist here, who, if I am a Type-A Friedman personality, Doug is a triple A-plus. At the ripe old age of thirty-four, in the midst of a massive coronary, he'd had his Bypass done at Houston. He said, 'Spike, I'm here to help you. There's no place for you to go except Houston. I know the surgeon personally. He's fantastic. I'm calling him right now and telling him to book you.' I said, 'Bless you, Doug. I'm putting myself in your hands.' It fit fine. I wanted to get away from the local scene. I went to Houston."

Who operated on you?

"A resident. Just a resident from Thailand. A young man you got assigned to by the luck of the draw. They did fifteen our morning. I was tucked in, you see. Everybody waited on a waiting list, which was almost a year. Because of the urgency, they slipped me in. They put me on hold, and I waited in the hospital for an opening. That was the *only* difficult part of the experience: waiting and not knowing when it would be done. The waiting was worse than the operation, worse than the postoperative period, which was a piece of cake."

How long did you wait?

"Four days."

Not bad, compared with some people's months of sitting around.[8]

"Not bad at all—in retrospect. You'd go at five o'clock and to-morrow's schedule would be posted; you'd check the list for your name. When my name finally appeared, the little nurses came in and said, 'Oh, you're so lucky to get Dr. S——. He has golden hands, better than all those famous names.' Who did it didn't bother me, just so long as we got past it. The quality of life was so bad that I would have welcomed being relieved of it by the Lord. I thought, 'Wow! They can do something. Finally, if I'm relieved, great. If I'm carried away by the Lord, what better setting could there be? It would be easy, no trouble to my folks or to my sisters.' That's the corner I was painted into.

"Once your name was on the schedule, their method was excellent psychologically. They took all of us identified as Tomorrow's Bypassers; they put us all together. We got to know one another. It was an interesting group-psychodynamics exercise. I was the only physician in this group of fifteen. In a strange way, I became known to the group as 'Doc.' I was the company doc. Afterwards, when anything happened postoperatively, because you got very little medical attention once you left the ICU, the group called me. Preoperative preparation and immediation postop ICU care was tremendous. After that, they sent you back to your room, and you were pretty much on your own. The nurses were busy. If any of the guys had something wrong, I'd go see him. Every day, I'd make rounds on each of my group. I'd push my I.V. bottles down the hall on my house calls, and check everybody. It helped me, to be practicing my craft again. For the first time in a long time, I felt like a real live doctor.

"I didn't have a venous Bypass. I had an internal mammary. At the time, I wondered, but now they tell me that the internal mammaries retain their patency much longer than the venous Bypass grafts. A lot of surgeons don't like to stitch internal mammaries. They're tedious, more technically arduous. I look back and say, 'I was in such lousy shape. Why did I do so well?' Some of our group

---

[8] Some hospitals require patients to remain in the hospital while they are waiting to get on the Bypass schedule. Sometimes, patients wait six or eight weeks in hospital, with Blue Cross footing the bill, until they are ready to climb the walls while after surgery, ironically, hospitals rush to discharge patients six to twelve days postoperatively to "free" the beds for "adequate utilization."

had problems. Some had repeat Bypasses. But I, I did remarkably well postoperatively.

"The night before the operation, this little priest came to see me—I'm Catholic—to give me the Sacrament of the Sick. He was so terrified. I felt like putting him in bed, taking his collar, and making his rounds. He was just a kid. So young—was I ever so young? I said, 'Father, I've had such a terrible few years. For me to feel that something can be done is exciting. I'm not frightened, I'm exhilarated. I'm prepared to meet my Maker, if that's the way it goes. Don't worry about me. See the other guy.' I felt accepting of death. I had worked to prepare myself. They'd told me straight out that my chances weren't good. There was none of this old-fashioned reassurance. They said, 'You've got terrible disease. We promise you nothing. Your left anterior descending is so bad that we don't know if there's anything to graft a vein onto.'

"In '74, with my angios, they weren't going to make me feel, 'Wow! this is easy, and I'll be relieved of angina.' And in fact, I wasn't. I was to find that I did have angina, but I became progressively better. Seventy-five was better than '74. Seventy-eight was much better than '76 in terms of what I could do without chest pain. The worst angina I ever had was immediately postop. Probably I overdid, but I know, consciously or unconsciously, I was pushing myself to see how far I could go."

Delighted, he laughs and claps his hands. "My *bête noire* always has been airports:[9] walking to Gate 22, carrying a bag. I could never do it. I'd always have to get a porter, take a pill, while everybody else was striding along, getting where he was going. Now I can walk to Gate 22 and carry my bag. I feel kind of breathless, a kind of giving out in my legs, the equivalent of nature telling me, '*Slow down, that's too much.*' Except for that, I've done extremely well.

"I was to wake up from surgery in this incredible Intensive Care Unit, almost like the Kennedy Center. The cardiac wing was brand-new, so their ICU was brand-new. Half of us, about eight of my new pals whom I'd met the day before, were lying in our beds. I awakened to see them all." Dr. Borget shifts in his seat and laughs

[9] Dr. Meyer Friedman is convinced that airports are the Bypassers' number-one threat. Dr. Friedman maintains that "once the Bypasser can cope with an airport, he has demonstrated proof positive that his Type A qualities are in control."

shrilly. "I felt all things. I felt pain. I could see the nurses hovering over me, I could hear them saying, 'Dr. Borget, Dr. Borget, blow into the machine.' But I had just come back from something that, never in my life, have I experienced before—or, sad to say, since. I had returned from a sense of well-being so extraordinary that I can only call it, if I had to choose one word, 'ecstasy.'

"I'd had surgery before. I've had it since, where I've felt comfortable and lazy, drowsy, and distanced from pain. What happened during Bypass was different; it was a plain and easy out-of-body experience. If I were to analyze it in Freudian terms, I might tell myself, 'Gee, maybe you were so hyper, you had worked your way up almost to the Hyperion. Or the end point.' Maybe. I've always been a psychoenergetic personality. I was always high. In practice, I would always try, Nancy, if you came into my office today as a patient, to make you"—Dr. Borget strikes the desk in four/four time to his words—"feel better. I'd say, 'Nancy, come on, snap out of it! Don't waste these hours feeling low! You're never going to be twenty-nine again!' "

Watch it!

Laughing, he goes on. "You know what I mean. I was always one of those. Maybe I hyped myself up, and maybe my brain, during this heart-lung machine trip, was storing or releasing or secreting biochemicals that— Oh, I don't know, but I had been somewhere, that much I know. It was as though I had been to a place, a place I knew, yet there were no familiar scenes and signposts. I couldn't identify anyone human, but there were people and towns, big long tunnels like something out of the movies, another world, another sphere somewhere. All I thought was, 'Wow!' As if by chance, I had verged beyond life. It was the most spiritual experience of my life."

You felt like this, coming to in the ICU?

"For an instant—an eternity—the joy! I felt, 'I want to go back there. Oh, shit, here's the ICU! Oh, my God! Now I have to get on with it. Oh, Dr. Borget, gung ho, chop, chop! Reach down, pick up those bootstraps. Pick them up, hear me? Pick them up, put them over your shoulder.' I kept saying, 'Oh, gee. Hey. Let me go. Just for five minutes, to . . . to test and see if there could have been this ecstasy.' I shall never forget it.

"If you had a choice, maybe if you just let go, maybe if you let your blood pressure go down, you'd be able to go back there. What you came here for is to make it, to wake up, to be in the ICU, to do all the things these *marvelous* people told you would make you well; then you could go home. But that— Never, ever, had I known anything like that.

"Needless to say," he adds flatly, "they didn't let me go back. I proceeded to get up and come home in an uncomplicated way."

He stops. For a second, he's run out of steam.

Have you ever done any transcendental meditation?

"No." He frowns at the interruption. "Anyway, I came home and did very well. If anything, I was a little hyper: 'Wow! I can move, I can do things!' My friends couldn't believe my recovery. But then I was to develop a fever, joint pain, kind of a Dressler's syndrome. I had pericarditis, and I thought, 'Gee! All *that* for *this?*' My nice high went crashing into the basement. For a month, I felt terrible. I took aspirin and I crept back under my rock, which was right there where I'd left it, at home, waiting for me. I felt tired and weak. I ached all over. And, as I told you, I had angina."

Were you readmitted to the hospital for the Dressler's?

"No, no. I'd had enough of hospitals. I don't like people here to see me sick. I stayed home in bed. My fever was about 101; I felt rotten. My associate came twice a day and checked me. We're very close. There wasn't much to do except ride it out. They weren't worried, and I, I got so fed up."

Were you on cortisone or Indocin?

"No, they do that now. We talked about it, but I elected not to. I thought it would go away, that it's self-limiting, and it did, and it was. With all that, I had the Bypass in May; by July first, I greeted my new house staff but I felt not so hot. Through July, I came in half-days. By September, I was back full tilt."

He sighs deeply. "I looked as though I'd been through the

wringer, and my friends worried about me. My color wasn't good. If I did too much, I got into trouble. While I was released from that awful grip of angina, I still had that postoperative angina; I felt pretty punk. I stayed on Inderal, my lifesaver since that miserable first angio. I can't get off Inderal. I think one gets addicted to it. Without Inderal, my pulse rate goes up; I feel uncomfortable. That's wrong. Strike that. 'Uncomfortable' is a doctor's word for somebody else's pain. I wish I could call back all the times I described a patient's pain as 'discomfort.' Without Inderal, I feel dreadful.

"I can't drink. I miss being able to take a drink with my friends when I go out. Alcohol affects my pulse rate, I get a sinus tachycardia, but Inderal quiets it down. If you want a balance sheet, I have improved dramatically, because I have developed collateral circulation around the areas of Bypass where previously I'd been ischemic. This collateral circulation perfuses my myocardium better than it did when Bypass initially was performed. I became better after Bypass. With each passing year, I've become increasingly better.

"Yet I will tell you this: I am so grateful. I haven't had a sick day. I haven't lost a day from work for nine years because of cardiac disability, but I will not let anyone do a second Bypass on me—ever."

Why?

"You know, people said, 'Wow! you were so lucky, you had it, you were a success, and it was done right!' But as I look at my life, and I have looked at it long and hard, I haven't been so impressed with what I did after 1974. It's all kind of crumbling and falling apart. As a personality, I so much loved being that gung-ho creature, always right up there and running with the kids, able to raise a crowd as I was able to do until 1967, that what I am now doesn't excite me very much. I'm not depressed about it. But it's a drag. I am a person who will not age gracefully. I will look at it and say, 'Oh, crap! Isn't this dreadful! Am I, Spike Borget, Dr. Borget, actually *this dreadful?*' Every morning when I shave, I will look in the mirror and see Dorian Gray after the picture was stabbed."

Isn't that better than the alternative?

"*Death?* Death to me is those two hours when I was coming to, those two hours which were the most *magnificent* moments of my life. At my most magnificent, when I was twenty-nine and first went into practice and thought I could cure *everybody*, not even then was I so magnificent as in the ICU. Are you ever a better doctor than the first year you are out of your residency? You think you know it all. Sometimes you let everybody else know you think that. You begin to have a practice. People can *depend* on you. Since Bypass, no matter what it's done for me, and it's done a lot, my life's never been *majestic* like those first years in practice—and that's what I like.

"Now I don't say I wish I were dead or I wish I hadn't had my operation. Don't get me wrong. But there's an ambivalence in me about my Bypass. Before I went to Houston, I talked to my associate, who is very close to me: 'Jim, I know I'm putting you in an impossible situation; I know you can't answer my questions, but I don't want to have a Bypass if I'm going to be left disabled. If something goes wrong, if the Bypass occludes, if I go into heart failure, if I stroke, then I'll be furious, just furious that I made the decision to leave my rock and go to Houston.'

"What could he say? I knew that. We talked for hours into the night, about everything, about the fallacy of informed consent. After all, *what are you consenting to?* You don't know. Nobody knows. We went through everything that could go wrong, through the way my life was then, what I could look forward to, if that's a properly chosen expression. Finally, I threw up my hands and said, 'Well, I'll give myself to them. Let's hope for the best.' Because I had been so limited, because of what they saw in my angiogram, which I didn't know, they were terribly concerned.

"Suddenly, I was in the patient's position. You don't know the whole story. They don't tell you everything, even when they pretend to. And that's wrong. Nobody has the right to withhold information from you, to play Little Tin God, to play 'Father Knows Best.' "

How do you like being a patient?

"I don't think it's so hard. The nurses were terrific. The service I got was great." Slowly, he adds, "If the doctors didn't see me, I understood why. I knew they were busy, too busy for me." Unexpectedly, his voice rises in white-hot rage: "I don't like being limited. I don't like being disabled. I don't like being sick. 'Disability' means 'no ability,' 'not being able.' I hate that. This American, maybe universal, impulse to extend breathing ridiculously beyond any meaning is immoral. Once, yes, for me; not again."

You say you wouldn't have Bypass again. Nothing, as you just reminded me, is going to make you twenty-nine again. You're sixty years old, and you don't like it.

"Well, I haven't any reason to like it. Have you got any reasons for me? I haven't any reason to dislike it either. If sixty-five were taken from me, I wouldn't be outraged or despondent. In my personal life, no one is dependent on me. Having said that, I know I have this old mother and, thank God—in a way—that I had these ten years. I saw her through this awful period where now, at last, she's at the end of the line. I wish the Lord would gather her."

Don't you have some close friends? What about your associates?

Slowly, softly, hesitantly, he says. "A few. Just a few. Actually"— his voice becomes louder—"I have thousands of friends."

No, that's acquaintances. I mean friends, real friends.

"Not any who are dependent on me. Define 'friend' for me. We use that loosely these days."

They care about you, their lives would be sorely diminished if you were gone. I can see where people would feel like that about you."

"No, nobody. Nobody. I have some old patients who still— With a practice like mine, they ceased to be my patients, but they remained my friends, as I promised I would be to them. My psychiatric practice goes on and on, more and more as patients don't get attention from their physicians. I've filled that function for them. *They* would be devastated. Yes, they would be devastated."

As the director of Medical Education in this hospital, don't you think you do good work? As a visitor from a foreign planet, I'm impressed.

"I have done good work. I have done. I am done, I guess. I would say, Nancy, that I wouldn't have missed these last ten years for the world, in terms of maturing, of looking at life. But if this is maturity, Nancy, the glass is upside down. I used to think, 'The glass is half-full, and with a little effort, we'll get it to the top.' No more. It's as though I turned and looked at life from a different perspective; now the glass is half-empty, and ebbing. It's kind of a cynical conclusion to a life, but it's the only one I know."

When do you think you changed? What changed you?

"In the interval since I stopped taking care of patients, maybe? Am I lost without that patient-dynamic? They say, 'Doc, do you miss your patients? Have you missed practice?' My answer is yes and no." He laughs ruefully. "I guess that's my answer to every-thing. Practice is done, it's over. I'm not going to look at it. There was nothing else to do.

"Hospital administration is a new challenge. But medical edu-cation is far less ego-gratifying than practice. Medical education in 1984 is worrisome. We live in a society which all around us is going downhill. We don't maintain standards. Our corruption is manifest everywhere. Perceiving corruption and idiocy, I wonder, 'Is this merely a function of getting older? Is it that, when I was younger, I only saw the Walt Disney parts of the world? Now that I'm older, it's all imperfect. Aren't both visions skewed?' Over and over, I've asked myself what it's all about.

"I'm part of the medical school. I've worked and worked for them, because that university did so much for me when I was young and didn't have the means. I can never work for them enough. It's brought me to young people. As an internist, the patients I liked best were the adolescents and the elderly. In between, the patients were kind of dull. Like me, maybe? What keeps me alive are the students, teaching, helping them with education loans.

"I keep asking, 'As alumni, how can we interface with the kids? How can we teach them not to forget how to communicate, not to get lost in the medical distance, not to lose themselves? Are they alienated because they have to learn so much, because their teach-ers are so busy trying to cram all this into them, so that the professors don't deal with them in a one-to-one, human way? Can't we, as people of the real world of medicine, stop this trend to dyscommunication?' By and large, with whatever satisfactions have come, it's been a bluish mood.

"My psychiatrist friends have put me and my experiences on the metaphoric couch. They laugh at me: 'Spike, so what else is new? This is where we all are. This is society. This is the world.' They must think me more immature now than I was before. It's interesting, I can't go to heart groups. Not any more. In the beginning, in '75, when the operation was new and people were terrified, I'd go up to see someone on the Cardiac Surgery floor in our hospital and say, 'You're not going to remember the pain. Yes, you'll have pain, but *you'll forget.*"

Do you remember the pain?

"*Oh, yes.* But the pain was worse when I got home and had this Dressler's. But in Houston, the pain was there, never fear. I'd give CABS patients a simple technique I'd used: lie there and repeat a litany: 'A week is only a moment in life. Other people felt like this a week ago.' Look out your door and see the guys who were operated on a week ago, and they're walking around, antsy to go home. Keep thinking, 'I'm going to take the eraser and erase my blackboard of pain today. The hell with today. I'm going to think of next Monday. Next Monday, I'm going to be walking around like those guys; this week will just be a moment flashed by. I won't pay any attention to today. I have pain. I'll tell the nurse, she'll give me a shot, and I'll go to sleep. And then, it will be Monday and I'll be walking.' Later, patients told me, 'Hey, I did what you said. It was next Monday and you were right!' I'd reply, 'Now, it's two years or five years since my surgery. I've had pain and discomfort, but wow! I'm functioning! I'm alive! I'm earning living! I'm paying Social Security! I'm going to the theatre, to the ballet!' "

What was the worst part of the operation?

"My cholecystectomy[1] was worse. To say it was hard is to exaggerate. I hated the endotracheal tube and not being able to talk, but I was so intrigued by what was happening to my new friends

---

[1] Surgical removal of the gallbladder.

that I didn't think about myself. Nancy, some of those guys smoked until midnight the night before, coughing their brains out. I was so tuned into them from the day before surgery that I knew whose lungs were acting up. I was so impressed with the nursing care. I knew how they were monitoring my potassium. I could see them overloading me with fluids to get my urinary output up. When I went back to the general hospital floor and went into a little pulmonary edema, I knew it was because they had put too much fluid into me and I didn't have to worry. My heart wasn't failing. It was just my fluid overload. As a doctor, it was easier. I could be much more objective about myself, if I wasn't personalizing."

What could doctors and patients do to make it easier?

"There are never single messages to give to everybody. We aren't unitary, we're all so different. What I was for thirty-five years before my surgery impacted on how I responded to Bypass. All my medical background is incorporated in what I am, so I can't pretend that I can tell a patient to be like me.

"At this hospital, we now have a social worker specializing in the needs of Bypassers. She works on a one-to-one basis; she has established groups"—he winces—"for people who like groups; she sees every Bypasser before and after surgery—and as many times as they want after they've gone home. She's extraordinarily dedicated, maybe because she's working off her own pains from a bad marriage and a rotten divorce. She's paid $20,000 per year, and the hospital is crabbing about her salary, even though Bypass alone keeps this hospital going. The hospital went out and bid for Dr. Ashberry, our cardiac surgeon, almost the way baseball teams bid for pitchers or football teams bid for tight ends.

"Anyway, if people who've had Bypass talk to prospective Bypassers and talk to them after the surgery, that's the best thing. When I could talk to Bypassers, I underplayed it. The skill of the surgeons is crucial. The nursing care and the availability of a residency staff is vital. Sure, it wasn't all fun and games. Sure, they don't all emerge like me, able to do everything except dance." His face darkens. "I wish I could dance, but I can't. I can't garden. I can't do much with my hands, yet I can do things with my legs."

Are your hands affected by your osteoarthritis?

"No, it's cardiac. It's work. They've proven in the laboratory physiologically that shoulder-girdle muscles undertake more cardiac work than just walking."

How long did you wait to drive a car?

"I drove immediately after I got home, but they hadn't told me anything different. Now they do, but it's nine years later."

Was your family still so dependent on you?

"Yes and no. The thing about this operation is that you feel better immediately. As soon as they have Bypassed you and have been successful, you're getting oxygenated blood to parts of your heart muscle which have been starving for oxygen for years. Even now, little changes in circulatory dynamics make the difference between a sense of well-being and ischemic symptoms in the heart muscle or even frank heart failure. In other words, the balance in nature isn't very great between the asymptomatic and the symptomatic. That's why you live for years with it and don't know. You make gradual accommodations, compromises without recognizing how much *you've* been compromised. The other side of the coin is not fearing every time you get a new ache or pain that the balance has been tipped."

How long did you wait to climb stairs?

"As soon as I went home. I was walking around the ward. At Houston, there is no anxiety about how much you do. After the ICU, you're on your own. My sister flew out to see me. I was fine. I made her leave after a day. Why hang around Houston? I remember walking her to the elevator and going down to the main entrance with her. I thought she was going to have a stroke when I did that!"

They let you walk her down?

"Oh, yes, they were very casual. In fact, on the general floor, I had an episode of heart failure. I came back and went to bed. I felt breathless when I lay down, so I cranked up my bed myself to be in the dyspneic[10] position. When I woke up dyspneic, I checked my pulse and it was clipping away at 180. I put my light on. For the longest time, nobody came. Eventually, this little nurse-clinician came in and said, 'Oh, Dr. Borget! You're just having a little left ventricular failure. They overloaded you deliberately; they give you lots of fluids. Everybody has a little ventricular failure. Don't worry about it. You doctors are all alike: all worriers.' I crawled under my sheet and said, 'I'm not going to let them hear from me again.' She said, 'I tell you what: I'll order a Lasix for you.' She gave me a Lasix, and, hey, I went to the john, and out it all came. My chest got clear. She was absolutely right."

No doctor came to see you?

"I didn't see a doctor. I was admitted to that hospital with only one name, a cardiologist's, and he had lost his only son the day before I went into the hospital. His twelve-year-old son walked up the stairs to his bedroom—and dropped dead. This guy was *zapped*. I thought, 'I will never see him.' He came in about the fourth or fifth day postoperatively, and he *apologized*. Can you imagine? He apologized. You looked at him and you knew something had been broken irreparably. Of all the ironies. To be a cardiologist and have your only son die of heart disease."

Since the operation, did you review your life and its course?

"Not much more than I would have under any circumstances. Sometimes, I think, 'How lucky, living and thinking when you live, and being part of a society changing so rapidly.' I always say, 'I wouldn't have missed it for the world.' But another part of me says, 'Until forty-three, you were a symbol of strength to a lot of people, to a community, to other physicians, and you're less than that now. If I were Arthur Miller and writing a play, wouldn't it have been better to end the play at forty-five? It would have made a better play, perhaps a better person.' As people keep closing in on me, this part of it is more sour, but I don't go round saying this.

"Since the operation, I went to Russia, and it was the most

[10] Dyspnea is difficult, labored breathing, shortness of breath.

horrendously dreadful experience. Again, I wouldn't have missed
it. I realized World War III had been going on for ten years, and I
never knew. The hostilities, the hatred, the structured zombiness
of a whole society, made me feel so hopeless. This is the only time
I have been anyplace where people never looked at me, where I
never established eye contact. Oh, I know, that's what people say
about doctors and eye contact, but this was different, or at least I
thought so. I wonder to myself, 'Is there something about you?
About your moods?' I'm a downer these days, and I was such a
upper!" Dr. Borget's bushy brows meet in a frown.

Is that since the operation?

"It seems so, and I don't know why."

*Did the hospital give you any instructions about when you could start
going out? Did they talk to you about how long you should wait to
have sexual intercourse?*

"Nothing. Nowadays, they're supposed to be better, but then, nothing."

Did you ask?

"No."

How long did you wait?

"A couple of months. If I hadn't had the Dressler's, I wouldn't have
waited so long. That's really much too long. Much too long."

Were you afraid the first time?

"No, because I had done a lot of things in my life." He stops, traces
patterns with his forefinger on his trouser leg.

Was your partner afraid?

"We didn't talk about it. Being a doctor and having yardsticks of
what I could do, I've never been afraid. Even in Yugoslavia, when

I had 'Class IX'[11] angina, I wasn't afraid. In Yugoslavia, I was embarrassed. I thought, 'You jackass! What are you doing here? Nobody knows you have angina.' "

What's wrong with getting sick?

"It *inconveniences* people. They're on a holiday. What in hell are *you* doing on a holiday when you know this could happen?"

You travel now and you're able to travel alone.

"For a long time after Bypass, I didn't. I found myself doing things, being functional, but sitting under the same rock which the first hospital told me to sit under till the Lord took me. It was the act, the aggressive act, of some friends with whom I'd traveled before I was ill, who said, 'Spike, get off your tail. You're just sitting. We're going to Egypt. Want to come?' I thought they were crazy, but finally, I went to Egypt. I toted that barge, I lugged that bale, I lifted that luggage, and they took care of me. They were monitoring me, but they didn't have to.

"Initially, I wouldn't go, but Theresa, God bless her soul, she's dead now, called me from New York. She'd been to Russia with us, and she said, 'Spike, I'm eighty years old, I'm hypertensive. I'm on digitalis. And I'm going. Why the hell can't you?' I said, 'Theresa, bless you. You've talked me into it.' And it was a marvelous trip."

What explicit questions would you advise a patient to ask his internist, his cardiologist, his surgeon, before and after Bypass?

"The only questions I could suggest are ones that any thinking, *communicating* family doctor, cardiologist, and surgeon would answer—without being asked: where you are in terms of your cardiac circulation, and more important, your myocardial function; what the quality of your life can be expected to be, within parameters. Nobody can give you an exact answer. Nobody knows for sure. If it's an honest place, they'll reject people who, they feel, won't have enough good-quality life to warrant the expense of money—and of

---

[11] Class IX angina is a doctor's way of describing his own severe angina, which is usually classified as I through IV.

spirit. If they have too much scar tissue on the myocardium, Bypass will change nothing. But some places are less scrupulous about whom they do.

"The other side of the coin is that the surgeons like to keep their statistics high; sometimes they reject people who might be good candidates. At our hospital here, they try to present the options to every patient; they inform him of both sides. But I'd be one of the patients who, being given a less-than-encouraging picture of what life might be, might decline, might say, 'Thank you just the same.' "

Supposing you were in that same bind as that awful period five years before Bypass, where you were not dead, but you were not vibrantly alive—

"My basic disease is not just coronary artery disease, but athero-sclerosis. It's progressive. Incidentally, I'm *terrible.* I don't exercise. I've gained weight. I haven't altered my eating pattern. I'm not a vegetarian. I use salt. I don't ride a bike or play tennis. I've never enjoyed it. Maybe I'm a good control. For going on ten years, I've lived, I've been comfortable, I've done more with each passing year, even though there's lots of things I can't do. What bothers me is—" He stops. "I'm not . . . I'm not as competent a person as I was ten years ago. When I tell my friends that, they say, 'Well, Spike, who is? You're describing me and I don't have coronary artery disease.' "

How can the operation, the hospital stay, the convalescence, even the present, be made better, easier, less traumatic?

"My Bypass was done very well. Here at this hospital, it's handled beautifully. Whatever could have been done better, we now do here, thanks to the special Bypass social workers and the organized pro-gram here. That kind of activity, its emphasis on communication when people are afraid to communicate, is most important. The cost-effectiveness argument is nonsense. My operation was cost-effective to society. It cost $10,000, and hell, how much Social Security and income tax have I paid since then? I've been a func-tioning heart of this medical-education world ever since. If I hadn't been able to go back to my job here, these nine years since Bypass would have been intolerable to me. People must be allowed to go back to their jobs. I couldn't practice internal medicine, but I like my job here.

"What distresses me, in young doctors, is nobody wants to work, nobody wants to be involved in responsibility for the needs of a society, so that the whole equation works better. As a role model, I'm irrelevant to these young doctors-in-training. Oh, I'm a great guy, they say, one of the most-unusual-people-they've-ever-met types, but no thanks. They want their thirty-hour week as doctors; what *I* want from them now is obsolete. I'm alienated.

"My generation gap is showing. They tell me they can't go to clinics and treat these old—what do they call them?—'dirt balls.' The indigent, the alcoholics, are 'dirt balls.' They're content to treat only the clean upper classes. If you have to take care of people and feel like that about them, you shouldn't have gone to medical school. It's a whole societal process. People can have a good time, a productive time, with the extra life Bypass gives them, *if they can do something worthwhile with that life.*

"In the end, there are no absolute answers. There are as many answers as there are people, which accounts for the complexity of your mission. I have had a brilliant Bypass result, and yet I would not go back for another one. My attitude has nothing to do with coronary artery disease or with the surgical approaches to coronary artery disease. It has to do with a life and a personality going through a process of vision and revision that he might have gone through anyway in evaluating what life is, what values are his."

Do you advise people to have Bypass?

"Absolutely. I tell them to ask themselves, 'How is my life? Am I able to do what I want to do? Am I functional? At the end of the day, do I feel, "I haven't climbed Everest, but it's all right. With all the pluses and minuses, it's been a good day?" ' Or is your day so limited that you think, 'God, I can't do anything. This isn't worth living.' I tell them: 'You'll come through it. Pretty soon, it will be a week from Monday, and it won't have been so bad.'

"With all my yes and no to life, it is not a bad experience. I'm glad I went through it, glad I had my Bypass."

14. Sister Cecilia O'Brien
Nun
Age at Bypass: 55

Sister Cecilia O'Brien has bright-blue eyes, short curly gray hair, and a wonderful smile. Dressed in a royal-blue cotton skirt and a white blouse, sitting on the edge of her chair, she often twists the ring on her third finger, left hand, which symbolizes her commitment as the "bride of Christ." She has come to talk, she says, "because if my experience helps only one other person, it's worth the time and energy."

How did you learn you had heart trouble?

"Five years ago, just after my fiftieth birthday, I began being tired all the time, always exhausted. I couldn't understand why—I took vitamins. After school let out, I went to the doctor, who sent me to a cardiologist. I ended up having a cardiac catheterization. It showed 25 percent blockage in one minor artery. That was it. The doctors said, 'It's a minor problem. Don't worry.'

"Then, last summer, I went on a long vacation. For me, three weeks is a long time away from responsibility. I visited all my nephews in Kansas and Texas. But I didn't want to do anything.

I was tired all the time. When I returned, I was more tired than when I went. In October, I started taking vitamins again. They seemed to help. By Christmas, I was waking up almost every night. No pain, only strange sensations in my head. I'd come home from school at night; I'd go upstairs to do some chores. I wouldn't know what I was doing or why I was there. My only living brother has Alzheimer's disease. I thought I was getting Alzheimer's. There's no proof it's not hereditary. In women, it comes in the middle fifties. I was sure I'd been doomed to Alzheimer's disease, but I was afraid to tell anyone. Even in confession, I never said a word. I kept awakening in the night with these strange sensations in my head. The Friday before Christmas, I gave in. I went to our nurse and said, 'I feel funny.' She took my pulse and ushered me home. The following Monday, I went to the doctor. After I told him my story, he opened my chart and said, 'Sister, this is exactly what you said five years ago. In the same words.' He sent me to the cardiologist for a stress test, which showed left bundle blockage. He gave me medicine; I took it religiously till March twenty-fourth. I felt absolutely horrid, but I didn't know what to do.

"On March twenty-fourth, as I was getting dressed for school, I got this terrible heaviness and tightness. No real pain. I felt as though a giant were choking me, with one hand crushing my wind-pipe and one hand pressing a rectangular area in the middle of my chest. My head felt so heavy, as though it would drop off my shoulders. I was very short of breath. I came downstairs and said to one of the sisters, 'This feels different. This is gonna cause trouble.' The doctor said, 'Stay in bed; call me back in the afternoon.' By the time I called him, left a message with his secretary—she wouldn't interrupt him—and he could get back to me, it was two-thirty. He said, 'Call the ambulance and go to the hospital.' I went. They catheterized me. I almost met the Lord on that one. I had no pulse, and my blood pressure dropped to fifty."

How long did that last?

"Long enough for the young interns to get there on a blue alert. I came out of it. I don't know why I survived, but I did. They said, 'It's still not enough blockage for surgery.' After two weeks, I was sent home. In ten days, I went from bad to worse. I couldn't function. I couldn't move to the table. I was bedridden. My internist

called the cardiologist and said, 'She can't go on like this.' Away
we went. Fast. In three days, I was admitted to the hospital again;
two days later, they did Bypass.

"The cardiologist was very kind. On Sunday, he spent an hour
explaining the operation to me and two of the sisters. I wanted
somebody else there. Not just me alone. I have no immediate family. Only nieces and nephews out of town. All my brothers and
sisters died of heart trouble, except for the one with Alzheimer's."
Sister Cecilia sighs. "So here I am. With the precipitous drop in
people taking vocations, I'm lucky to have three friends in the
community—really, two—who are super. They're my family."

*Even though you knew you had heart trouble for four years, you did
pretty well. In the year before Bypass, did your stresses mount?*

"Stress and strain could bring on these funny feelings, but my
trouble is hereditary. If they hadn't done the Bypass, I might have
had a stroke. Not enough blood was getting to my brain. That's
why I was functioning so poorly."

*Five years ago, when they didn't want to do Bypass, were you dis-
appointed?*

"I was relieved."

And this time?

"I was terribly disappointed. I never told anyone before. I kept
seeing myself go down, down, down, with no help. I'm a lively,
vibrant, action person. I couldn't live like a vegetable. There was
no future for me."

Did you get depressed?

"Inside, I was depressed, but I wouldn't show it. Nobody must ever
know what's churning inside. That's the way I am. Finally, I called
my internist and said, 'If I'm going to need Bypass in the long run,
let's do it. I can't go on like this.' I'd been home for ten days, trapped
between the bed and the chair. The bathroom was like a trip to
Europe. One way."

You said stresses accelerated before Bypass. What were they?

"I'm a special-education teacher, which means I should have a small number of children. My mouth doesn't know the word no. I kept taking more. They needed me. I was the only one who could help, so there I was. That was one stress. My sister died very unexpectedly. I'd been down in Florida with her. Because she seemed better, I came home. In two weeks, she was back in the hospital. They called me: 'She's dying. She's asking for you.' I called her doctor who kept saying, 'They're just panic-stricken. Don't worry.' The next night, she died. Alone. I had to go to Florida, bury her, put her house on the market, have everything packed up to come back. Besides"—her cheery, open face winces—"my anger at being abandoned, the last one of the family, left all alone. Six months later, my closest brother-in-law died of cancer. That Christmas, I was called about midnight. My sister-in-law, always my good friend, had been found dead of a heart attack. For almost thirty-six hours, she'd been lying there dead on the floor. Nobody knew. In two years, I buried four of them. In the four years before, I buried five of them. One thing piled on top of another. The anger of being a sole survivor assaulted me. I don't feel it now, but I did then. Being left alone is one of the prices paid by the youngest child. I had one brother who had Bypass. After his Bypass, he lived one month shy of five years." She frowns, "He smoked. He had emphysema. We couldn't get him to stop smoking. I never liked smoking. It's too smelly. Not smoking may be one reason for my rapid recovery."

What are the special stresses of being a nun?

"Did you ever see ten women living together? Communal living is fractious. Women are women. Some you like; some you don't care for; some you endure. Nuns or not, they're women."

What about the stresses of a church in transition?

"Oh, they talk about women and the church, fire in the thorn bush. I'm not a nun with any desire to become a priest. I'm one who's perfectly contented to be a Sister of St. Jude, with all it entails."

Do you ever regret not having children or a husband? Aren't there stresses in celibacy?

"For me, no. When you're young, when you're in the convent about ten years, you begin thinking, 'What's on the other side of the wall?' The turmoil is terrific. I've talked with priests and other sisters embroiled in that same drama: 'Oh, let me get out of here! I don't even know the person who got me in here. That woman is dead. Why must I live by her decisions from the Dark Ages of long ago?' Generally speaking, we all live through that terrible conflict. These days, I can honestly say it doesn't bother me. I don't know if I'm glad I went into the convent. But I'm no longer sorry."

Do you believe in God? Do you think He was in the operating room?

"I certainly do. When I was taken down to that operating room, I was positive I wasn't coming out. This sounds strange coming from a nun, but I'm afraid to die. I've always said I was afraid to die. Yet when I went into that blue alert on the catheterization, I was as calm as could be. When I went into that operating room for Bypass, I was calm. The night before, they gave me a sleeping pill. I wondered whether I should take it, how I should spend my last night. But I took the pill, and slept all night. I set a little alarm for four o'clock in the morning, because I knew they'd come for me at five. I thought about my life; I prayed. Only faith and prayer could have soothed my unquiet spirit. My nature is uptight, tense, and scared. Yet before my Bypass, I was peaceful. Let me add this: I went into that operating room at eight-thirty. They started the surgery about nine-thirty. At that very moment, our parish had a mass for me with six hundred children. One teacher said, 'You had to get better. Sixty-five first-graders believed it was their individual prayers alone making you well.' The children with whom I work argued with the other children about whose prayers brought me through. Only prayer could have made everything come along so perfectly. My faith and everybody else's faith was working overtime."

I asked a priest I interviewed if he believed in God. He said, "Yes. But I'd make sure I had a darn good surgeon."

"I had faith in my internist. We know each other well. I had to put my faith in his judgment. I knew he'd get me the best doctor available. He did."

Yet you said you were sure you wouldn't come out of the Bypass. Why?

"Almost everyone in my family has died in his fifties. Only my mother lived to ninety-one. I felt this was my time."

Between the Bypass decision and the Bypass, what could have helped you?

"Opening up the relationship between these sisters who are my close friends and me. If you live with people for ten years, you become part of one another. For better or worse. I could not or would not open up to them; I couldn't tell them how I felt. Nor would they face it with me. They were facing Bypass, but not openly with me. We didn't communicate our fears, even our hopes. When I'd start to talk about the Bypass, when I'd start to talk about dying, I could see them freeze up, pull back. The one prescription for prospective Bypassers is, 'Talk about it openly. Don't withdraw. Don't let other people withdraw from you.' I don't communicate well; perhaps they took their cue from me. My looks will convey my anger, but I don't say much about what's roiling deep inside. I acted as though Bypass was happening to someone else, someone out there someplace. I even talked a good game to myself. Until the morning of surgery, I didn't permit myself to recognize Bypass was happening to me. As for the sisters, to some I wouldn't have talked. To others, I wanted to spare their sensitivities. It's a mistake. If we'd talked about living and dying and Bypass, it would've been better for me and better for them. I knew the sympathies of my three close friends. I didn't know how all the other sisters were reacting. Maybe they wanted me out of the house. I went on with my big-hurrah smile and my everything-will-be-all-right big lies."

At a few Bypass centers, a psychiatric counselor is a member of the team. Would that have helped you?

"Probably not. To speak my mind, and my heart, I have to know somebody well. I'm this free with you because I want to help other Bypassers."

What about peer counselors? Having Bypassers talking to you?

"The hospital didn't have anybody. Two men from the parish talked to me. Nobody said anything about that deep depression which comes four or five days after Bypass. I got over it, but then I sank back. Despair is a cardinal sin. Father John, the Catholic chaplain, helped. In the hospital, the father of one of our teachers wrote me: 'I know what you're going through now. In a week or two, you'll feel like a million dollars. Don't let the blues get you down.' That card turned the tables. Afterwards, he came to see me. Surprisingly, I have so much in common with other Bypassers: yet they're male; I'm female. They're married; I'm a nun. Even now, after the fact, it helps to talk to each other. It helps me to aid and comfort people confronting Bypass. There's a bond between Bypass veterans."

After Bypass, did you review your life?

"To a degree. I was overwhelmed by the love and gratitude given me. One friend said, 'Never tell me again that you haven't any friends.' I don't cry easily, but I fill up"—Sister O'Brien wipes her eyes—"because it's so deep. Words are just words. They can't say what I feel." Blowing her nose, she apologizes, "I'm sorry."

Since Bypass, do you get misty-eyed more readily?

"Definitely. I'm not glad when tears overcome me. Still, they show other people that I can feel deeply."

Did Bypass make you more aware of your mortality?

"If Bypass doesn't, what will?" she retorts sharply. "Not just Bypass, but heart disease. Yet before the operation, when I was feeling terrible, I'd think, 'This can't be happening to me.' Afterwards,

Bypass *did* happen to me. It has happened. Before Bypass, I felt so awful. I knew I was suffering. I knew my name was O'Brien. You can't be an O'Brien and not have heart disease. But I pushed the awareness outside of me. These last few weeks since Bypass, I've let the knowledge seep into my bones."

Are you self-conscious about your scars?

"The scars don't bother me, but I'm aware of their impact on others in the house. They look, then look away. Sometimes, they flinch."

Since Bypass, have your personal relationships changed?

"My nieces and nephews are much closer. I come from a family with the slogan 'If I see you, fine. If I don't see you, no problem.' Now, suddenly, everybody calls. My nephew in San Antonio never called me in his life. Since Bypass, he's called three times. He's only forty-six, but he's got the O'Brien curse. He's had two minor heart attacks. The others know they're susceptible. Their father and their mother dropped dead. They've stopped smoking, they exercise, they watch their weight, they try not to react so hotly to minor provocations." She sighs. "I hope it works."

After you came home, were you depressed?

"Only a few times. When the physicians' assistant talked to us, I insisted two of the sisters be there. She told us, 'You'll get depressed. You'll want to take somebody's head off. You'll say anything. You'll cry. You'll hate yourself and cry some more. You won't know why.' About ten days after I got home, it hit me. I recognized the signs. I said to one of the sisters, 'Now I know what she meant.' Mary said, 'Yeah. We do, too.' Other people should be there to hear what will happen. You hear, but you're sick, you're worried. How much will you remember when you go home? Nobody had told me about the hospital depression. Father John came to see me on that lousy fifth day. I was cranky and crying. I said, 'John, what the h—— is the matter with me?' He said, 'It's the fifth postop day. Everybody has the blues. It's a kind of postpartum depression.' Doctors may be afraid to tell you. They might think it's a self-actualizing prophecy. They're wrong. If you're prepared for the depression, if people around you are prepared, you'll pull out of it more quickly."

Did Bypass change your attitudes about being a nun?

"I've always been happy as a sister. Everyone has the normal temptations of wanting to leave; everyone wants to get out. That's normal. I've loved being a sister. I'm grateful for the chance to continue, grateful there's more work to do."

Why have you always loved being a sister?

"I wish I could tell you. Whenever we seek words, we're the most mute. Being a nun is a special privilege, a special gift, given to me. There've been hard times. But I love people; I love the chance to go out to people. I'm outgoing. I'm not the shy, backward kind."

Yet you keep Cecilia O'Brien hidden.

"You're right. I do. A friend said to me, 'I wish you'd let people see what you are inside.' I said, 'It's none of their business.' Now I'm finding out they see through me. Bypass has made me want to show people how much they mean to me."

Did Bypass make you feel old?

"For a while, before Bypass, I *was* old. Not now. I feel young. At fifty-five, I don't always feel young, but I've been given another chance. After all this, I don't know what the Lord's got in store for me, but I'm ready to do His work. When I came home from the hospital, I hadn't walked upstairs since March twenty-fourth. In the hospital, we didn't practice stairs. The physicians' assistant had said, 'When you get home, go upstairs. It'll be like climbing Mt. Everest, but walk up those stairs. After this first day, get dressed early in the morning and stay dressed all day.' That night, we postponed those stairs as long as possible. They put a chair on the landing. It took me ten minutes to go up. But I made it. I wasn't as exhausted as I thought I'd be. We four went to my room. My windows were open. The sun was setting. The sky was crimson and lavender, all streaked with pink and gold. The four of us stood together. Rivers of tears cleansed our cheeks. I said, 'I never thought I'd see anything so beautiful.' We hugged each other. Then they helped me to bed. To see that sunset, to see the sun rise every day, the light streaming through the windows, has intensified my joy in being alive."

After Bypass, how did you feel when you awakened?

"I remember trying to say, 'My arm is hurting,' just as the doctor was exulting, 'The operation's over. Your Bypass is a success.' The next thing I knew, they were taking out the tubes. When the tubes came out, I was scared I'd stop breathing, that I wouldn't be able to breathe on my own. Removing the tubes didn't hurt a bit. I started breathing; I started talking. I never shut up. They nicknamed me 'Motormouth.' "

What was the worst part of the operation for you?

"The worst was being lifted onto a scale and weighed. I shook and I fought because I was afraid they'd drop me. They said, 'We won't drop you, don't worry,' but I didn't trust them. I wish I'd known more about being filled with all the tubes, what they were for, about all their procedures. It's easier if you're forewarned—and thus forearmed."

What was the worst part of the convalescence for you?

"It's only five weeks since Bypass. I worried about how long I'd be laid up. I dreaded being alone. When I was able to go out but couldn't drive, people thought I was still recuperating. Nobody offered to take me anyplace, even for a drive to the park. I missed getting out, but I don't like to ask people to do for me. Nevertheless"—suddenly her pert Irish face is lit by a smile—"school starts next week. This morning I went to the surgeon's partner and was discharged."

Happy discharge.

"I still have to take it easy. I go from being full of beans to being dead-tired. There's no in-between. This bone-tired fatigue is different from before Bypass."

Who cooks your meals?

"The cook comes in and prepares dinner. We put together the last-minute fixings. We don't have it as soft as the priests—dinner is served to them. Yet I don't have the responsibilities of a wife and mother. I'm one who likes to cook. I still can't go in the kitchen and fuss; they told me no beating and no mixing."

Did your surgeon restrict you?

"That's one thing I mind. Very much. I haven't seen Dr. Vinod since the Bypass. In the hospital, the junior varsity comes around. Afterwards, you see whatever doctor's in the office. It's like having a love affair, giving someone your heart, and being jilted."

What did Bypass do for you?

"Gave me more years, good years. I couldn't live like that. Gave me more insight into myself, into my spiritual life, my prayer life. Bypass has intensified my prayer life."

What do you mean by your "prayer life"?

"My meditation, my prayers, my relationship with the Lord. You can get into a routinized rut. You go through the motions. Did you ever read the sermons of John Donne, the English poet? He prays to the Lord for forgiveness because his mind wandered during meditation. As he prays for forgiveness, his mind again wanders. If you're not careful, human relationships get stale. A relationship with the Lord is even harder to keep fresh."

How did your insight into yourself intensify?

"Even as a young child, I remember my mother telling me, 'No matter what, you should be polite and kind.' And she was. My mother was sick for seven years. When a son walked out at noontime, I watched her say, 'Drive carefully. I'll see you tomorrow.' She died that night. With two alcoholic daughters, one who never spoke to her for five years, an alcoholic son who went for rehabilitation, got better, and ended up with Alzheimer's disease, she never complained. With all of them having heart attacks, she never winced or cried aloud. Always with a smile, she was courteous and patient. Lord! she was so patient. Bypass taught me to be like my mother. I've been lucky. Bypass helped me beyond my expectations."

Has your having had Bypass affected any of your relationships in the house?

"They don't stay away from me, nor do they treat me with kid gloves. When I came home, everyone was great. Now they let me do a lot. If they see me going too far, they'll pull me back and say, 'Hey. You're not sick; you're in-between, at that fork in the road of neither sick nor well.' Last Saturday, I was at a party with some sisters with whom I entered the convent. They started in on me: 'You shouldn't do this. You shouldn't do that.' I had to say, 'Hey, would you people shut up and let me alone? I know what I can do.' A few minutes later, they began asking, 'Are you getting tired?' I said a little sharply, 'When I get tired, you'll know.' This in-between stage where I am now is the hardest: not sick, not competely well. Some people will let you do more than you should. If you hold yourself back, they think you're shirking.

"It was strange. One sister who never shows any affection—she was raised without any affection—came up to me last night, put her arms around me, and said, 'I'm glad you didn't die.' I said, 'Yeah, so am I.' The sisters, even the ones whose lives touched mine only tangentially, were enriched by my Bypass. Of course, *they* didn't have to go through it."

When you saw the surgeon this morning, did he suggest any cardiac rehab program for you?

"I thought he would, but he didn't. I figured if it were important, he'd send me. I've read that it's important."

Why didn't you ask him?

"They're busy. They're in and out the door before you have a chance to formulate a question. For a motormouth, I'm not assertive enough around doctors."

Now that you're a Bypass veteran, what are your greatest fears?

"That it'll happen again."

If it happens again, will you go for a Bypass?

"Yes"—she lifts her chin defiantly—"and I wouldn't wait so long."

Before and after Bypass, what explicit questions should people ask their internist, their cardiologist, and their surgeon?

"People should ask their doctors to *sit down* with them, to explain step by step what's going to happen. Nobody's a seer, but doctors should predict the odds, as best they can. They never told me my leg would hurt a heck of a lot worse than my chest. I complain and complain about the leg. Until I came home, I didn't have any feeling in my right chest. Even now, it's like Novocaine's injected there. In my left chest, it feels like I'm having a coronary. They should explain about the chest pain from the muscles and bones knitting together. They should give more explicit instructions about diet. Surely they should let you know what you're in for with the depression. The doctors didn't warn me about the pitfalls. Father John did. If I'm prepared for depression, the tears don't bother me so much, because I know they'll go away.

"Bypass fixed my heart in more ways than one. When I'd have chest pain, I'd think, 'If anything happens to me, who's gonna care anyway? Comes Christmastime, I haven't anyplace to go. I'm so alone.' It's only Memorial Day now, yet already I have four or five invitations for Thanksgiving and Christmas. I'm lonesome. That's the nature of the beast. But now I know I have a place in the sun."

15. Willard Dreiser
Shoestore owner-operator
Age at Bypass: 58

Willard and Orville Dreiser are twins. For thirty-eight years, they've eked out a living from their jointly owned shoestore in Flint, Michigan. In their early days, living and working with a mirror image was tolerable; now, that tolerance is gone. For the past ten years, they have "hated each other's guts." Lately, they hate their customers, too.

The shoestore is losing money. Since their teens, both have been three-pack-a-day smokers. Orville, a POW for two years during World War II, a chronic alcoholic since his twenties, still smokes his three packs. Defending his brother's drinking, Willard apologizes, "Maybe the prison camps made Orville an alcoholic, I don't know. We're half-Irish and half-German, so everybody drinks pretty good, but nobody hits the bottle like Orv. I never have more'n a pint of Seagram's a day." Like his brother's, Willard's clothes exude the acrid stench of tobacco, yet Willard claims, "I've cut down on the weeds. I'll bet I don't smoke more'n a pack a day."

The last seven years have been lean for the Dreisers. Willard had a blood disease—"some kind of blood cancer"—treated with chemotherapy and a splenectomy. Shortly after his spleen was removed,

"I had a heart attack. And another. And another. Since then, I'm always so tired. It's hard to drag around. For four years, my heart behaved itself. Then, it started in again with one attack after the other. Finally, they did an angiogram, which showed four blockages. They kept me in the hospital till they could get an operating room for my Bypass. Took 'em seven weeks. That's a long time to sit on your duff in a hospital. The muckety-mucks get taken first. If I sit in a hospital waiting for my turn at Bypass like some broad in a bakery with her ticket, everybody's Blue Cross rates go up."

Willard snorts, "I'm not like my poor father. He respected doctors like they were little tin gods. Even though he had chest pain, he wouldn't call a doctor in the night. It was '36. Maybe he didn't have the dough. He'd had heart trouble. Nobody seemed to know what to do for him. So he died. Orville and me were just twelve when he upped and died on us."

What did you do for money?

"Orville and me are the babies. My mother never worked. She was an older mother, but she was a doll. We all lived in a big old house. My two sisters and three other brothers worked. We got by. The family used to be so close. Now, there's only four of us seven kids left. And Orv and me are fighting. Everybody used to tell me, 'You'll never have a heart attack. You yell and scream at everything. You get it all out.' Just shows how much people know. I'm very excitable. I never can just sit."

Do you eat fast?

"I probably haven't eaten at a table at home in three years."

Why?

"Now that there's just my wife and me, we eat in front of the TV set. That way, we don't have to talk." He stops. "But I'm not like Orv. When my wife talks, I listen. My wife's okay. She's got a good job; she's workin' for Rite Aid Drugstores. She's not just a cashier either. Lately"—he frowns—"she makes more'n me. That bothers me. She babies me too much. That irritates the hell out of me."

What things irritate you most?

"TV irritates me. I can't hardly watch it. Lately, people irritate me. The customers drive me crazy. I been there too long. Nothing big, just all the little things drive me up the wall. My brother's not a worker, never has been. He gets in late, goes in the back with the paper, a cigarette, and a bottle. I'm stuck with the customers. I'm so listless. I drag my wife down. She likes to run and go. Yet she never says, 'Why are you such a deadhead?' "

Do you both get home at the same time from work?

"I get home first. Business is lousy."

Who makes the dinner?

"My wife. Who else? She has everything ready anyhow."

Who does the dishes?

"The dishwasher."

Who puts the dishes in the dishwasher?

"She does, of course. Say, what do you want from me? I work hard all day."

Before and after your Bypass, did your surgeon talk much to you?

"I never met him before. Afterwards, I had a sore throat. His hired help said it was from that damned tube. They sent me home with the sore throat. That night, I had a fever of 105 degrees and had to come back into the hospital. I had a staph infection; I had to stay in the hospital for a month. My wife wrote the doctor a letter saying, 'How come you let them send him home?' She didn't say anything about suing, but after her letter, he came in to see me. He's a good-looking fellow, all dolled up, with his followers walking ten paces behind him. They all had little pencils and papers and serious looks. Only he didn't have a pencil. By that time, I didn't give a damn about talking to him."

Before Bypass, what did you worry about most?

"The store. There's a shoestore on every corner. I can't compete with the big discount stores. Orv's not much help. While I was in the hospital, my son pitched in. Just as I was getting back in harness, Orv keeled over with a heart attack. Right in the store. He ended up with a Bypass."

When your twin brother had heart surgery, how did it affect you?

"I didn't like it. When they sent him for an angiogram, I thought for sure Orv would never need a Bypass. Why should they do that to him? I hated it."

Why?

"It made me sad. Knowing what he had to go through."

I thought you didn't like your twin brother.

"That's different. You don't understand how it is with Orv 'n' me. Twins are different from the rest of the people. I could kill him, but I can't stand for anybody to hurt him. Before my Bypass, the thought of it was terrible. The anticipation was worse'n the surgery. Then, havin' Orv get racked up was too much." He shakes his head. "Just too much."

Before your brother's Bypass, what did you tell him?

"I said, 'Orv, there's nothin' to it. With my blood problem, I got through it. You're strong as an ox, even with everythin' you do to yourself.' I was wrong. He minded the operation even more'n me."

Did he ever ask you, 'Why did you let me have Bypass?'

"Nope. We never talk about it. Never. We don't talk much. If I talk, he talks."

If you don't talk?

"He won't talk. That's just the way it is."

Did you see your brother while he was in the hospital?

"Sure, I saw him before and after his Bypass. The night before, I said, 'Orv, I'll come see you in three or four days. Before that, you won't know me anyways. When you see me in the door, you'll know you're getting better.' I couldn't go up much because I had to mind the store. Before my Bypass, I would've liked somebody to talk to me, tell me what to expect. I never saw the doctor before my heart operation. It would've been a comfort to me if somebody had said, 'This is what somebody else went through. You have four blockages, but we're optimistic.' "

What questions should Bypassers ask before the operation?

"In the first place, I asked none. I didn't have a chance. I would've liked to have asked, 'What are my odds? Better than Vegas? How much suffering will I have?' It's funny; you expect to suffer, but you don't. They keep you under all the time. Afterwards, you're down a little, you're weak, but that's all."

By 'down,' do you mean depressed?

"Absolutely not. I was thrilled to have it over and done with. In two or three days, I was walking. Every movement thrilled me. Bypass is a lot easier than a splenectomy, no matter what they tell you."

Did your brother ask you any questions?

"Not a one. I told him, 'Orv, you're stronger'n me; that'll help.' "

When you were in the hospital, did your brother come to see you?

"Not so much. He was busy with the store. When I asked for him, he'd come in so I could check on the inventory."

Did he see you with all the tubes?

"No. I told my family I didn't want anybody in until I was back in a room."

Was it hard for you to see Orville after Bypass?

"Not at all. Mostly, we have gotten the same breaks. Except I got a blood disease 'n' he didn't. He got captured by the Nips and I didn't."

If your sons had to have Bypass, how would you feel?

"I'd pass out. *I love them.* Yet . . ."—he scratches his head—"if the doctor recommended it, I'd want them to go ahead. God, I hope my sons don't need it. I'd sooner go in their place. Still and all, everybody who has it seems to be better than before. Even I'm better. My appetite's better. Even Orv's better, although I doubt he'll talk about it. Booze makes it hard for him to concentrate."

Now that you're a Bypass veteran, what are your greatest fears?

"I don't fear anything until it happens. I don't want to be a burden on anyone, to be lying around somewhere in a home, so sick I couldn't get up and move around."

What are your greatest joys?

"My kids and grandchildren. Even my wife. Just to see them every-day. Nothing special."

What's been your greatest disappointment?

"I can't think of anything. When I got the first heart attack, I said, 'If I go, I go. I've had everything I wanted.' I never wanted to be rich. At least I achieved *that* goal." He laughs hollowly. "Don't get me wrong. I'm an optimist. My wife says I'm a perfectionist. If we go to a restaurant, I rearrange everything so that it's right. She'll say to me, 'Are you happy now?' At the store, I have to have every-thing perfect."

Is your brother like that?

"Naw. Just the opposite. The odd couple, that's us. I don't know what he'd do without me to run things."

Before you went home from the hospital the first or the second time, did anybody instruct you about when you could resume certain activities?

"Nobody. They were just glad to get rid of me."

Did they tell you when you could lift, when you could drive, when you could resume sexual activity?

"I can't lift. I haven't been able to for years. Orv useta do the lifting. The doctor made me wait a couple of months on the car. I didn't like that, but I did as I was told."

What about sexual activity?

"They didn't say anything. Since my blood problem, I haven't felt like doing it very much."

What is 'not very much'?

"Nothing. Not for a few years."

Does doing without bother you?

"It doesn't bother me."

How does your wife feel about sexual abstinence?

"She doesn't say anything."

Did you ever discuss your loss of sexual desire with your internist?

"No. He doesn't ask and I don't ask."

Would you like him to talk about sexual matters?

"I useta wish he'd ask me. Now, it's too late. A few drinks put me to sleep just as well, and it's not so much trouble. Our sex life is like Orv and me." He sighs, pulls on his earlobe.

I don't understand.

"Orv and me useta be good pals. When we wuz little, we always had each other, we never hadda learn to talk to anybody else. Lately, we hate each other, but we don't know how to talk to anybody else. That store's got slices of silence in it as thick as liverwurst. I don't hate my wife, not like I hate Orv. She's not a bad kid, but we rub each other the wrong way. We been doin' it too long and too much. It's like we know the right places to nick. That takes the fun outta goin' to bed together. Maybe if the doc had talked to me about sex, it woulda been different. But he didn't and I didn't. Anyway, I'm just too tired. Too tired to fight, too tired to mess around with my wife, too tired to get up in the mornin' and face Orv every day."

Are you identical twins?

"Naw, fraternal. Yet we had identical angiogram pictures, we had identical blockages, we each have identical twins for grandchildren—I got grandsons, Orv's only got granddaughters—and lately, the more we fight, the more we look alike. People get us mixed up. God, I can't stand that!"

Why do you hate each other so much?

Will Dreiser stares at me: "Don't you understand? How would you like to spend the rest of your life with someone just like you? What could be worse?" His voice rises angrily. "When I hate myself, I hate my brother, which makes me hate myself more. When I yell, I'm yelling at myself and hollering at my brother at the same time. My wife says I treat Orv the same way I treat her. She's wrong. Orv is the worst."

Since Bypass, do you fight more?

"Not any more. Not any less either. I told ya, he's always in the back room with a cigarette and a pint and the paper. If I holler, he just puts the paper up higher." Willard Dreiser scratches his nose, taps his thin fingers on the table. "That reminds me. You got all you want from me? Orv's alone in the store. We been tryin' to sell the place, but nobody wants it. Since his Bypass, he can't lift those heavy cartons neither. If I'm there, I take one side and he takes the other. It's too soon for him to be liftin' by himself. I gotta run. If Orv'll talk to you, get the rest from him."

16. Orville Dreiser
Shoestore owner-operator
Age at Bypass: 58

Six months later, after three broken appointments, Orville Dreiser shows up one rainy day. Taller than his brother Willard, he too looks like a bony, beaten version of Fred Astaire, but without the jauntiness. Although the Dreiser twins are only fifty-eight, they look older. Before Orville Dreiser sits down, he lights a cigarette with a shaky hand. His first heart attack was five years ago, he tells me. "After my first attack, I was okay for four years. Then, I had one heart attack after another. Six months before, Will had had Bypass, so"—he smiles mockingly with half his face—"they decided not to cut me out of the fun and games."

What did you think caused your need for Bypass?

He shrugs. "I'm a heavy drinker. I smoke heavily. Heart killed my dad. My older brother and sister died of heart. I assumed those three things did it. My cholesterol level was all right. Bypass didn't particularly scare me. I didn't want to go through it, but I figured I'd better listen, follow orders. I asked Will about it. He said, 'It's not too bad.' He didn't give me any advice not to have it. He didn't tell me to have it either. He wouldn't commit himself one way or the other. When I told him I'd need Bypass, Will said, 'Lemme show you my scars,' He was very noncommittal. He said, 'It didn't bother me none. I don't even remember what happened.' Once they rode me to the operating room and put me under, I don't remember much either, not for seven or eight days. No pain. It was nothing."

What did the doctors tell you about Bypass? How did they prepare you?

"After the last heart attack, they kept me in the hospital until they could get me on the operating schedule. A long time. Maybe six weeks, I hung around the hospital waiting for Bypass. Nobody told me much. Then it was over."

Because you knew what your twin brother had gone through, was it harder or easier for you to face your own Bypass?

"A little easier. He was in worse shape than I was with his blood trouble. His white corpuscles were bad, but that's been arrested. So far. I figured if Will could make it, I could."

Before Bypass, did you want Will to talk to you about the operation?

"No. I was more interested in whether Blue Cross would cover it all. Besides, Will was busy running the store. Once a week, while I was waiting, Will would run in and see me. He'd read the paper. We'd watch football. We didn't discuss Bypass much."

How did you feel when you woke up?

"Relieved." Patiently, he explains, "It was all over. I wasn't suffering any pain. They all convinced me it came out good. The tube was out. My brother had had a terrible infection in his throat. They said it might've come from the tube. He suffered so much from that infection. It almost took his palate away. They never should've discharged him from the hospital. I saw his palate. Any doctor who took the time to look at him should've seen it. How could they let him go home?"

Did you have the same doctors as your brother did?

"The question was, 'Do you want it done in a hurry? If you do, you take whoever you can get.' You don't get much choice of doctors. Whoever is handy. They made me sign papers saying I knew the dangers, but they never described the operation. I had seen part of it on TV. When they opened up the chest, I turned it off."

When you came to, when you were convalescing, what was the worst part?

"The coughing they made me do, bringing up all that glop to clear my lungs. My whole chest hurt. They had me hold a pillow, but it still hurt."

How was it when you came home?

"Pretty good. They wanted me to walk, but it was winter outside. Winter in Germanville is bitter, blowing all the time. They didn't want me to walk outside. They wanted me to go to a mall and march up and down like when I was a POW. I didn't go much for that. Since the Nips got me, I'm not much of a walker. For a couple of months, I could tell my chest wasn't feeling right. I didn't know whether it was from them spreading my ribs apart or if I was getting another heart attack. After I went back to work, those pains came fairly constantly. Not sharp. More like bruised flesh on the inside. They lasted a couple of months."

How long after Bypass did you go back to work?

"Maybe three months. But I worked only a couple of hours a day for a whole month. I couldn't drive for the first three months. That was difficult because my wife doesn't drive. My daughter had to do all the shopping."

Usually, who does the shopping?

"I do. It's a real pain."

How long after Bypass did you wait to climb stairs?

"My bedroom's downstairs, so there's no reason to go up. I wouldn't climb just for the fun of it."

How long did you wait to resume sexual activity?

"That's a sore point. I hadn't had any sexual activity for five years before Bypass."

Why?

"I don't know. I went to doctors. They said it was in my head. I went to a psychiatrist. After a year's worth of going every week, he told me to walk a mile every day. I gave up on that."

Do you have difficulty getting or sustaining an erection?

"The last one."

Did Bypass help you maintain an erection?

"It didn't change at all."

Do you mind?

"Sure, I mind. I'm not dead yet."

Does your wife mind?

"Elsie's my age. She doesn't say anything. I don't ask. I assume sometimes she minds. It's a big nothing."

Are you on any heart or blood-pressure medication?

"Just heart medicine. One kind or another."

How long have you been on heart medicine?

"Five, six years. Since the first heart attack."

After you started the heart medication, did your sexual desire and erectile function diminish?

"I asked Doc Williams, my internist, about it. He thought no. I asked him, 'What about trying a different pill for my heart?' He said, 'Better not to monkey around.' That's what I tell my brother about selling the store: 'Better not to monkey around.' Will wants to sell the store in the worst way."

Have you sold it?

"Almost. Will's cooking some kind of deal, if nothing goes wrong."

How will you feel about selling the store?

"Sort of bad. Thirty-eight years we've been there."

Why are you selling it?

"My brother isn't up to it any more. We can't lift the cases any more. We have to hire people to help us. The store doesn't make enough money to support us and help, too. We have to do it ourselves. All our lives, we've done everything ourselves. Will's sort of tired after thirty-eight years. I don't know."

How do you feel about the customers? Do you enjoy waiting on them?

"Enjoy? I don't know if that's exactly the word. I'm a good floorman. My brother's temper is too short now. He can't take waiting on people any more. If they don't take his advice, he blows his stack. I always got along with the customers. I don't have any particular fondness for any of them."

Since Bypass, are you more short-tempered?

"I don't know. More the other way. I'm more easy to get along with."

What does your wife say?

"God knows what she says. Sometimes she likes me . . . sometimes she doesn't."

Probably you feel the same way about her, don't you?

"Definitely. We've been married thirty-eight years, since I got back from prison camp. Before the war was over even. She doesn't drive, she doesn't like to go out any more. Now, she's got a problem where she can't swallow. Food just sticks in her throat. She has to drink about a fifth of wine to eat dinner. She's been to seven doctors. She can't eat in the morning, she can't eat at noon, she won't go out to dinner. The wine relaxes her so she can eat."

Has she lost weight?

"Originally, she lost an awful lot of weight. She was trying to drink milkshakes, but she couldn't get them down. She wasn't drinking, she wasn't eating. I told her: 'Go ahead and drink. If you don't, you're not going to live.' Now her weight is back. One meal a day is all she can do. With the wine."

Are you still drinking a fair amount?

"I drink a lot less. Medicine and alcohol don't go together. I was always a heavy drinker but never to the point where I couldn't drive. One time, on the medicine, when I'd had a little too much to drink, I couldn't even get in my car. I couldn't do anything. I went sort of crazy. I don't drink much with the medicine. My doctor says, 'Whatever you drink is too much.' "

How much do you drink a day?

"The last few weeks, I haven't been drinking at all. Just a couple of beers, some wine with Elsie. Usually, I drink a pint of peppermint schnapps, a few beers, not much. If we're having a party, getting together after golf, I'll have a few beers. It all depends on the time I got. Sometimes, at night in the store, when it's really quiet from seven to nine, I'll drink. I shouldn't do it. I shouldn't be drinking at all. The doctor says drinking is partly why I had three heart attacks."

What do you think Bypass did for you?

"Not much. I felt as good before Bypass as I do now. I felt as good before I had my heart attacks as I did after Bypass. I always felt good before I had a heart attack. In between and after the big operation, as soon as I was on my feet, I was playing golf, walking and talking, waiting on customers. I feel the same."

Since Bypass, have you had any heart trouble?

"Not a bit. If Will weren't so dead set on selling the store, I'd say Bypass had improved my life." He frowns. "The doctors say Bypass will prolong it. I don't know for how long. Without the store, if I live longer, I don't know how we'll get by. The new owner might hire me as a floorman. Maybe I can get work at some other shoe-store. I don't know any other business. Will started the store and got me to come in with him."

If you had to have another Bypass, would you have it?

"That's a toughie. They'd have to convince me how much good it would do. I don't know. I don't want to go through it again."

You said it was nothing.

"Did I say it was nothing? It's not. It's months of lying in bed, eating sawdust which the hospital passes off for food, pains here and there, worrying. I'd have to think it over pretty much, before I said yes to a second Bypass. If they said, 'You're going to die without it,' I'd probably say, 'Go ahead. Open me.' "

Would you go to the same doctors?

"I didn't like Raman, the surgeon."

Why?

"I don't know. Too brisk and too offhand about it. Before the operation, he breezed in for five minutes, then waltzed out. After the operation, I never saw him again. One of his lackeys checked my scars. I didn't think much of him. I liked the cardiologist. I wish I could think of his name."

Do you think your twenty-year-old self would be proud of what you've accomplished?

"Running a shoestore is not the greatest thing in the world. I should have taken the GI Bill and gone to college after I got out of the war. I'd planned to. But after prison camp, I couldn't sit in school. I came home, I got married, I drifted into the store. I'd prefer to be more educated. I like to read. I like to golf in the summer and read in the winter."

What gives your life pleasure?

"Pleasure? Well, I like it when my kids get together at Thanksgiving and Christmas. I get pleasure out of reading. Pleasure out of drinking. That's taken for granted. I don't know about pleasures. I'm sort of set in my ways."

Did Bypass make you more willing to stop and taste the sweetness of everyday life?

"Not especially. I'm either going to work, coming home, watching TV, going to bed. Nothing new in my life. No change."

Now that you're a Bypass veteran, what are your greatest fears?

"I don't have any fears."

What's been your greatest disappointment?

"Myself." He is annoyed. "I just told you a little while ago. I achieved nothing special. I've lived an ordinary life. I haven't done anything for anybody particularly. Or for myself. I'm not too good a father.

When I was young, I was never around. I was always playing golf, playing cards, drinking. That's no way."

In those days, did you have fun?

"I thought I was having fun. I was a young man who'd saved up a lot of oats."

Are you sorry now, or glad?

"I'm just as glad. Except I could've been a better father. I could've given my daughters more attention. Since I've gotten older and they've grown up, I'm close to all of them. Not when they were young."

If you'd had to pay for Bypass yourself, would you have had it?

"I couldn't afford it. I wouldn't have had the money. Those doctors want their money up front."

After Bypass, did you get depressed?

"Not any more than usual. I get in the dumps when things aren't going right, when I don't know how I'm going to support Elsie and me. The cost of living is so tough. I don't know what I'd do if I had young kids around. I couldn't support 'em."

If the store is sold, can you get along?

"Just barely. Nobody's got any cash. The 'maybe' Buyer wants us to take a lot of paper back. The down payment's small. My house is still mortgaged. We'll get back maybe six hundred dollars a month, split down the middle. That's not enough to live on."

Does your wife work outside your home?

"She's never held a job. In the old days, I didn't want my wife working. Now I think I made a mistake, but it's too late."

Are you close to your twin brother?

"We've been together fifty-eight years. God, we suffered three years being apart in the Army."

Yes, but twins either like each other a great deal, or they don't like each other at all.

"We're incompatible, if that's what you mean. We get along, but we're nothing alike. He doesn't like to read. He's a Republican. I'm a Democrat. He's conservative, really. He believes people ought to do for themselves. I think not everybody can help himself. Sometimes, everybody else has to help. Even in high school, we had different sets of friends."

You're as different as . . .

"People who aren't twins at all, aren't even brothers. But we belong to each other, that's what you don't understand."

Will you miss seeing him every day in business?

"It doesn't bother me one way or the other." Defiantly, he adds, "If Will wants out of the businss, then we sell, that's all! You watch! He'll miss it. When it's too late."

If you had Bypass to do over, would you want them to change your care in any way?

"I had good, nice nurses, nice doctors. Except for Raman, the surgeon, or whatever his name is. I didn't like him. Everybody else made it as easy as possible."

If you had a friend who'd been told to have Bypass, what would you tell him?

"It's nowheres as frightening as you think. For several days after it's done, there isn't any pain. You aren't even with it. You don't even know who's visiting you. When you finally come out of the medication, most of the pain is gone. It's all over. When the doctors first say, 'You need Bypass,' you're frightened. Anybody would be. You get over it. Unless you're frightened of dying."

Some people are.

"I suppose. Being afraid of dying never occurred to me. During the war, I was so frightened. There's no comparison. That's ten times as bad as Bypass. The missions over Japan were murder. I was a bombardier. When we had to bail out, my blood ran cold, I started to shake. Turned out I was right to be terrified. When I got out of the Army, I began drinking. I turned into a heavy, 'disturbed' drinker." He shakes his head, lights another cigarette. "After Bypass, I didn't drink or smoke for ten months. As soon as I got back on my feet, I'd have a beer, then a few more. Doc Williams got so sore at me."

Why did you start smoking again?

"It's a vicious habit, that's all. Nicotine is a drug. You ought to know that. I'm addicted."

Which habit does Dr. Williams berate you more for? Cigarettes or alcohol?

"Alcohol. He won't even mention cigarettes. He smokes. He knows I smoke. He figures, 'What's Orv Dreiser going to do if he can't drink, can't smoke, can't get it . . . have sex?' I might as well go over the bridge."

Did he tell you that drinking might be a factor in your not being able to have intercourse?

"He told me."

Wouldn't it be a good trade? Giving up drinking for sex?

"I don't know. At twenty, it's worth it. Now? Well, I've sort of become asexual." He stops, stares moodily out at the lines of rain beyond the window. "Funny. I don't like drinking the way I used to. I don't want to drink heavy. It ruins my golf in the summertime.

We don't have the parties we used to have. Elsie and I always had a gang over at the house with martinis and Manhattans and that stuff. Everybody's moved away," he laments, "everybody but Will and me. When I was younger, I drank a lot more, what with raising the kids, than I do now."

We all have insecurities. What are your insecurities?

"I don't know how capable I am of taking on a big job or following through. Since I got out of the Army, I've been kind of a goldbrick, just going along with things. I used to be a leader. No more. I've not led or outdistanced anybody. Not even myself, let alone my brother. Will thinks I shirk my duty, that he does most of the work. He does the bookkeeping. I do the lifting, the floor work, the selling, refilling shelves, cleaning the place. He's not as strong as I am. He's always tired. But don't misunderstand: he's selling the store because he's sick of it, not because he's too sick to run it."

Could you run the store without him?

"When he was out sick for six months, I ran it. But permanently? There's no way I could buy him out. I couldn't get the money. Besides, what's the store without Will? I wouldn't want that."

Is it harder to be the one who had Bypass or the one who is the family member? You have been both.

"The one who has Bypass has the easiest part. The person who takes care of the Bypasser has a tougher time. It's a pain taking care of sick people. What's worse is worrying about them. Caring about what happens to them. When you realize how much you're concerned, you hate them for putting you through all this worry." Lighting a cigarette from the one dangling from his lips, Orville Dreiser stands, tries to smile, but fails. "No doubt about it. It's better to be the Bypasser than the Bypasser's twin."

17. Phil and Bernice Milard
Engineer/Housewife
Ages at Bypass: 50/49

Phil Milard is fifty, thin, with a thin face, straight gray hair, steel-rimmed glasses. Well dressed in a gray suit, a blue oxford shirt, a blue-and-gray rep tie, he smiles rarely; his thin lips and right eye twitch frequently. Bernice Milard, forty-nine, is perky and talkative, with brown hair, deep-set blue eyes, and an engaging smile. If Phil Milard looks professional, Bernice Milard is suburban-casual in her white trousers, pink print overblouse, and white canvas shoes. A passerby might dismiss them as an average middle-American couple in Wichita, an average middle-American town. So much for the passing glance: both Bernice and Phil Milard are Bypassers.

Who was Bypassed first?

"He was." Bernice points at her husband.

"She should be Italian, she talks so much with her hands," Phil Milard objects.

Would you like me to interview you separately, or do you prefer to answer together?

"Go ahead and see what happens," Phil advises. "We don't always agree."

"Sometimes," Bernice notes, "we can't agree on anything."

"Bypass sure didn't help our fighting any," Phil remarks. "Since our Bypasses, our argumentativeness has intensified."

"And our hostility," Mrs. Milard says acidly. "When Phil had Bypass at Christmas, I never dreamt I'd have heart surgery by the following Mother's Day. Some Mother's Day present. Considering the stress from our son, I guess it's appropriate. When the doctor sent me for catheterization, I thought, 'Much ado about nothing.' During the cath, I had a heart attack. That same day, they did Bypass."

"From the time of your heart attack," interrupts Mr. Milard, "to the time they plunked you on the operating-room table, it was less than an hour."

To what did you attribute your illness?

"Stress," Bernice replies. "For seven years, Jason put us through hell. His learning disability became a severe personality and behavioral disorder. He was using drugs, drinking, in trouble with the police. After Phil's Bypass, Jason might have had a nervous breakdown. I don't know. He went out, got drunk, got himself arrested, tried to commit suicide in his cell. We took him to the hospital to dry out. They kept him for six weeks. When I had my Bypass, Jason was still in the hospital. He'd gone off the handle many times, but that was the worst. We'd fight so; Phil and Jason would be ready to trade blows." Embarrassed, she twists a lace handkerchief. "A couple of times, they traded blows. The idea of physical violence in the house was appalling, but I can't blame Phil. Jason is bad news. Now that he's twenty, he seems to be settling down. Lately, we haven't had such big battles. I'm not superstitious, but every time we say, 'Things are going smoothly,' he goes off the deep end. The school couldn't teach him. Nobody can." Her hands flutter helplessly.

Do you have other children?

"Our daughter Melanie has a learning disability, but she's never been a behavior problem. Melanie's tugged at her bootstraps; she won't admit defeat. She's twenty-six, worked as a receptionist; she just got laid off. For a girl with diffuse brain damage, she's come a long way. With Melanie unemployed, we'll have to help out. It's endless. Only our eldest, Michael, is fine. We should have quit when we were ahead. He got his doctorate in electrical engineering from Cal Tech, is happily married to another electrical engineer. They don't want children. Michael used to love children, but after what we went through with Jason, he's not interested in a family. He stays out in California, nice and far away"—her voice is bitter—"calls once a week, keeps his life neatly self-contained. I don't blame him for not wanting children. I just wish he'd want to see us, even once in a while."

If there's no family history, why is he afraid?

"Who knows? The doctors say, 'Maybe both children fractured their skulls in severe falls; maybe they had high fevers; maybe Mom's and Dad's genes are defective.' Doctors don't know very much. When I'd complain about my chest, my doctor would say, 'You can't be having heart pain. At forty-eight, still menstruating, a woman doesn't have heart disease.' My husband had Bypass, even my doctor had Bypass, but nobody figured *I* needed Bypass. That's my fault. Partly. Phil cares more about his heart and his health than I do. He cares more about hanging around. I don't. I was so mad at the doctor. About three weeks after my Bypass, it hit me: if they hadn't interfered, I would've . . . Well, you know. If I have to sit around and think about dying, then I don't want to. Not yet. But if I've got an engraved invitation, what right do they have to butt in? Funny, we've both been through the same hell, but Phil wants to live forever."

Tell me how you went for catheterization.

"For a year, I'd had these funny feelings in my back and under my arms. Phil insisted I see Dr. Fox. I told the doctor about these pains. I was fairly skinny then, down to 115 pounds. He said, 'It sounds like angina!' I said, 'You're nuts. I'll bet it's my pinched nerve acting up again.' Dr. Fox did a stress test and nothing showed. He said, 'You're right. It must be a pinched nerve.' He didn't order any further tests. I didn't press him to go further. My blood pressure was 190 over something or other. Dr. Fox said, 'With what you're going through, a little blood-pressure elevation's understandable. You're having battle fatigue.' I agreed. Then, Christmas Day, Phil was despondent because he was in the hospital. I went out in the hall and cried, but I wouldn't let him see me cry. He was too blue on his own. He's one who thinks one shot of painkiller will addict him for life."

Tell me about your Bypass.

"Jason and Phil are part of my Bypass. In April, Jason got terribly drunk. I picked him up, arguing and swearing. Suddenly, he opened the car door, jumped out, and ran towards the bridge. I followed him. I said, 'Jason, please get in this car and come home.' He wouldn't answer me. He wouldn't look at me. I said. 'Okay, I'm going home.' To myself, I said, 'If he jumps off the bridge, that's his problem, not mine.' After I came home, he burst in, broke the door down, ripped the phone off the wall, began pushing Phil around. When he walloped me in the chest, I didn't think anything of it. When we got him quieted down, we took him to the hospital. The next night, I got this horrible pain in my back. I tried to hide it, yet Phil could see. He wanted me to go to the hospital. I said, 'Honey, there's nothing wrong with me.' After the aching became torment, I said, 'Okay, I'll go to Emergency, but first let me take a shower.' The hot water made the pain go away. I figured it wasn't heart; it couldn't be heart."

Why did you take a shower?

"I wanted to be clean. My mother always said, 'Never go anywhere unless you're clean.' After the shower, not only was I clean, I was better. I said, 'I don't have to go to the hospital. The pain's gone.' I didn't go. For the next month, I went every day to see Jason in the hospital. He was laying a lot of guilt on me. Everything that ever went wrong with him was my fault. I tried to make things better, took flowers into him, took him for walks. During that month, I saw Dr. Fox about the pains. He kept saying, 'It's nerves, not heart trouble.'

"After Jason came home, I was hit by a bad attack. I'd asked him to get me some cigarettes; I was all out. Coming back up the stairs, I said, 'Doggone it, that pain is starting again.' When I lay down, it went away. Jason said, 'Do you want me to stay here with you?' I said, 'No, please get my cigarettes.' When it got too bad, I called Phil at work and said, 'You'd better come home. I'm in trouble.' I'd never done that before. After Jason came back with the cigarettes, I told him: 'Jason, I'm having a heart attack. I think I'm going to die. Tell Daddy I love him.' Even though I thought I was dying, I was so mad at Jason that I couldn't tell him, 'I love you.' I couldn't lie. He was holding my hand and saying, 'I'm not going to let you die, Mom.' I thought, 'If I'm having a heart attack, what the heck can he do?' By the time I got to the doctor, the pain was gone. Repeatedly, I'd get myself to the doctor, because the pain was so awful; I'd be so faint and sweaty and cold; when the nurse took the cardiogram, it'd be normal. He'd act annoyed because I'd interrupted his office hours. Finally, Phil called the doctor and said, 'It's time to quit screwing around. Bernice should see a cardiologist; I want her to have an angiogram. She can't go on this way.'

"They took me in, did all these tests, finally did the catheterization. Right in the middle, I told the doctor, 'I'm having a heart attack.' He gave me massive doses of nitro, but nothing helped. He said, 'We're going to have to do Bypass. Right now.' I was stunned. I said, 'Can I see my husband? I'd like to kiss him good-bye.' I kissed him, and cracked some kind of joke. I figured, 'Okay, I'm dead. So what?' The next thing I knew, I woke up. Everybody was saying, 'It's all over. You're fine.'

"I was wishing they'd shut up. I didn't want to be fine. I was so tired. I'd been all through it with Phil only five months before." Suddenly, she stops her story, points her finger at her husband: "Why don't you ever ask *him* any questions?"

However you want to do this . . . Were you both emergencies?

Quickly, Bernice answers, "Yes," while Phil says, "More or less."

"More or less!" she explodes. "Phil had pericarditis. He didn't even know he was sick. Suddenly, he was in the hospital. And they went from there."

Phil picks up the thread: "I was at a sales meeting, when I felt funny in my chest. I thought coffee and doughnuts would help. They didn't. For three days, I worked and stalled that pain. The third morning, I called the doctor, who did an EKG in his office. He said: 'You've got pericarditis.' I said, 'What's that?' 'An inflammation of the heart sac,' the doctor said. But he wouldn't let me go home. He wouldn't even let me drive myself to the hospital. He called Bernice; she came over and took me. I didn't think it was serious till they popped me into the Coronary Care Unit. After that, I was in and out of the CCU three times." Phil Milard asks Bernice: "Is that right?"

"He was in and out of the CCU like it was a revolving door," Bernice agrees. "When they felt Phil had stabilized, they took him up to the fifth floor. Five hours later, nobody had even come to see him. One nurse brought pills and didn't bring any water. He went from total wiring, all that monitoring, to absolute indifference. Here I fault the hospital and the doctor. When I started making waves, they took him to the intermediate floor, where he was monitored. Because he seemed better, they took him to a rehab class. It was his first trip out of that room; he got kind of excited. He said to me, 'I feel dizzy.' "

Phil interrupts: "No, no. The nurse asked, 'Does everyone feel all right?' I said, 'I feel funny right here,' so she handed me a nitro, the first nitro I'd ever taken. I went out like a light."

"His eyes rolled back in his head," Bernice notes. "I told the nurse, 'He's gone.' Three nurses came running. They threw him on the bed. It was funny: one nurse was under him when he landed. Just then, he sat up in bed and demanded, 'What's going on around here?' They rushed him back to the CCU. He was petrified, so scared he'd have a heart attack and die. He'd made up his mind it depended on him to keep his heart going. I told him, 'Honey, you've got to settle down. Don't be so terrified. You're your own worst enemy.' Who isn't, tell me that? But he wouldn't listen. He'd watch that little pulse counter. He felt he had to watch it, to work on keeping his pulse rate down. While he was working so hard on his pulse, he'd forget to breathe. To humor him, I said, 'Phil, I'll sit here.' I put my hand on his stomach. 'When you don't breathe, I'll tell you. I won't let anything happen to you.' We sat like that all night. When I saw the first gleaming of the day, I said, 'It's dawn. The sun's coming up.' He said, 'Good. I always sleep better in the daytime.' " Clapping her hands delightedly, Bernice laughs like a little girl. "He slept for twenty-four hours."

Phil interrupts: "They'd indicated I hadn't had a heart attack, but the intern told me, 'You only have a little heart muscle damage,' and she upset me. To this day, my doctor insists it was pericarditis. He won't admit I had a heart attack."

"Dr. Fox told *me* Phil had a heart attack. He said, 'That's why he needed Bypass.' "

"Well," Phil admits, "maybe I never asked him outright, maybe I wanted it left unsaid."

Since your Bypasses, have you reexamined your lives, tried to make them better?

"Phil's satisfied with his life as it is. He wouldn't change it if he could."

Phil says mildly, "I'm not a complainer. I'm not a millionaire, but I'm not a pauper. I figure I've done halfway decent with my life, done what I've enjoyed doing."

Have you changed priorities since Bypass? Do you value human closeness more?

"Human closeness? No. Bypass has complicated my life because we argue so much."

"And now," Phil remarks, "I get my feelings hurt; she gets her feelings hurt . . . very easily. Neither of us will stand much guff from anyone, especially each other. Since my Bypass, I tell her: 'Hey, I don't have to take this nonsense from you.' We've lost our good will."

Do you think, 'I've been touched by death. I don't have to take this'?

"I don't consciously think I was touched by death," Phil asserts stoutly. "I fought death. And I beat it."

Do you feel Bypass was an ally in beating death or that you licked it with some inner strength?

"If the Bypass hadn't been performed, probably I wouldn't be here today. Whether there's any truth to that, I don't know. But I'm convinced if they hadn't operated, I'd have died. Consciously, I don't think, 'I defeated death.' But I don't want to die. I fear death. Bernice doesn't."

Do you think men are more afraid of death than women are?

"Possibly. There's no way I want to go," Phil replies.

"When I was young," Bernice remembers, "I used to dream everybody in my family was dying but me. I'd be left alone. I'd call my mother long-distance and tell her to drive carefully."

After Bypass, were you both depressed?

"Definitely. Even now, Bernice is despondent. Hitting bottom doesn't bother me as much any more. It's longer since my Bypass. I came through better, although she won't admit it."

"Let's qualify this, Phil. Before Bypass, I'd never had surgery in my life. Afterwards, I was doing fine, exercising, feeling on top of the world. Four months later, I had emergency gallbladder surgery. I haven't come back from that one. Phil has a good job. I don't. He leaves Jason and Melanie behind. I don't. If I had job skills before we married, I've forgotten them. Phil never wanted me to work."

"She's right. Going back to work definitely helped. When I sat around the house, I bellyached about every twinge. When I go to work, I forget my troubles. Work is the only place where I'm free from my heart's shadow. There I have too many other problems; I forget my home and my heart."

Has your Bypass changed any of your work relationships?

"The guys realize I'm grouchier."

"He always used to be even-tempered. That's why I married him."

Does your grouchiness bother you?

"It sure does. I never was cranky before. If I'm crabby at work, it's bad for business, bad for me."

Is it possible that both of you are striking out at the universe?

"I don't feel angry at the world," Phil replies. "Deep down, maybe I am. This irascibility is a definite side effect of Bypass."

"Every Bypasser complains about his black moods, his surliness. Not just us," Bernice says.

"It's leveled off some, but my I-I—my Irascibility Index—hasn't returned to its pre-Bypass level. I doubt if it will."

On the other hand, you're under tremendous pressure at home.

"Not as much as we were," Bernice says. "Things have eased."

"They were better," Phil corrects, "but with our daughter coming home, with all her bills, we're back to square one. That's why we're skimping now—at least, *I* am, Bernice isn't so careful—to put money away. If anything happens to us, I'm putting money away to help take care of them."

"We've done it all our lives," Bernice retorts hotly.

"Listen, Bernice, the more we skimp, the less we put away. The cost of living keeps going up. I make more, we have less. When I was a kid, I never thought I'd make $40,000 a year. If I had, I would've thought I'd be on Easy Street. Some Easy Street!"

"He makes me feel guilty if I spend too much money on groceries, if I don't save coupons, if I talk long-distance on the phone to my mother. After we got married, he wouldn't let me work any more. Now there aren't any jobs for fifty-year-old women with no job skills and heart disease."

Since Bypass, do you concentrate as well?

"Absolutely not!" Phil responds. "I get confused easily. It makes me angry; I forget what I'm supposed to do. The top brass remarks on it. That scares me."

"I get mixed up so bad, I don't know what to do," Bernice says softly.

What were your own roles in getting yourselves to Bypass?

"Smoking," Phil answers flatly. "Even back when I knew I shouldn't be smoking, I was. Bernice smoked two packs a day till after her Bypass. Other things, too. Inside, I seethe at my family for putting me through all this."

Do you mean your son?

"Well, yes. And we resent each other at times . . . because we get . . ."
    "He means I'm a nag."
    "She's a terrible nag. She'll latch on to a subject for days; she won't drop it. She'll go on and on—if you'll let her."
    "When he gets mad at me, I cry. My son puts blame on me, my husband puts blame on me. It's been a joke in our family: proving me wrong. Jason and his dad never make a mistake. If you've never lived with a person who never makes a mistake, you don't know what you're missing. After a while, you feel you're wrong about everything. After a while, everything hurts. When he gets mad at me, I take it that he thinks he's right, that I'm being nasty and mean. When I start to defend myself, I cry. The crying makes me mad at myself for not being able to come to my own defense, and mad at him for needing a defense in my own home, where I feel like an enemy alien."

Do either of you have heart disease in your families?

"Phil's the first one in his family, but my side's polluted," Bernice says brightly. "My dad, my uncles, two aunts, all have angina. My aunts both had Bypass."

At a young age?

"Not any younger than I am."
    "That's young?" Phil asks sardonically. "Not in my book."

Do either of you have nightmares about Bypass?

"It happened so quick," Phil replies, "I didn't have a chance to dream evil dreams. If I'd had to sit and think about it for a month, like some people, I'd have been haunted by 3-D Technicolor phantoms. I don't like to think about Bypass. Even so, I'd go through it again, although I'd be a nervous wreck before they came to get me."

"Not me," Bernice remarks. "I told the doctor, 'If I need another Bypass, you'll need an Olympic runner to catch me. When I went for my six-week checkup, I told Dr. Orr: 'I'm mad at you. I'm alive, and it's all your fault.' I hurt his feelings so bad. Nobody ever said to him, 'Why did you interfere in my life?' Funny, he was so shook up. He thought everybody should kiss his hand."

Did Bypass make you more aware of your own mortality?

"I know I can drop dead any minute," Bernice answers. "I don't really care. In a way, that knowledge is a comfort. If I do, I don't have to keep worrying about my kids. I'm out of it."

Did Bypass make you more alive to the sweetness of daily life?

Bernice frowns. "That's why I'm so depressed. I hate to complain, but life is the same old drag. There's not much 'happy' left for us."

Do you believe in God, Mrs. Milard?

"I used to. But the more you pray to God, the more trouble you have. If there is a God, I've told Him: 'Hey, look, I've had enough. I can't take any more.' I told Him years ago. He keeps proving that I can take more. After a while, you begin to wonder if anybody is up there."

Do you believe in God, Mr. Milard?

"We ask the same questions, she and I. I was brought up to believe in a Supreme Being; but if He's such a merciful God, how can He permit all this nonsense? When the chips are down, I guess I believe in a God, yet I can't for one minute understand His actions."

"Once I made up my mind," Bernice declares, "that when you're dead they stick you in a hole and that's the end, I quit worrying about dying. There aren't any curtain calls."

Mrs. Milard, do you think much about your Bypass?

"Why should I? I'm not afraid of dying, I'm not afraid of dropping dead. I *am* beset by the devils of depression, always reminding me that my heart was fixed but my soul's in the same lousy shape. If Phil gets a twinge, he panics: 'Oh, my goodness, am I having another heart attack?' If I have pain, I ignore it. The doctor would ignore it, too. When I had angina, he missed the diagnosis, yet I can't fault him. It was back pain. He may have five hundred people with back pain; he can't run them all through the cardiology lab."

"Dr. Fox never monkeyed around with me," Phil asserts. "He put me right in the hospital."

"I'll tell you this about doctors," Bernice observes. "A man could go in looking as lousy as he feels; the doctor will pay attention to his complaints. If a woman wants medical attention, she'd better have her makeup on, her hair fixed just so. If she looks sharp, the doctor will look at her. If she looks like she feels, the doctor will bawl her out for bothering him."

When you awakened from Bypass, Mr. Milard, how did you feel?

"My worst memory is gagging with the tube in my throat. When the nurse came over and turned on the suction in there, I was petrified. Then I said to myself, 'Looks like I'm still alive.' Nothing is worse than that tube."

"For me," says Bernice, "the worst was not being able to breathe. My head was too high. I tried to tell them that. They pulled the curtains right up to the wall. No air got through. I tried to write, but it came out 'Head's too hot.' The nurse said, 'If you're too hot, I'll take off the covers.' Then, I froze. I said, 'No, no, no,' but she couldn't understand. With the tube, I found that if I kind of bit on it, the tube went back into place, and I didn't gag."

"You didn't have phlegm down there," Phil replies angrily. "I was gagging on it. You don't know how bad it was for me."

"I was there every minute with you. I knew. Biting on the tube worked for me, which is all I cared about. What I hated was being tied down."

"The I.V.'s are there," Phil tells her. "They have to keep you from flailing around. If just once, you could be more patient."

Would it have helped if there'd been a psychiatrist or a counselor, before and after Bypass, to talk to you?

"Primarily afterwards. Neither of us had any time between diagnosis and operation. People who wait six or eight weeks for Bypass would benefit from counseling," Phil replies.

"Not me," says Bernice. "I've had it with psychologists and psychiatrists. Look how they loused up the diagnosis and treatment of our son."

"We don't have any faith in psychiatrists," Phil remarks sadly. "Too little, too late, and too apathetic."

"What people need, and don't get," Bernice comments, "is a cardiologist whose sideline is psychosomatic medicine. A whole doctor for a whole patient."

"Look," Phil interrupts, "they don't have to tell you how you feel; they need to explain *why* you feel so blue. They should sit down and try to get you out of it. You know you're depressed; but you don't know why you're depressed. You think, 'Jeez, I went through this terrible operaton, I really suffered, I ought to be feeling fine, but I'm feeling lousy. I hate myself, I hate my wife, I hate my doctors, I hate this hospital. What the hell did I have this operation for?' They shouldn't tell you cheerily, 'Buck up! Chin up!' Slap you on the back, and all that jazz. Most doctors are depressives, so depression in patients makes them run ten miles in the opposite direction. They're scared, but that doesn't help the patient. He's scared, too."

"You know all those valentines?" Bernice asks. "The ones saying, 'Love is from the heart'? There's a connection. You can't put your finger on it. You know your heart's not right; you're not right. You don't know how much depression is caused by the operation and how much is caused by medication. Mostly, around here, they give Inderal, which can cause depression. I wonder how many other doctor-given pills can carry depression as part of the baggage."

Which was worse, being the patient or being married to the patient?

"Being married to the patient," Bernice replies promptly. "I kept thinking, 'If Phil dies, what'll I do? I can't stand it.' "

More slowly, Phil reflects. "I'm not sure. I was afraid I'd die. I wanted Bernice well, but I never feared for her life. I've always known I'd die first."

Why?

"It's the way of the world."

What did Bypass do for each of you?

"Other than keeping me alive, not much," Bernice answers.

Phil shakes his head. "They talk about the 'quality of life.' Until the day I walked into the hospital with pericarditis, I wasn't handicapped. I did anything and everything. I'd never had a heart problem. I got tired a lot, I'd stopped working on the house, but I didn't have the faintest notion about heart trouble. Nothing's changed."

Despite your depression and memory loss following Bypass, would you be willing, if necessary, to have a second heart operation?

"Of course," Phil answers quickly. "Assuming it's better than the alternative: death. It's better than being crippled in a wheelchair."

Shall we hear from the opposition?

"I told Phil on the way over here, 'I don't know if I'd have it or not.' If I get a heart attack, I hope I'll have the good grace to drop over, and that'll be the end of it. If another attack means being an invalid, feeling bad, all alone somewhere, I don't know what I'd do. I don't like feeling bad. After Bypass, the back pain was horrendous. Every four hours, I'd have my rear in the air: I couldn't wait for the next morphine shot."

The aftermath of two Bypassers in the family is more fights?

"Five minutes later, I forget what we've fought about," Bernice says. "It has nothing to do with how much we love each other."

"The fighting doesn't mean we love each other less," Phil agrees. "But love doesn't mean I won't fight with her." He laughs a little. She edges closer to him on the small love seat, and tucks her hand under his arm.

After your Bypasses, did the doctors talk to you about sexual relations?

"It was never a topic of conversation," Phil replies. "I asked him, 'When can we resume?' He said, 'Whenever you feel like it.' It was a month or so, I guess."

"It wasn't long," Bernice interjects. "You started patting me on the rear in the hospital."

He laughs affectionately with her.

Maybe you fight because you like the making up so well.

Phil frowns and pulls away from Bernice. "There's very little making up. She's . . . ah . . ."

"That's been the one thorn in our marriage," Bernice notes.

"That's been *the* big thorn in our marriage," Phil corrects.

Quickly, Bernice says: "Before I got married, I never knew I didn't like sex."

How long after your Bypass, Mrs. Milard, did you wait to resume sexual relations?

"It's only been what? Twice a year," Bernice replies. "I know, I know, that's terrible. That's another of my guilts. I've felt bad about it for a long time."

Since the Bypass, are you less sexually responsive?

"When we were young, I didn't get anything out of sex. I worked very hard at it until finally I could achieve orgasms. To me, it's not worth all the bother. Which I've told Phil many times before. He's not hearing anything new."

And for you, it's worth 'the bother'?

"Oh, yeah," Phil says good-humoredly. "Did you ever know a man who thought it wasn't?" They both laugh, as though this is an old story. "That's another thing: if this God up there in His heaven had created men and women the way He should have, they'd *both* want it. Apparently, women don't have the same . . ." He laughs uneasily. "Oh, well, that has nothing to do with this."

"Phil would prefer the new generation of females to my generation. Most of the girls I know are like me. We were taught, 'Nice girls don't like sex.' "

"It's the way they were brought up, I guess," Phil muses.

"It's down there in the deep recesses of our minds," Bernice chatters nervously. "It's nothing we can overcome, no matter how much we understand or have self-diagnosed."

Since Bypass, do you feel more sexually deprived?

"It's always been a loss, a deprivation," Phil mourns.

"But more since Bypass," Bernice reminds him.

"We haven't done it *as much* since surgery, so it's one more big thing between us. I feel the loss more. Where can I find solace? What comfort is left for me? But I wouldn't blame it all on Bypass. It's only gotten worse since Bypass."

"Long before our Bypasses," Bernice says, "it was hard for me to say yes. Every time, I'd say to myself, 'Okay, I won't resent it. I won't hold it against him. I'll let him make out tonight, I'll make a point of it.' The year before my Bypass, every time I made up my mind to let him, I'd have angina, heart skipping, pain in my back, from apprehension." Bernice hesitates. "We have separate rooms. Sometimes, I've pushed myself all the way up the hall, stood outside his room, and thought, 'Okay, I'll be a nice wife. I'm going in to my husband. I'll force myself.' I'd stand there for twenty minutes, have palpitations, turn around, and go back to my room. I know. I probably need a psychiatrist; but he can't help me any more than I've been able to help myself."

Have you always slept in separate bedrooms?

"The last ten years. Phil was on the road for a whole year. We got used to sleeping apart. Every morning, he'd wake me. Putting on his clothes, bumping into my bed, asking me where things were, he'd wake me. I suggested he put on his clothes in the other room. When he refused, I moved into the other room. If he's asleep at night, I'd never put on the light to undress and waken him. If we slept together, that might help." She stops, plays with tiny pearls at her neck. "It's the truth. If we had that—you know, it would help. A good sexual relationship has to make married life easier."

"If it weren't for *that*, even with all our problems, we might have a happy marriage," Phil notes carefully.

Sometimes, just sleeping in the same bed is comforting.

"It wasn't," Bernice answers quickly. "We fought each other all night long. He was always pulling the covers off . . ."

"Being in the same bed probably would help."

"He likes the covers tucked in, and I like them all out." Spine rigid, she faces Phil defiantly. He shrugs, looks away.

Since your Bypasses, are you both feeling well?

Bernice purses her lips. "Okay, I guess."

"Most of the time," Phil observes, "I feel pretty good. I haven't had any angina—that I know of. Right after I came home, I went flying back in because of this terrible pain. They were afraid of more heart trouble, but they decided it was pleurisy."

"You had pneumonia, too," Bernice reminds him gently. "We worried."

Phil frowns. "I can't tell the difference between another heart attack and tension. I worry, I stew, I hem and haw. Finally, I have a cardiogram. When it's unchanged, I wonder if it's accurate." He forces a wan smile. "Lately, that pressure occurs less often. Time must be healing my fright—as well as my patched heart. I'm getting back to my normal preoperative state. But I'll never get back completely; I'll never have that blissfully ignorant peace of mind. You can't go home again, that's for sure. No one can. It's always 'afterwards.' " Twiddling his thumbs vigorously, he looks up half-smiling. Tears stream down his cheeks. "Other than these occasional love letters from my chest, I feel pretty good. I enjoy getting up in the morning, seeing the sun shine. Just living."

"You're fine till you get home."

"Yes," he agrees soberly, "fine until I get home." Suddenly, Phil puts his arm around Bernice. "That's not true either. The worst day of my life was when they came out of the cath lab from doing her angio. I'd expected her to have the cath, come home, and everything would be fine. Here she was, lying so small in that bed, being rushed to have a heart operation. That hit me hard."

"Nothing's ever come easy to me. Not even a Bypass. If I have a heart operation, my wife has it, too. I'm smart, but I have trouble learning. I work hard to grasp things, and poof! they disappear. I'm an engineer, a manager, yet I have to read and reread things three or four times to retain them. I'm a troubleshooter, a problem-solver. When the company sends me to solve a problem, everybody else sits back and relaxes: 'Let Phil do it.' My office is small; that isolates me from the big boardroom. I'm lousy at company politics. They're worse'n state politics, honestly. I have a terrible time carrying on a conversation about anything but my work. That's all I know.

"When I was thirty-eight, I was transferred from my hometown. I couldn't go and make new friends. We don't see our old friends any more, just gradually drifted apart. Their interests changed, ours changed. Every time I got promoted, friendships were broken. If I liked a guy from the company and the president didn't like him, well, we didn't dare be friends. What galls me is that some people don't work as hard as I do, yet they accomplish more, they make more money, climb the ladder higher. I'm a darn fool; I spend twelve to fourteen hours every day at that company. Before Bypass, it used to be more. No wonder I don't know how to talk to anybody. She's the fast talker." He points an accusing finger at his wife, draws away again. "I like to *think* before I speak. When people interrupt, that really gets me. What irritates me most is that parking lot at work. When I see people taking two and three places in the lot because they won't take time to park right or because they've got a fancy new car and don't want anybody getting close to them, I could clean their windshield with a sledgehammer!"

As suddenly as it erupted, Phil Milard's outburst subsides.

"Phil used to be so even-tempered. This impatience is only since Bypass. I don't know what to do when he starts spouting like this. That's one reason I'm depressed. Mostly, all these years, we looked forward to the next step, the next achievement. We had our children; we were building a home and a life. Now we don't have anything to look forward to. When we moved into this house, we were going to get another one or remodel in five years. It's twelve years."

"I didn't start making decent money until recently. A big chunk of that was taken away by Jason's tomfoolery. He's cost us not a small fortune but a large fortune. Medical expenses, tutors, damages."

Have you ever consulted a marriage counselor, a sex therapist, to help you with each other?

"I keep telling Phil, 'Let's run away from home.' "

"And I keep telling you," he says angrily, "I still have to work. We can't live on what we've put away. My pension is a joke. We've got to look after Jason, too. Maybe even Melanie. That's all part of it. We feel fine when we're not home."

"He worries all the time. I say, 'Why worry? We never had to seek out trouble. It's always known where to find us.' "

You both have a very strong sense of responsibility.

Phil and Bernice Milard lock arms. "They're our kids, we brought them into this world. If we don't take care of them, who will?"

18. John Boggs
Retired Army colonel, retired hospital administrator
Age at Bypass: 55

John Boggs is tall and cheerful, tanned, with an open face, wavy gray hair, deep-gray eyes, and a Cary Grant cleft in his chin. A one-time lawyer, he had served in the Army in World War II and remained in the reserves, so that when he was called back to go to Korea, he decided to stay in the Army. Finding the judge advocate's office "boring," he became a hospital administrator. When he retired as a colonel, he became a civilian hospital administrator, a job he hated. The job was "a pressure cooker": "I was working seventy or eighty hours a week. Everybody was jumping down my throat. I was smoking two packs of cigarettes a day. I had some money put by in good investments. I had my retirement pay from the Army. I was fifty-two then. Time to live a little. So I quit. But I didn't quit the weeds. The stresses were awful.

"Our son had had cancer of the colon, with lymph-node involvement and metastases to the lung. The guys at Walter Reed saved his life with all kinds of experimental monkey business. My son had chemotherapy and radiation therapy. But he lived. He's okay." John Boggs raps the coffee table. "It's six years now since he got sick. He finished medical school, is interning. He's a great guy."

Boggs's eyes mist a little. "I owe my life to my wife and son. It was he who got us gung ho on CPR.[1] Because if we had not been CPR instructors, I wouldn't be here.

"Jack had been at a medical meeting where the professor of anatomy had had a coronary. In a room full of doctors, not one of those guys knew CPR, not one of them knew what to do except call the ambulance, put his stethoscope on the guy's chest, and say, 'He's dead.' Nobody *did* anything. They just watched him die. Jack came home and said, 'You learn CPR. I don't want anything like that to happen to either of you.'

"We thought he was overreacting. He'd been through so much with this cancer, we'd been through so much with him; we were pleased he cared so much about us, and we wanted to please him. First we took the CPR courses. Then we became instructors. By then I was retired; we liked being active in the Red Cross here in Fort Lewis.

"A year after I quit my job, we went on a trip across country with my wife's folks. We were staying in a motel in Nowhere, Texas—literally. I'd never had any heart trouble, I'm not your typical heart patient.

"I never had chest pain, shortness of breath, any definable symptoms of heart trouble. My family, especially my mother's family, lives to their nineties. Lots of times, they're not so good upstairs, but you have to arrange a contract on them for their hearts to give out. Anyway, I woke up about five o'clock in the morning. I had this funny pain in my right chest and down my right arm. I've never had left-sided pain, never. I sat up on the side of the bed. Fortunately, my wife woke up because we had set the alarm for five. Army people like to get going early; we wanted to get on the road and beat the traffic.

"Mary opened her eyes and shut them again, murmuring, 'You okay?'

"For an answer—" John Boggs laughs loudly. Not hilariously: "I keeled over—on top of her, which was a good thing, because she was 99 percent asleep. She tried to do CPR on me on the bed, but it was too soft. Tugging and yanking at me, all 100 pounds of her, wringing wet, trying to lift 216 pounds of me, dead weight, she was pushing me on the floor. At that moment, her father came to

[1] Cardiopulmonary Resuscitation.

the door to check that we were up and getting ready for the drive. He helped Mary get me on the floor. Then she sent him to the office to call the ambulance.

"For twenty-five minutes, which is one helluva long time, Mary gave me CPR until the ambulance and the paramedics arrived. Her mouth was all swollen and bleeding, but she kept pumping that air into me. She couldn't get my heart started, but she maintained the flow of oxygenated blood to my brain. I had three more cardiac arrests on the way into the hospital: one more in the room and two in the ambulance. Luckily, those Texas ambulances have well-trained paramedics, usually guys who've served on the front lines in the Army. I'd trust them a lot more than any intern—but don't tell my son.

"I was unconscious for twenty-four hours, often a sign of major brain damage after cardiac arrest. When I awoke, I was scared shitless. I didn't know where I was or how I got there. I only knew that I wanted to get the hell out of there as fast as I could. Finally, I had to be restrained with a straitjacket and lots of sedation. I guess I settled down after a while, but my short-term memory was gone. I didn't recognize Mary until late that week. I'd ask her questions, she'd reply, then the next morning, I'd ask the same questions right over again. I remembered nothing about the trip to Texas. I still don't. I couldn't keep track of what day it was or what had happened to me. Mary eventually made a diary for me and added to it each day. It's funny. I couldn't remember things she'd told me, but I could remember where I'd put the diary. When she'd gone back to the motel, I'd get it out of the drawer, I'd look at it and say, 'Yup, today's Tuesday. Yesterday was Monday!' Reading the diary reinforced my memory and helped me get my bearings."

Calendars and diaries help people orient themselves in the hospital.

"After two weeks, they flew me back to Indiana with Mary as my medical escort. My gut and my old kit bag were packed full of drugs. I wasn't feeling much better, but they had to unload me. In Indianapolis, they stuck me in the CCU for 'further evaluation.' I had one arrhythmia after another. The chest pain was wild. The only way they could control the chest pain was with I.V. nitroglycerin. My head kept pounding like blazes the whole time from the nitro, but every time they'd cut back on the nitro, I'd have more angina and more arrhythmias, so there I was."

Why did you go back to Indianapolis? Why didn't you go to an Army hospital? Brooke in San Antonio was nearby, Walter Reed in Washington, Letterman in San Francisco, all have excellent, well-trained staffs. All give good care.

"I thought I was going to die. I figured it'd be too tough for Mary to get this carcass of mine home, too hard on her to stay in a strange city with me in the hospital. It was better to come home.

"They decided to do a cardiac catheterization. I could hear them talking about me outside my room. Y'know, doctors and nurses treat you as though you can't see and can't hear, and besides, what difference is it to you? I hated that cath. No, it didn't hurt, I didn't have that flushing feeling they warn you about. *I felt invaded, vulnerable, unnecessary.* Three vessels were blocked from 50 to 90 percent, but they couldn't figure out why I'd had all those cardiac arrests. As I lay on the cath table, one doctor said to another: 'Beats me why he arrested all those times. He's probably got Sudden Death syndrome.' All very reassuring.

"In any case, they recommended triple-bypass surgery for the end of May. The longer they waited for surgery, they explained, the better were my chances of surviving the operation. They didn't pull any punches about whether I'd survive or not. The trouble was my heart wouldn't cooperate with the doctors' plans. The continued arrhythmias and unstable angina made them decide to perform the surgery on an emergency basis. When I had another severe heart attack that Saturday morning, I was glad to be in a hospital where doctors will do Bypass on a Saturday. If I'd been in one of those stop-dead-on-weekend places, I might not have been here today.

"From that point, things moved like a house afire. I felt so miserable and discouraged that I didn't care what they did to me so long as something improved my condition. Suddenly four nurses descended on me and started shaving my whole body from my neck to my toes, all four grimly intent on what they were doing. Two weeks later, I discovered that they had missed the right armpit completely. For some strange reason, seeing this bush under my right arm struck me as hilariously funny. I looked in the mirror and laughed out loud for the first time since Texas.

"I signed the consent forms without reading them. Look, I'm a hospital administrator. I knew what the risks were and I didn't want to be reminded. Besides, a part of me felt so awful that I didn't care. One of the four nurse-shavers gave me an injection in the butt. I was wheeled to the operating room, where I met the surgeon for the first time, all decked out in his scrub suit with a small lamp affixed to his forehead. He introduced me to the anesthesiologist, who explained how he was going to put me under—but I didn't listen. He put a needle into my arm. Out I went.

"My first awareness that I was still alive occurred at about eleven o'clock the next morning when a group of people started yelling at me—at least, to me, they seemed as though they were yelling. For some reason, I refused to open my eyes. In fact, I'm not sure I could get my eyes open. I remember trying to open my eyes and feeling as though they were stuck shut. I tried to talk, but I couldn't. The endotracheal tube was still in place. I didn't know that the tube was keeping me from talking. I thought I had had a stroke. Nobody had told me about the tube beforehand.

"A woman's voice said, 'We're going to take you off the machine now and let you breathe on your own.' I nodded. I figured they'd do what they wanted anyway whether I 'consented' or not. Then she said, 'You're breathing on your own now.' We're going to take out your tubes and send you back to your room.' Again, I nodded. There were tubes and things in every orifice, and where nature had failed to put in an orifice, such as in my chest, the surgeon had carved out his own. The chest tubes were left in, but everything else came out without event, except for the endotracheal tube, which I was the most anxious to have removed. I felt so isolated because I couldn't talk. When I coughed while they were pulling it out, I paralyzed my vocal chords. I couldn't speak above a whisper for a month. What's a lawyer doing whispering? I think that they were afraid I'd institute malpractice proceedings, the way they pussyfooted around that month. But malpractice suits were the last thing on my mind. I was so tired of hospitals.

"Much to my surprise, after they took out the tubes, they placed me in a wheelchair and wheeled me to a room on a general nursing floor. My wife and son were waiting for me. Boy, were they shocked to see me sitting up after less than twenty-four hours since having Bypass! So was I!"

John Boggs stretches his long legs, locks his knobby hands in back of his head.

"I'd begun to think I was out of the woods. For five days after the operation, I seemed to be improving. I was delighted. On the fifth day, I had another heart attack, which depressed me so; I was ready to give up the ghost. They transferred me back to the CCU and monitored me closely. The medical resident suggested that it might be necessary to perform another cardiac catheterization. I refused; he was much miffed. 'It's just to satisfy your own medical curiosity,' I told him. 'Even if there were another blockage, I'm sure they wouldn't try surgery again so soon, and I'm very sure that I wouldn't let them.' Afterwards, I could hear the resident fretting and fuming to an attending, a doctor closer to my age, who probably felt fear for himself as well as concern for me. The older doctor told the young one to drop it.

"This last MI was a blessing in disguise—or so I like to think. It apparently 'killed' that part of my heart causing the arrhythmias and the unstable angina. After a few days in the CCU, I went back to my regular room in the cardiac wing. From there on, my recovery was rapid, I started a gradual walking program within the hospital, followed by an exercise stress test. Finally, thirty-two days after the operation, I was discharged. What a relief!

"My greatest complaint, pain-wise, was with my legs. Except for that first sneeze, my chest gave me very little grief, but, oh, how my legs ached! My ankles were swollen continually. They still swell. Both of my legs were incised because the surgeon could not get enough vein from one leg alone." He rolls up his pantleg and shows me his scar.

Now John Boggs is back working in his garden, woodworking, carving chess tables and duck decoys, back teaching CPR. "For her actions in saving my life, my wife received the American Red Cross Certificate of Merit, their highest award, signed by President Reagan, and presented by our local congressman. Had it not been for her cool head, skillful, never-say-die application of CPR, I wouldn't be sitting here talking to you today—unless you've got a special WATS line to the nether regions, because they sure as hell wouldn't have sent me anyplace else.

"I speak about what she did to every group that asks me. I'm the best living example I know of the benefits of CPR."

Does it bother you to talk about it?

"Not usually. It bothers Mary, though. You know, this winter I've started having angina again, just on the right side of my throat. At first, I thought it was yard work and too much swimming, but then I noticed that when I stopped doing too much, it stopped. That's been a real disappointment. After all we went through, I thought we had the angina licked. I've been trying to prepare Mary that she's going to have a lot of years as a widow, that she'll be living without me—unless she gets hit by a bus or run over by a car. Mary won't accept the idea of living without me. That worries me about her."

Maybe that's why she kept going for twenty-five minutes with the CPR.

"Probably." His face clouds over. "Since you called me, I've been thinking about what I'd say to you. The biggest question I have to ask myself is, 'Have I changed since all this?' " His hearty laugh fades hollowly. "No one can experience that kind of trauma and still be the same. I've accepted my mortality—even if Mary has not. I don't fear death. I think. I've been there—and back. I tend not to put off things I want to do, and to put off things I don't want to do. I'm less inhibited and more outspoken than before. I'm proud of my children. I love my wife—and we have fun together. I sure as hell am not about to get into an argument with her. After all, she's my oxygen. She's my lifeline."

And the operation? Would you have another if it were recommended?

"Maybe. I'd have to wait until I was in real trouble before I'd consent to go through that again. But I don't want to be a cardiac cripple, skinny and hunched over, shuffling around with purple lips . . ." He stands up and imitates his idea of "a typical cardiac cripple of fifteen years ago." Sitting down again, his face grows grim. "This angina scares me. You wake up in the night and you don't know if you've got some arthritic pains or if it's your heart.

The pain's on the left side so you say to yourself, 'It can't be my heart. My pain is always right-sided.' Then you wonder, 'What if my pain is beginning to be left-sided chest pain?' You go around in circles. That doesn't help the stress any." He stops, looks searchingly at me: "Do you know CPR?"

I'm afraid not.

"I thought so. Whether you know it or not, you've just signed a pact with me. In exchange for this little talk, when you go home, go enroll yourself in a CPR course at the Red Cross. Not just Bypassers go into cardiac arrest from ventricular fibrillation. Sometimes, even people who never knew they had heart trouble have their ventricles freak out. If your heart stops, it's a crying shame if nobody can administer CPR and they stand around watching you die. Better to administer CPR than last rites. In Seattle, bystanders gave early CPR and twice as many people lived. And the life saved may be your own. Ask me. I was there. Is it a deal? Will you learn CPR?"

It's a deal.

"And every year"—his smile dims—"as long as I'm around, I'll write you a note to have a CPR refresher course."

And every year, John Boggs has sent his little CPR reminder.

19. Kevin McDonough
Time-study supervisor
Age at Bypass: 36

Kevin McDonough is broad-shouldered, with a round face, short brown hair, and a bushy brown mustache. Looking younger than his thirty-nine years, in jeans and sneakers, a cotton sport shirt, and a red plaid mackinaw, he shakes my hand hard and sits down heavily on the black vinyl sofa. In a strangely old voice softened by an Oklahoma twang, he tells me he's a time-study supervisor at a local factory. "Before Bypass, I was in a managerial position, moving right up. When I came back, my old job was gone. I was working toward my pension, so I took what I could get. It's better'n shift work. Jobs are tight here in Kenosha."

How did all this happen? How did you come to Bypass?

"It started in November '81. One night I went to a fifties dance. Trying to relive my teen-age years, I made a fool of myself. I danced all night, drank like crazy, smoked two packs of cigarettes. The next morning I had terrible heartburn, or what I thought was terrible heartburn. Through the week it got worse and worse, started radiating down both my arms. I didn't pay any attention to what aggravated it. Looking back, I realize when I'd walk from the parking lot into work, it'd hurt so bad I could hardly stand it. As soon as I got to my desk, sat down, put my feet up, and relaxed, it'd go away. By Wednesday it had got so bad, I went to Medical. I told them, 'I'm having awful pressure in my chest and pains down my arms.' They did an EKG. The doctor said, 'It's fine. A hiatus hernia could cause these symptoms.' Then he made a statement no doctor should make: 'I can guarantee you it's not your heart.' He really set my mind at ease. But the pain didn't get any better. He gave me some antacids, which didn't help. They seemed to make it worse. Finally I said, 'To heck with this.' I left work early for the first time in twenty years.

"Thursday, I called a new doctor in our area. When I told the secretary I wanted an appointment, she didn't ask me why. Secretaries should ask. Nicely, not snippily. She gave me an appointment for Saturday. The next morning the pain was real bad, so I called the doctor's and said, 'I can't wait till tomorrow.' The girl said, 'We have a cancellation for eleven-fifteen; you can see him then.' About ten o'clock I thought I'd better take a shower before I saw the doctor. My mother always said, 'You should be clean for the doctor.' As I walked upstairs to the second-floor landing, it was like an invisible person was hiding and hit me across the chest with a baseball bat. Oh, I had the worst pain and pressure! It almost knocked me down. I staggered back, hit the wall, rolled across the floor into my bedroom, and fell across the bed. The burning was radiating right up my chest and down my arms.

"For a few minutes, I lay there. I remember looking at the clock. When I hit the bed, it was two minutes past ten. That time will stick in my mind forever. To make it even worse, it was Friday the thirteenth. I propped myself up with pillows. During that week, if I used pillows, the pain seemed to go away a little bit. But this pain wasn't going anyplace. It kept getting worse.

"I'll never know why I did what I did next. My father died when I was an infant. He'd had a heart attack at thirty-four—and just died. I never knew my father. I was only four months old when he died. I never think about my father or what my life would've been like had he lived; but I lay in that bed and talked out loud to my father. Even when I was a child, I never talked to him. As I lay there with this awful pain, I kept begging him, 'Please don't let me die. Please, please don't let me die.' I knew I was going to die,

I was sure I would die. I started praying out loud, I started crying, all the time talking away to my father, 'Don't let me die.'

"I broke out in a cold, clammy sweat. I tried to get out of bed, because I knew I had to get to the doctor, but I couldn't move. I couldn't raise my arms. They felt like they weighed a ton. I couldn't get up, but I knew I had to. Finally, out loud to myself, I said, 'Kevin, if you don't get out right now, you are going to lie here and die.' I threw myself off the bed and rolled onto the floor. Because I couldn't stand up, I crawled over to the phone. The phone was unplugged. I was so panicky, I didn't realize I could plug it in. I crawled and rolled out the bedroom door. As I grabbed the stair rail and tried to stand up, I had so much pressure and pain that I couldn't stand. I sat down and slid down the stairs on my butt. When I got to the bottom, I crawled to the front door, grabbed the doorknob, and pulled myself up. Somehow I got the door open and staggered out to my car. I drove to the doctor's office. I don't know how I got there, how I missed having an accident. I knew the doctor was my only chance.

"When I walked in, I must've looked like death warmed over, because the girl said, 'My gosh, what's the matter?' I couldn't talk, but I clutched my chest. She took my blood pressure on my right arm. She looked puzzled, and took it on the left arm. I wanted to say, 'Get the doctor, please get the doctor,' but I couldn't talk. I heard her holler, 'Doctor, come quickly.'

"The next thing I remember, I was on a table. He was standing over me and reading an EKG strip. Knowing he was there, I felt better. I said, 'It's my heart, isn't it?' He said, 'You're having a heart attack. You'll be all right. I've called an ambulance. We'll take you to the hospital. You'll be in Intensive Care for a few days, then everything will be fine.' I remember telling him, 'Call my wife, but don't tell her I've had a heart attack because she'll panic.' The nurse put nitroglycerin under my tongue. It helped a lot. I remember them putting me in the ambulance and taking me to the hospital, but I've lost the next four days.

"Sheila, my wife, said they were shooting morphine in me every twenty minutes. I'd tell her I didn't want to see the kids because I didn't want them to see me like this. Then I'd say, 'Where are they? Get them up here.' I'd say, 'I want my mom. She knows what this is like.' To this day I can't remember my mother being there even though I talked to her. I told her, 'You raised five of us all by yourself. You worked as a seamstress. You made a life for us with a lot of love and a little money. You'd never marry or see any man. It was only us kids. You should tell Sheila how to do it.'

"When I got home from the hospital, my family doctor sent me to a cardiologist. He examined me and set up a stress test several weeks later in his office. Around here, everything takes a long time to get done. During the stress test I started having bad angina. He gave me a nitro and asked me if I could continue. 'Sure,' I said. I went the full nine minutes. I was determined I'd do it. I was exhausted. But I had to prove I could go the stress test's entire nine minutes. After I got off the treadmill, I lay down. He said, 'How're ya doin'?' I said, 'Fine,' sat up to show him how fine I was, and passed out. He said, 'Kevin, I don't like what I see. I want you to have an angiogram.' They couldn't get an angiogram appointment for another month. I went home and was having chest pains all the time. I was taking nitroglycerin like crazy. They'd told me to walk, to exercise. Every time I walked, the bitter cold air would make the angina worse."

Did anybody tell you to walk in a shopping mall?

"No. I was so dead on my feet, I didn't think of it. I had no strength. Before the heart attack, I'd always been an active guy. Suddenly I was a weak old man. Anyway, the month wore itself out. Even before the angio I knew I needed Bypass. I know the look. I know the stories people told me. Something had to be done. After the angio, the cardiologist set me up with a cardiac surgeon at Community Hospital. Funny, he didn't know which member of the surgical group would be operating on me."

Did you like your surgeon?

"No."

Why?

"The man never talked to me until the day before Bypass. I didn't like their attitude, any of them, the whole group. I'd been put in the hospital ten days ahead of schedule. The cardiologist thought I could be managed on medicine until the end of June, when they had an opening. I wonder if they move any faster for big shots than for guys like me. He had me on more drugs than a junky. Despite all his pills, one night, just watching TV, I started getting real bad chest pains. It took eight nitros to make them go away."

Did your cardiologist ever tell you how many nitros to take before calling him?

"Yes, but I didn't want to call. I kept thinking, 'Just one more nitro and the pain'll be gone.' After two nitros, if the pain still hung around, I was supposed to call, but I didn't want to bother anybody. I was afraid they'd stick me back in the hospital. The next morning I had a regular appointment with Dr. Eugene, my family doctor. When I told him about the night before, bingo! I was on my way into the Emergency Room. Those surgeons came in and out; I just didn't like their attitudes. They paraded around there like they were some kind of tin gods, especially Dr. Shah, my surgeon. He walked in and said, 'I'm Dr. Shah. I'm going to do your surgery tomorrow. I'm here to tell you what are your chances of living. You're a young man, but you've had a lot of damage. You've got between 80 and 90 percent chance of living through the operation. Any questions?'

"I said, 'I don't know what this operation involves. Can you explain it? Tell me which arteries are blocked. Why do I have this? I'm a young man.'

"He said, 'We'll go into your chest, we'll see exactly how bad your heart is, we'll see how much of the blockage we can Bypass, and we'll do it.' That's all he said. I just didn't like him. Period. He's an excellent surgeon. I thank the man for my life, but I don't care for him."

How did you do after Bypass?

"Excellent. They did four Bypasses. They'd wanted to do five but one was too small. You always wonder about the one that got away, but they said not to worry. I recovered fast. By Tuesday morning at 6:00 A.M., when my wife stopped by on her way to work, I was sitting up drinking a cup of coffee. Seven days later I walked out of there. I wanted to leave after four days. They wouldn't let me.

A friend of mine recommended a new rehab program at St. Joseph's Hospital. That's been great."

To what did you attribute your heart problems and need for Bypass?

"Mainly heredity. I couldn't do anything about my genes. At St. Joseph's they talk about risk factors. My cholesterol count was up. My work was stressful. I'd gone thorugh a tough divorce. We're happy in this marriage, but this setback with my heart has been hard on us.

"Since the Bypass, money's been tight. A year after our marriage, we'd fought a huge custody battle for my five children. We won, but the adjustment's been hard on my wife, because she's only twenty-four. Life at home is stressful, but the main stress was at work. I worked seven days a week in a small satellite lab. As a first-line supervisor, I was responsible for a lot of work from very few people. We worked under deadlines all the time because we dealt with fresh information on products. On the double, they needed to know—bam!—'Was it good?' The other two bosses didn't give a damn, didn't care whether the work got done or not. I'm not like that. I care. I was trying to carry their load as well as mine. I couldn't stand their goofing off."

After Bypass, did you review your life and its course?

"Bypass changed my life. It slowed me down, made me stop and smell the roses. When my wife drove me home from the hospital, we drove past the factory. I saw the smoke coming out of the chimney, even though I hadn't been to work in months. That smoke made me stop and think, 'Hey, those guys don't need me. They'll manage.' I appreciate my family more. I don't worry like I did before; let someone else worry. I don't even worry too much about the bills. I'm making less money now. It doesn't bother me in an ego sense, not in the least. But it sure bothers me at the end of the month."

Does it bother you that your job has less status?

"Changing jobs, my doctor said, was the only way I'd live to be an old man. That's ironic because *he* died. He was a runner training for a marathon. Early one morning, he was running beside the lake and he was hit. I cried so. That man was only forty. I tell you, I miss him more than my best friend. When I got to his office, if he hadn't been there, I wouldn't be here today. Literally, he saved my life. He wasn't a stiff doctor, he was such a nice man."

Did you ever write his family and tell them?

"Just the other day I thought about it. I figured I'd let them get over it. What's the use of writing them a letter? It won't bring him back."

Did Bypass make you aware of things you wish you'd done with your life?

"Oh, yeah. I wish I'd spent more time with the children as they were growing up. I'd always thought about what's best for my wife and children, not me, but when you work a seven-day shift, you're busy all the time. You keep thinking about what you need to get done. When you go on at midnight, you need to get chores done in the afternoon, so you don't see the kids. When you're on the afternoon shift, you're at work when they come home from school. When you come home from work, they're in bed. Before you know it, the chance at a life with them is gone. They're grown. You're left behind.

"Bypass helped me with family life. Now, I work like a normal person and get off at four in the afternoon like the rest of the people. We go cross-country skiing. We all go to the Y for exercise programs. Before Bypass, if you'd said, 'Join the Y,' I'd have said, 'You've got to be kidding. I don't have time.' Now I have all kinds of time. I want to do things while I have time."

Did Bypass make you feel old?

"Hell, no. It made me feel young."

Did it make you more aware of your own mortality?

"You better believe it. Not so much Bypass as the heart attack. When I went in for Bypass, I knew I might not wake up. I wasn't the least bit afraid."

You said Bypass changed you. Tell me some of the ways.

"I don't smoke. I exercise. I enjoy my family. My fuse is a helluva lot longer than before."

Did you have a short fuse?

"I'd let things boil, but, boy, when that fuse was lit, you'd better look out. I'd fume inside, but nobody would know until I erupted. I've broken a couple of noses in my day. What got to me before doesn't irritate me any more. I won't let stuff aggravate me."

Before Bypass, did you have any preoperative fantasies or nightmares?

"Not before the Bypass, but before the angiogram. Aw! I feared that more than anything. I have a terrible fear of needles. They'd told me I'd be awake, that they'd put Novocaine in my leg. I didn't care what they did to me afterwards but, man, don't stick that Novocaine needle in my leg! For weeks I worried constantly about that needle. When they took me down to that cath lab, I was so nervous. The nurse held my hand and said, 'Kevin, what's the matter with you?' I said, 'I'm scared to death.' She said, 'About what?' I said, 'You're going to laugh at me, but I'm afraid of the needle for the Novocaine.' She just smiled and said, 'Don't worry. Lots of people are.'

"She told the doctor; I couldn't catch what he said, but she told me, 'I'll make you feel better.' She injected something in my arm, my head started swimming, and I took off into outer space. When I came back down, the doctor said, 'Can I give you the shot now?' I said, 'Give me anything you want.' He said, 'I already did.' After that, everything was fine. In hospitals, nurses save you. I'm on a campaign for nurses. They're underpaid and overworked."

Since Bypass, how well have your family and friends stood by you, given you support?

"My family was great. Is great. They're really on me about taking care of myself. Up North here we don't have any real close friends. My first wife drove away all our friends. Since I've been married to this wife, it's tough to make friends because of our age difference.

Her friends are her age. They accept me, but they're just not close. Fifteen years is more than you think. She's a kid. I'm not."

Before you went home from the hospital, who talked to you about when you could drive, resume sexual relations, go back to work?

"I don't remember, because lately sex is a problem for us. Since Bypass, I have absolutely no desire for sex."

Before Bypass, how was your sexual drive?

"I've never been like those guys you read about who want it five nights a week. I didn't even want it once a week. Really."

What about your wife?

"Being as young as she is, yes, there's lots of times when she makes the first move. I think, 'Aw, God, I'm dead. I'm so tired, I want to get to sleep.' After six months, I spoke with the cardiologist. By then, Dr. Eugene was dead." McDonough blows his nose fiercely. "The cardiologist said, 'Kevin, it's right here,' and tapped my head. 'There's nothing wrong with you. You're afraid something will go wrong, that you'll strain yourself during intercourse. Nothing will happen. It's okay.' He didn't recommend a counselor or a psychiatrist. He's a good man, but he's cold. He just said, 'You're going to have to work this out for yourself.' I guess he couldn't help me. I said, 'Why am I doing this?' He said, 'I've seen this problem in many of my patients, more after heart attack than after Bypass. Usually, people are better after Bypass.' Subconsciously, I'm afraid. The more I stay away, the more afraid I get."

Would you like to see a psychiatrist or a sex counselor?

"This disturbs my wife more than anything. Before we got married, we discussed children. She didn't want any children of her own. She only wanted my five children to raise. They were fairly well grown anyhow, so raising my children wasn't so tough. *Now* she's decided she wants a baby. I can't have children. Before we were married, I had a vasectomy. After discussing kinds of birth control, we decided on a vasectomy. *Now* she wants me to have it reversed.

Our big arguments are about this. I love kids, I'd love a dozen more, but I'm not going through an operation like *that* again. No more operations for me! I suggested artificial insemination. I said, 'This would be as much my child as yours. Absolutely. I wouldn't even think about it not being my own child.' Finally, she agreed. Next week we're seeing some doctor, I don't even know his name, about artificial insemination. She made the appointment . . ."

In a handful of American hospitals, there's a psychiatrist or a psychologist as a member of the team. Would such counseling have helped you?

"If the counselor were good, yes. It's not like I had such problems, I had doubts. Fear of the unknown is number one. Nobody knows how his body's gonna react. Even now, if I'm sitting there quietly and, aw, God, I get chest pain, right away I start thinking, 'What's going on?' When I was in the hospital, I saw three guys who'd had Bypass three years before going back under the knife again. It bothered the hell out of me. Even in the hospital, I kept thinking, 'God, in three years, will I have to go through this again?' "

If you needed a second Bypass, would you have it?

"I'd have to, wouldn't I?"

Would you go to the same doctor and the same hospital?

"He's a bastard, but he fixed me up. I'd go to him, but I'd hate his guts."

What did the operation do for you?

"Gave me a chance to live. If I hadn't had Bypass, I wouldn't have lived very long."

How long do you want to live?

"Forever."

What was the worst part of Bypass?

"That damn tube. I wanted to breathe for myself. When I'd breathe on my own, I'd inhale a little bit; then the thing would kick on and make me inhale even more. I had a heck of a time. The nurse came over and said, 'Quit fighting the respirator. Let it do the work.' I hated that tube."

After Bypass, were you depressed?

"After the heart attack, I was very depressed. Not after Bypass."

Since Bypass, have you had memory loss?

"The memory loss is rotten. It goes from bad to worse. The cardiologist said, 'It should go away.' To begin with, my memory was never great. It's hard for me to concentrate, to get my mind on what I'm doing. What bugs me more'n anything else is when I'm talking to you and all of a sudden my mind goes blank. I can't remember what I was saying. That bothers the hell out of me. The doctor said, 'After six months, it lifts.' He may be right. It's easing off, but it aggravates the hell out of me. I wish I'd known about these lapses and that they'd go away. I wish somebody who'd been through it had sat down and talked to me. Since my Bypass, I'd have been happy to sit down with any guy facing a heart operation. Nobody ever asked me.

"Let me tell you what I'd tell people. I had a terrible fear of hospitals. I thought a hospital is the place to go to die. I hate hospitals. Anyway, what was I saying? You'd hate hospitals a lot less if you knew what to expect. But I never knew how I was going to feel. I didn't anticipate I'd lose my sex drive. I didn't expect this memory loss.

"Even so, I feel better today than I have in ten years. This probably has been building up for an awful long time. Physically, I'm taking care of my body because I feel better and I want to go on feeling better. I'm exercising. If you exercise, you feel better. Mentally, I feel better because I don't worry about the factory. To hell with them. There's 65,000 people working there. Let the other 64,999 worry. Not me. They don't pay me enough money to fret about their quality control. They didn't pay me enough before either, but I stewed because it was my job. No more."

Since Bypass, is your marriage better, the same or worse?
"Much better. That's why I don't understand my lack of desire."

When did your wife decide she wanted a baby?
"The year before Bypass."

Was that a stress?
"No, but we had some wing-ding fights. When I had the heart attack, I began telling myself, 'Hey, if you don't start taking care of yourself, brother, you're not gonna be here, not for your kids, not for your wife, not for anybody.' Bypass was the major step in beginning to take care of myself. I know guys who had Bypass; some still take Mason jars of heart medicine. Since I came out from under the knife, I haven't taken a pill. I'm not even taking aspirin." McDonough's face darkens. "I don't understand about the aspirin. Almost every Bypassed guy I know takes aspirin, and what's that other stuff—Persantine? Nobody told me to take anything.

"When I went for Bypass I wanted them to video-tape my operation; they wouldn't do it. Said it wasn't allowed. If they could do it on TV, they could do it with a little video camera."

Why did you want it video-taped?
"I love seeing stuff like that. To me, it's interesting as hell. They did it on me; I wanted to see it."

Since Bypass, do you and your wife go out more, less, the same?
"I told you, we don't have that many friends. We used to go out to dinner, but we can't afford it. We're strapped right now. We're hurting. I'm not ashamed to say it. I had a helluva setback going from $750 a week to $500 a week. People keep calling us. That chews me up inside to have these damn people call: 'You're a week

late with a payment.' Hell, if they'd leave me alone, I'd pay 'em as soon as I can. *I don't have the money."*

That's tough.

"I can understand why they have to call. It's their job. Look, I can't complain. My cup's overflowing. Right now, I can't get enough of life. For the first time, I realized I could've lost it so easily. I almost did lose it. I love life, I love going to work, I love coming home. If they call, so they call. I wouldn't want to change and be someone else."

If you'd been William Schroeder, would you have done what he did?

"The man didn't have any choice—if he wanted to live. He was taking a big chance, but he's a pioneer. If I could be a pioneer, I'd be one tomorrow. Look at those people who had Bypasses in the early days. They were pioneers, too."

If and when William Schroeder gets better, he'll be tethered to a machine.

"He isn't dead, is he?"

Do you think your behavior had anything to do with your heart attack?

"Plenty. The way I lived, the way I acted, had a lot to do with it."

All of us have insecurities. What are yours?

"Only financial insecurity. Otherwise, I'm not insecure about anything. I'm me; I can't be you or anyone else. I can't live anyone's life but mine. I don't let things bother me. I took rehab therapy with guys who didn't like that scar to be seen by anybody, not even us other guys with the same scar! To me, that's insecure. I can't help it that I'm scarred for life. That scar is a sign boasting, 'Hey, look at me, I'm fine now.' I go to the Y. I walk right into that pool with my bathing trunks on. Everybody looks. Kids even have asked me what happened. At one of my son's baseball games, I had on shorts and a kid asked me, 'Hey, Mister, what happened to your leg?' I have four individual scars on my leg instead of one long one. I told the kid, 'A polar bear attacked me.' He thought that was great. 'Jeez, I never met anybody,' he said, 'who fought a bear.' "

In a way you did fight a bear.

"You're damn right I did. But now that it's over, it wasn't so bad. My life's better. I don't keep inside what burns me. I never in my life sent back food not cooked to my liking. I do now. I'm not trying to carry more'n my load at work.

"I have only one dream I'd like to come true. It's stupid, but it's not stupid. I'm a country boy and I love country music. My favorite group in the whole world is the Statler Brothers. I would give anything to be able, just once, to get up on the stage with those guys and sing!

"As for the rest of my life, today might seem bad, but tomorrow morning I won't even remember what happened yesterday. Why worry about it? I hate my job, I hate making less money, but now that we've cut down on going out, once we get paid off, we'll be able to live on what we're making. I wish the surgeon had settled for what Blue Shield paid him, but he didn't. Blue Shield only allowed 80 percent of his fee. He keeps dunning me for the rest. We'll get it paid. How do other Bypassers manage their bills?"

There are support groups, like Mended Hearts, where Bypassers can meet and compare notes even on balancing their reduced budgets.

"I wouldn't like that. I don't want to dwell on my heart operation. I don't want it to be such a part of my life that I go to heart meetings all the time. What I'd love to do is go to Community Hospital and talk to people who're gonna go through Bypass in the next couple of days. When I was laid up there in that hospital, I had no idea what it was going to be like. And nobody told me. I'm sure people are up there right now thinking the same thoughts, worrying the same worries. If I went up there, I could sure put them at ease, because I feel like a million bucks." He frowns. "I just don't want another baby."

20. Bill Doell
Advertising executive
Age at Bypass: 54

Bill Doell is a red-faced Irishman, with white curly hair, bushy golden-white brows, bright-blue eyes, and a cherubic smile. Dressed in a gray silk suit, with a blue chambray shirt and a brown-and-blue Countess Mara tie, he looks like a sartorially splendid teddy bear. On hearing that his name and address, even his occupation, will be fictionalized, he laughs. "The way business is going, I'd as soon you changed it, before I do. But let me stay in Rockville."

What's your occupation?

"Advertising."

What's your title?

"Senior vice-president."

Do senior V.P.s have one account or many?

"Since Bypass, I've whittled it down to one account. Pierce-Arrow. It's a good account, but the automobile business has seen better times. They've been my account for the past ten years."

Then you've seen better times, too?

"Over the years I've had a lot of automotive accounts."

If you had your life to live over, would you have been an advertising man?

"I sure would. For the first ten years after college, I was an automobile dealer. Because I got so interested in automobile advertising, I went into the advertising business. If I'd had my life to live over, I'd have eliminated the first ten years. I've always loved this advertising game, because that's what it is for me: a game, which I've played well, and which has been good to me."

How did you learn you needed Bypass?

"I had no pain at all, just some chest pressure and shortness of breath for two or three years. It got so bad that I decided to quit smoking. I quit for eighteen months, and then started my three packs a day again, as though I'd never stopped. When I was so short of breath, I quit again on a business trip to Mexico. Even on the beach at Ixtapa, I'd have to stop walking and fabricate some reason so nobody would know I was so winded.

"When I got back from Mexico, I tried to walk the ten blocks from the Metro to the office; I had to stop three times for breath. I got to the office, I called my wife and told her, 'Get me an appointment with Dr. Cheeft. I'm coming right home.' By then, I thought, 'Maybe I have angina. My father had it.' I always remember him with the little nitroglycerines in his pocket. I saw Dr. Cheeft; the next thing I knew I was in Intensive Care. After they got me stabilized, they sent me home.

"Like a bad penny, I turned up in the Emergency Department, in trouble again. This time, they decided they'd better find out what was wrong in there. They did a stress test, the only test I've ever flunked. Took thirty seconds to put me on the ropes. During the catheterization, I knew I was in trouble, because instead of the promised forty-five minutes, I was in there for two hours.

"That night, they came up to my hospital room and said, 'We've got good news and bad news.' " Doell laughs uproariously. " 'The bad news is you're lethal, really lethal, and you need surgery immediately. The good news is we think you're a surgical candidate.' My wife said, 'If he needs surgery, I want God in the operating room; no lesser archangels will do.' They said, 'We'll make arrangements for you to go anyplace you want, Texas, Boston, Milwaukee, Cleveland, but we happen to have God right here in this hospital.' I wondered if they were being arrogant; now I'm convinced they were right. Dr. Rogers came in and talked to me for an hour. He said, 'You're sick enough for me to operate tomorrow, but I want to give your heart a day's rest. I'll operate the day after.' I waited one day and then I got Bypassed."

You never went home?

"By the time the experts finished talking to me, I was a little concerned about moving in bed. They told my wife, 'Until the Bypass, feed him.' The only time I moved was to get up and take those three showers."

Did stresses or your responses to stresses intensify in the year before Bypass?

"Sure they did. The automobile business was atrocious. Now that I've made my mark, I'm in this business for fun as much as anything else. My clients have become friends. Seeing what these automobile dealers were going through, trying to find the nonexistent magic bullet, the cure for their financial cancer, was stressful, even though it was harder on them than on me. Then, my wife's kid brother was killed in a car accident; she had been very close to him. And . . ." Doell pauses, "in the past, I've had some tough deals which sometimes come back to haunt me in the night."

Such as?

"Back in the war, my war, World War II, I was a fighter pilot and was shot down. I was a prisoner of war in Germany for eighteen months. Then, I was president of a big ad agency. The CEO owned 60 percent of the stock and sold it. There was fraud involved. Within a year after the sale, the agency went bankrupt. It cost me about half a million dollars. I'd just been divorced. I'd made a bad first marriage, one of those war marriages. Supposedly, we stayed together for the children. By the time I was divorced and the ad agency went kaput, I ended up with a four-year-old Mustang and my clothes. I had to start all over again. Because of the bankruptcy and because I'd been president of the agency, my salary was published. Everybody said, 'We can't afford you. You're too experienced, overqualified.'

"It was two or three years before I found an agency willing to give a fifty-two-year-old guy a chance. Even though its causes are pretty much gone, the stress remains in the wings. Strangely, this monkey business didn't start till two years later when I'd gotten things squared away. It was as though it was stored up, waiting to pounce. I'd married Valerie. Things with her are as good as the other was bad. An unbelievably great marriage." Doell stretches his long legs, and laughs comfortably. "In the tradition, I s'pose, of second marriages where you're longer on tolerance and shorter on the back of your hand."

Do you have children?

"That's my one regret. I had three children, but only one sees me. Since the divorce, only Danny is my friend. Even he stayed away for the first year. Now, we go sailing together. Val has two daughters; they're daughters to me. I've a grandchild I've never seen. It's painful, but not painful. I don't dwell on past history."

When you learned you needed Bypass, what did you think caused your heart trouble?

"A combination of things. First, I'd been a heavy smoker. I always thought, 'Someday, I'll die of lung cancer.' I never thought about what smoking does to the arteries. And I went right on smoking. Second, diet. When I came out of that prison camp, I weighed 120 pounds. I began eating, and I've been eating ever since. I've been fighting the battle of the bulge ever since I stopped fighting the real Battle of the Bulge. I'm like my father. I love to dine. I don't like to eat a meal and call it quits. I thoroughly enjoy dining. I love to go out to dinner. Other than squid, there isn't a single food I don't like. I eat lots of rich foods. I've lost twenty-five pounds, and I've another fifteen to go, but it's murder. My family history's good. Mother died at seventy-four, of heart, but it was a pretty good age. Dad lived to eighty-four, eating nitro pills for as long as I can remember. At eighty-four, he was as young-thinking and spry as some people my age. I'm an only child with no cousins, so there's nobody in my generation to compare notes with."

When you were told you needed Bypass, how did you feel?

"Nervous, apprehensive, and relieved. At last, we'd zeroed in, now we knew what's wrong and could fix it, instead of all my self-diagnosis. Val's a young girl. She's five years older than my Dan. I wanted to be made young again for her."

You found out very suddenly. What helped you?

"Number one, I'm extremely happily married. I had fantastically perceptive, intelligent support from my wife. No histrionics, just calm confidence. Second, I've been so lucky in my choice of doctors. It was dumb luck, but they've been so personally interested. I never felt I was a number on the docket. They made me feel, 'These people are looking out for *me*, not for some patient in the hall.' Everybody in my business has one of these zippers. They say, 'Where did you have yours done? Texas? Milwaukee? Cleveland? Boston?' When I tell them about my community hospital here, they're stunned. I'm not knocking those other places, but nobody else got the special care I did, care from the heart."

Are you on any medication?

"After the surgery, my blood pressure went up. The doctor put me on a beta blocker, which wiped me out. I couldn't work, I couldn't think, I couldn't make love. And if I could, I didn't want to. Finally, I complained to the doctor. He said, 'Let's see what you do without it.' I bought one of those little machines; I take my blood pressure twice a day. It's fine. Right now, I'm only on Persantine and aspirin. I take three of each a day, because they're supposed to keep the Bypass open. So far, so good."

After Bypass, did you become more irritable?

"I'm getting over it. I'm still a little irritable, but nowhere near as cranky as before. That first month, I was a bastard." Doell roars with laughter at himself. "More to my wife than to anybody. She was overprotective, really overprotective. I kept saying, 'Val, I can't do everything at once. I can't diet, stop smoking, and learn to take life easy in one fell swoop.' If I even glanced sideways at an ounce of animal fat, she'd be all over me. My first wife wouldn't have cared. We don't have any problems now. In fact, the only time in our marriage we've had problems was the year *before* Bypass. I was so cantankerous, because I wasn't feeling good. I was too tired. I didn't ski, I didn't sail, I was crabby in the office. I still blow in business. I'm trying to get hold of that.

"In business, I'm a perfectionist. A good boss shows his workers how to solve their problems; he gives them a fishing pole instead of fish. I tell my guys that, but it's hard to practice what you preach. In my work, I'm extremely dedicated and professional, but I'm unbelievably short with people who goof for no reason. That's where Bypass has made a big difference; for the first time, I'm looking forward to retirement. Not because I want to stop working. I love my work. I can't believe they pay me for doing what I like so well.

"But I've so many things I want to do. I want to develop my painting. I'd let it go. When I went for this heart, I started to paint again. I love to travel. I want to do more varied consulting work, where I can pick my time and place. I'm crazy about Val; I'm exceedingly jealous of any time away from her. When I retire, I can spend much more time with her. Bypass taught me that: with the CABS and the mending time afterwards, I was with her constantly. We got along better. We got on each other's nerves, but that's ten minutes, and it's over. No lasting grudges. When I get scratchy, Val blasts me back. Then, we're done."

After Bypass, did you get depressed?

"No, but I had the feeling somebody was trying to make me into a cardiac cripple. Every minute: 'Take it easy. Don't do this. Don't do that.' I was more impatient than depressed, but I was fortunate. I went home from the hospital a week from the day of the Bypass. Two days later, I walked a quarter of a mile. Slowly, mind you, but I did it. I got my strength back quickly, because I made up my mind I'd do anything they told me to, even though it hurt. I've a friend who got Bypassed out of town. I said, 'Paul, you've got to follow their orders. You'll get better faster.' He didn't like the breathing, because it hurt. He didn't want to do this, he didn't want to do that. He's paying for it."

After your Bypass, could your wife see you right away?

"No, they'd just instituted the same rule as at Cleveland Clinic, that the family can't see you till you're out of Intensive Care."

How did you feel about not seeing your wife for three days?

"It made sense to me. Afterwards, when I was ready to be moved from the ICU and there wasn't any room for me on the step-down floor, I felt bad because I wanted to see Val. When she brought boxes of candy to all the nurses, they let her peek into the ICU, but she couldn't come and talk to me. She said, 'It'd have been better if I could have been with you after Bypass.' "

Since Bypass, have you changed your work pattern?

"I leave earlier. I don't work so aggressively for new accounts. I do it, but I don't go out of my way."

Does the firm object?

"A little. But without me, they'd lose the Pierce-Arrow account, so they only mutter under their breaths. Whither I goest, Pierce-Arrow goes. That's five million in billings. I have to fly to California every month. I used to catch the red-eye. No more. Now, I take Val with me. She gets to see her mother out there; I get to see Val."

Since Bypass, have you changed your play pattern?

"I'm playing harder. I wasn't playing before. My cardiac status wouldn't let me. I was too tired. Bypass made me feel young again. Val used to say in that year before we knew what ailed me, 'Sometimes, you act like an old man.' Not any more."

Did Bypass make you more aware of your own mortality?

"The war taught me that lesson."

Before Bypass, did your surgeon talk at any length to you?

"He amazed me. He talked to me on several occasions. I don't know where he got the time."

Before Bypass, what concerned you most?

"My wife. She was great, but it was awfully hard on her. She'd just lost her brother; now, she was facing Bypass for me. My affairs were in apple-pie order. I keep them that way."

How did you feel when you awakened?

"I guess I started to panic, because they put me under again. Because of the rush to Bypass, they'd told me everything I was supposed to do in a hurry. I was trying to remember all the instructions. When I came to, my bed seemed locked in a traffic jam. I couldn't get my bed to the head of this pack of beds, to have Bypass. I thought, 'If I don't get up there and get this operation, I'll die, because they told me I'm lethal. I'm going to die, I know I'm going to die,' and I panicked.

"When I came to again, with all the tubes in me, I couldn't talk. Finally, I got hold of a nurse and signaled for a pad and pencil. I remember writing, 'Is it all over?' I didn't know. Nobody told me the Bypass was all over. She said, 'Yes. Doing fine.' When I started coughing, she said, 'Don't cough.' I wrote on the paper, 'They told me to cough.' She smiled and said, 'Not yet.' Amazingly, she could read my writing. They should have the pad and pencil right there and offer it to you, before you have to go into a song and dance to act out what you want."

When you awakened, did you have much pain?

"Yes, but not unbearable. I only took pain medicine once. When I was shot up in the war, I got burned, I got shrapnel in the back. The British doctors captured at Dunkirk operated on me. They did a good job, but they didn't have anesthesia. When they took out those damn tubes in the side and belly"—Doell whistles—"that hurt. That's when I asked for pain medicine. The resident said, 'This is going to smart a little.' When he finished, I said, 'I'll buy you a dictionary. You can look up the definition of "smart." ' He just laughed and went on to the next guy with the same line."

What was the worst part of the operation?

Doell thinks for a while. "There was no worst part. Bypass wasn't as bad as I thought it would be. My back hurt from lying there. My first sneeze was hell on wheels. I'd no time to grab a pillow. After the sneeze, I looked down at my chest. I thought I'd split open. The CCU's a bad place. It needs fixing up. It needs some light. There's no windows, no anything. I'd ask, 'What time is it?' They'd say, 'Two o'clock.' Two o'clock when? A.M. or P.M.? That makes you disorganized, disoriented. If I'd doze off, when I'd come back, I'd no idea what time it was, whether it was night or day. CCUs need windows and big clocks, visible to every patient, with the time, the date, and whether it's night or day. That's my one complaint. I've been thinking about donating clocks to that place."

What did Bypass do for you?

"I hope it put a lot of years on my life. It's given me more life, more pep. It's changed my diet, but I've adjusted to that."

Do you cheat?

"Of course I cheat! Though I'm trading off more sensibly. Before and after I cheat, I go straight. I'm not such a straight arrow, but I go straight on the diet. Mostly. My cardiologist makes me toe the line."

You seem to like your cardiologist.

"I have to. I see the younger one regularly, but if I got into trouble, if I started to have pains again, I'd want the older one to sit in on the decision making. He's more mature; he's seen a lot more. With the snow on my roof, I respect a man with experience."

You probably had white hair in your thirties.

"I did. So did my father. I don't care, so long as I keep it. No Johnson's Glo-Coat for me. I want my father's vigor, too. I'd hate to be a vegetable."

Does the "snow on the roof" or the Bypass affect your work relationships?

"The Bypass does, although people are getting over it. The first time they see you, after Bypass, they act as though you're going to start to bleed on the spot. They pussyfoot around. They keep asking, 'Are you sure you're all right? Do you feel good, Bill?' Sometimes I say, 'You should see how good I feel.' Every now and then, when I talk to the clients, I have to say, 'I want a straight answer. You're not going to get me upset. I'm doing business at the same old stand. I'm better than I ever was.' "

Does Bypass affect your job itself? Your ability to be promoted?

"I'm as high as I can go. I've had offers. I had an offer last week to head up an agency. I don't want it any more."[1]

You must be good. "Snow on the roof" is unusual in the ad business.

"In the field of automotive advertising, I'm one of the best in the country."

Since Bypass, you said, your marriage is better.

"We took a great marriage and we made it better. We're both more aware of what we have."

At a few hospitals, there's a full-time psychological counselor as a member of the team. Would such counseling have helped you or your wife?

"Only once, but that would have been enough; just before I went home, I needed to talk to someone. I needed a professional ap-

---

[1] Since the interview, Bill Doell has started his own ad agency.

praisal of what the healing process would be like, physically and psychologically. It would have helped to know I'd be irritable. When I was churlish, I knew, but I couldn't stop myself from making everybody miserable. After people go home, there should be a small post-Bypass group to relieve anxieties and depression, to answer questions. Guys like me know how busy the doctor is. I hated to impose, so I wouldn't call with a question. In the office, I wouldn't hold him up with questions, because I knew other people were waiting. When I'd leave the office, I'd be sorry I didn't ask what was on my mind."

How long did you wait to drive a car?

"Six weeks. Whatever they told me."

How long did you wait to climb stairs?

"Right away, when I went home."

How long did you wait to have intercourse?

"As soon as I got home. The last day in the hospital, a little student nurse came in. God! was I ever that green and eager? She said she had a bunch of questions to ask me. 'Fire away,' I said. 'Do you have any trepidations about sex?' she wanted to know. I said, 'None at all.' She asked, 'Do you have any idea when you'll first have intercourse?' I looked at her, and said, 'My wife's picking me up at ten o'clock. By the time she pays the bill, I get checked out, and we drive fifty miles home, it'll be noon. I'm a little slow from this Bypass, so probably not until twelve-thirty.' Flabbergasted, she ran out of the room." Doell laughs delightedly, remembering. "Kids that age never think anybody over thirty has intercourse.

"When Val and I were getting married, and she was twenty years younger than I, my dad came up to see us and wish us well. After my mother died, he'd married my mother's kid sister, a widow, who later died of a heart attack on a cruise, when my dad was eighty. He was having brunch with me, and he said, 'Bill, I don't want you to worry about the age difference between you and Val.' I couldn't figure out what he was getting at. He was hemming and hawing around, because he'd *never* discussed sex with me. 'Don't be concerned,' he said, 'because Rachel and I had relations the night before she died.' I told Val afterwards, 'I don't know if the old gentleman was trying to reassure me or to brag.' "

What explicit questions would you advise people to ask before and after Bypass?

"It's hard to talk in generalities, because people need such complete understanding of what they can and cannot do—every step of the way. More than that, they need a crash course in what it's like in the ICU when you come to. If I didn't know, it would have scared the hell out of me. Everything's blinking and buzzing. You see your life going by you on the monitor. Usually if you've had Bypass, you've been to Intensive Care before, you've learned to watch your own monitor to see if they're telling you the truth. You get so you know your own blood-pressure reading.

"One time, after Bypass, I looked at the monitor and, boy, the blood pressure reading was terrible! I thought, 'I'm dying, and nobody wants to tell me.' I called the nurse. I didn't want to die alone." Doell laughs at his own fear. "I asked her about the blood-pressure reading on the monitor, and she explained it was a different kind of reading. She came when I called; she explained carefully; that's important. But Bypass wasn't anywhere near as bad as I thought it would be, which is why I said I'd talk to you. The fear is lots worse than the operation, an awful lot worse."

What can help those fears?

Doell grins. "Your book. I'm serious. People with Bypass saying, 'It's not wonderful, but it's not so bad as you think.' When I can go out and get a testimonial from an owner, I've got a great way to sell."

As a car-owner, I can tell you about antitestimonials. Not every Bypasser is a satisfied customer. I'm not out to sell Bypass. I want to help people get through Bypass and back in their cars again.

"People need to have an understanding with their internists, their cardiologists, their surgeons. They need to lay it on the line, to say, 'Look. I'm not interested in being a number.' Medicine is a business too. The physician needs to be nice to the customer, to give his service. He's not doing the patient such a favor. Just as people can buy another kind of car, they can go elsewhere for their medical care. Prospective Bypassers should tell their doctors, 'While you're taking care of me, pretend you're Jean Hersholt, the kindly old country doctor. Treat me like a whole human being. If you're too busy, no hard feelings. I'll try the dealer across the street.'

"People refer to my cardiologists' office as 'the factory.' Those guys are organized. I *respect* the businesslike way they run their office, but once I'm in a room with the doctor, it's very personal. He acts as though there's nobody in the world but me. Yet he knows what's happening in the office. His secretaries don't yak to each other. They dress neatly. They don't call me or my wife by our first names. God, but I hate that kind of pseudofriendship," Bill Doell reflects. "When things tick me off, especially in business, my wife tells me to quit being a fighter pilot and take it easy. Bypass gave me a hand in putting away my pilot's wings.

"Heart disease sneaks up on you. I don't know when I began not feeling well. Since Bypass, I feel great. I've got so many things planned, so much we're doing together now, so much we can do. I don't mean to sound like a testimonial, so I'll leaven my praises: I've a great friend, a one-time all-American. He had his Bypass in Texas. The day before my operation, he called me long-distance and said, 'Hey, Champ! Don't worry about a thing. It's a piece of cake.' After I had the Bypass and they sent me home, I caught a cold and started those God-awful sneezes. I called *him* on the phone, and said, 'Say, Jack, about that piece of cake . . .' " Bill Doell laughs his wonderful laugh. "Going too far the other way's a mistake, too. Nevertheless, for me, Bypass was worth the cookie and its crumbles."

21. Moira Kitt
Editor
Age at Bypass: 50

She's a senior editor with a major Boston publishing firm. In her office, high above Boylston Street's Friday afternoon busyness, we talk. Our appointment had been for one-thirty, but she had called that morning to postpone it to two-thirty.

"I can't spare you an hour," she had warned on the phone. "A half hour is too much." She had never completed the second questionnaire I'd mailed her.

At two-thirty, Moira Kitt appears in the waiting room. An ash-blonde, her short wavy hair is not "styled," but frames her white, tired face with its arc of freckles across her nose. A wan, weary, late-fortyish woman, she's harassed by too much to do on a hot Friday afternoon.

"I'm afraid I'm going to be late," she explains, curiously courteous yet ignited to a hot-eyed curtness by my questioning.

"I've got to get to the country," she replies shortly, eager to be rid of me.

The big glass doors close behind her, as she disappears. An hour later, Moira Kitt reappears, leads me through a maze, as people pull at her skirt: "Moira, luv, just have a look at this review."

"Moira, if we change this promo tour . . ." Her office is unpretentious, cluttered, with no photographs on her desk. Curling up in her desk chair, she displays her very good legs, the saphenous-vein scar nearly invisible beneath her stockings.

"I'm afraid all I've got left for you is fifteen minutes," she apologizes. "You'll just have to come back another time."

Once we begin talking, we connect. She's not in her late forties, but fifty-two. The fifteen minutes stretch to two hours.

How did you come to surgery? What happened?

"Suddenly, one day, I had chest pains. I was perfectly fine. I had no symptoms, none whatsoever. I walked home from work one night, as I had all my life. I live in town. The next morning, I got up and walked to work as I had for years, up the hill to the office. Halfway up, I began getting chest pains! Pain in my chest, pain in my arm, pain along my chin. I stopped; it went away. I resumed walking. The pain came back. People probably know more what heart symptoms are like than any other problems, so I was suspicious. I'd just had a physical. I'd had, I thought, a thyroid problem for many years. I was taking thyroid medication; the doctor had told me the thyroid wasn't functioning properly.

"The main pain was in the base of my throat . . . in the back of the throat like you used to get when you were a child and you ran too fast and your throat would ache. I thought something was wrong with my thyroid, but in some part of my mind, I knew it was more.

"Anyway, I didn't do anything for a couple of days. It happened every time I went up that hill. Finally, I called the doctor. I said, 'I think the thyroid is the problem.' He said, 'It sounds more significant than that.' I went back to see him, but I wasn't satisfied with his responses. My best friend is a physician who doesn't live here any more. When I mentioned my problems to her, she got upset and said, 'You need to find out more right away.' She put me in touch with a cardiologist, who gave me a stress test. Just from my symptoms, he had no doubt I had some kind of coronary artery disease. But after the stress test, he said, 'It's only garden-variety coronary heart disease—nothing to worry about.' Do you want me to go on with the whole story?"

Yes, but one question: are you still menstruating?

"Not now. I was at that time. I was edging up to menopause. My periods were tapering off.

"I had a falling-out with the doctor over something unrelated to my heart, so I had to find another cardiologist. It took me about three more weeks to get an appointment with an internist who specializes in cardiology. In the meantime, the symptoms got worse. I was taking five milligrams of Inderal, which is like nothing."

I know.

"Do you have this, too?"

No.

"But you know so much about it. Why are you doing this? Why should you care? When I got to the other doctor, he accepted the first cardiologist's stress test because it was recent. He was going on my symptoms. He said I needed more Inderal. Suddenly I went into a state called 'unstable angina.' Before it had been a normal thing, triggered by exercise or emotional upsets. Then I began getting it for no reason at all. Sitting at home at night and reading the paper, suddenly I'd have an angina attack. Or I'd be awakened in the middle of the night with angina, not an intensely crushing pain, but it was frightening. I was taking nitroglycerin. Then I started putting nitroglycerin paste on my chest to go to sleep at night. By this time, I was getting so I couldn't walk more than half a block without getting pains. It'd be brought on by the slightest little thing—playing Ping-Pong, for instance. Just moving the paddle would give it to me. The doctor I have now said, 'This is a very serious situation. You may have to be operated on right away.' So, better late than never, I began doing my heart homework. I read an American Heart Association heart book that said, at this stage, either you're hovering at the edge of a heart attack or you're going to return to a more stable condition. The doctors decided I should go into the hospital and have an arteriogram. They found three arteries blocked—one 95 percent closed, two 65 percent closed. Luckily, they were mobilized occlusions, they were accessible, which made me a good candidate for Bypass surgery.

"Then I had to decide whether to do it or not. The first pain was in December. By February, I had the arteriogram. Once started, the heart trouble took over my life. Then, I did not know quite whether I wanted to do it or not. I should say, I suppose, 'whether I wanted *them* to do it or not.' I said, 'Let me see how I go on medication.' So I did. Then I said, 'Let me go through the summer and see how much limitation this imposes. I've a house in Maine. I want to work in the garden. Let's see how the summer, a much more physical time for me than winter, when I sit reading manuscripts, will go.' By the end of summer, I decided I wanted Bypass, not because I was so handicapped, but because I felt too young to be handicapped at all.

"When the summer was over, I told Dr. Holmes; he set up an appointment with a surgeon. Bypass was the surgeon's advice, too. Neither of them pushed me. Meantime, I stabilized on medication. Now there wasn't any urgency about the operation. What decided me were two factors: number one, I didn't want to be limited; and number two, I wanted to do it now. They said I should do it while I was young and healthy, while my heart was strong and uninjured by a heart attack.

"I'd been going with a psychiatrist, a man I no longer see; he was enormously supportive. He was a great help in getting me to see Bypass as a way of making an easier life for myself: 'If it's heart trouble, *use it* to make a freer life.' At that time, I was director of the Trade Department, a more demanding position."

What's your title now?

"I'm executive editor of the Trade Department, a notch down, which means I took myself out of the running for the presidency of the company, something I'd been working towards for years. A director has lots of administrative responsibilities, which are taxing, which test—and prove—your mettle. My friend's feeling was that I should make a less-pressured life for myself. Yet when you're on the merry-go-round and you've got a chance at the brass ring, you hate to step back to those safe horses on the outside"— she smiles self-deprecatingly—"the ones that don't go up and down."

*Did your psychiatrist-friend advise any psychological counseling pre-
and postoperatively? In a few places, such psychological services are
routinely included on the Bypass team.*

"It depends a great deal on what kind of support you have to begin
with. If you're a person with a supportive family, you might not
need it so much. But if you're by yourself with no one to turn to,
it's a good idea. I'm interested in talking about what, to me, were
the biggest psychological aftereffects."

That's what I want.

"The biggest surprise to me was the regression I went through
. . . regressing to a childlike state. I've been on my own all my adult
life. I've always considered myself a strong, self-sufficient person.
I've heard this happens to people who become seriously ill or have
an operation—they revert to this dependent state. I couldn't believe
it would happen to me. But it did. I wanted to be taken care of; I
became very dependent; I had zero interest in my job. I was incapable of concerning myself with other people's problems. I went
right back to a child's level, which persisted much longer than any
physical limitations. That dependency was the hardest aftereffect
to cope with. If I had to have Bypass again, I might seriously
consider going to one of those halfway houses for the first few weeks
after the hospital. I live alone, but my family—my sister-in-law in
particular, a wonderful person—came to stay with me for the first
week. My brother stayed for three days, and then had to go back
to Washington to work. That was wonderful. But after they left, I
had to depend on friends, who were very good, but it's different.
They weren't there all the time.

"I was crotchety. I wanted to be waited on, to be taken care of.
At the same time, I didn't want people around all the time. It
became difficult. *I* became difficult, yet childishly, I felt I had a
right to be pampered and indulged. I would go to the refrigerator,
look in and make no sense of anything in the refrigerator. I was
incapable of thinking of meals or cooking for myself.

"It's not physical limitations at all. The most important thing
people have to think about in their recuperation is having a real
support system there for them *all the time.* For married people,
that's different. They're lucky. They have that. But for people on

their own, they need to arrange that for themselves. For me, that was the hardest part."

How long did that last?

"Months and months. After two months, I got out of the house. The dependency began to lift a little, but I wasn't able to muster full involvement in my job for about six or seven months.

"I went through a period of depression, but I'm not talking about depression. This was something else all together. I felt depressed, but I understand everybody gets depressed postoperatively from the effects of the anesthesia or the isolation or whatever makes you feel like Mrs. Kitt's little lost girl. I've heard all surgery leaves you feeling desolate. What was it Pope said? 'The world forgetting by the world forgot.' Ha! We literary types have literary allusions to remember—but no fortresses to keep us secure."

The depression occurs in 30 to 40 percent of Bypassers. Doctors argue about why it occurs.

"I'm not going to be able to say why either. I've always been given to depressions. Whatever causes it, I get depressed now and then. I don't get blue. I go through downswings."

How long do they last?

"They can last three to four weeks."

That's a long time.

"It can seem an eternity, and there's nothing you can do about it. Maybe I've a tendency to depressive reactions to life events. But this dependency wasn't depression. I've been much more depressed than I got after Bypass. In my case, I got so much attention, it helped my depression. It helped a lot. I did go through a phase of feeling bleak and forlorn, it's true, yet it wasn't acute depression. I've been there, I know."

Have you ever been married?

"No."

Because a lot of married people have the same sense of forsaken isolation when they have Bypass. Often, unmarried, divorced, or widowed people do what you've done. They believe if people are married, it's different.

"My father had a heart attack. I remember what he went through afterwards. His moods were terribly exaggerated. He was depressed and impossible to get along with. I've heard this about other people after heart attacks."

How old was your father?

"Let's see. He was in his forties somewhere."

He was young.

"He died of a heart attack when he was fifty-six. He didn't have even ten years after the first attack."

Is your mother living?

"No. She died at fifty-two of a massive hemorrhage."

You have a family history on both sides. Do any of your siblings have heart disease?

"Both my brothers."

Where are you in the family?

"I'm in the middle. Both my brothers have arrhythmias. My younger brother takes Digoxin, I believe it is. My older brother, I don't know if he takes anything now. He did for a while. They both have the fibrillation."

Do they live in Boston?

"No. One lives in Maryland, the one who works in Washington. The other lives in Pittsburgh."

You don't have a family support system?

"No. I have none. Friends, yes, but no family. How my mother'd snort if she could hear me mouthing this cliché, but it's true: blood *is* thicker than water—it's even thicker than martinis."

To what causes did you attribute your illness and your need for Bypass?

"It never occurred to me until afterwards, but I did absolutely everything wrong. There are seven risks; I embodied every single one except maleness. I had heredity, probably the major factor, because I have circulatory-arteriosclerotic histories on both sides. I am an absolute Type-A personality. I smoked two packs a day for twenty-three years. I thought my diet was terrific, but now that I know what heart diets are supposed to be, it was all wrong. Every day of my life, I ate a poached egg on toast, smothered with butter; I drank five cups of coffee. My life was difficult, I had to struggle to get where I am—or where I was before I stepped down a notch. I've lived an enormously stressful life. I've been under stress since I was thirteen years old. Because I was a restless, high-strung person, I thought I was active, but I never was. I never exercised, never did anything. I just sat in a chair and worried. If you name the risk factors, I had them in spades. Which accounts for me having a heart operation at fifty. In fact, I think I had heart trouble much earlier."

Did you ever think, 'Why me?'

"Of course. You think, 'It isn't fair.' You feel your life is coming to an end. You get resentful. I got old in my ways because I started thinking in terms of limitations, of options closing down, old ambitions I could never accomplish. The end of my life was in sight. I felt like an old person.

"After the operation, I didn't buy any clothes. When I was able to do things again, all of a sudden, I started thinking, 'Maybe someday I'll move to southern France,' and I bought new clothes, I got my hair done again. There's a difference between thinking of life lying ahead and thinking of it as closed off—closed out. Now, I'm back in between." Her face clouds. "I've had some angina again.

"But the first year after Bypass I was a brand-new person. The good part of that kind of thinking, of thinking you see the end, is *you stop postponing life.* You stop saving your money for when you are going to be sixty-five. You say, 'Maybe I'm never going to be sixty-five. I'm going to enjoy it now.' Before, I felt I had to save, to be careful, because I have no family, I had no security. I'd think, 'I don't want to be one of the "baggies" on the street, those bag ladies cadging the trash cans. I have to take care of myself.' Now who knows whether I'll make it or not? I splurge more readily. I have a freer attitude about lots of things; at the same time, I've a less open view of my life, of whatever life lies ahead."

Do you still value your work as much?

"I like this work. It's wonderful work. I like the people I work with. I like the way their minds operate. I like why we do what we do. I've been enriched by spending my life working with people I enjoy and admire, in doing work of some value. The people here are crazy idealists, most of us. We're doing this not just to sell books, but because we genuinely want to address issues in a way helpful to the country and to its intellectual life. I like the ideas we deal with. I love working with words. I've been fortunate with my job. It's not the glamorous life that people imagine. Yet I've been lucky to work with people who think, people I respect."

Since Bypass, have any close relationships changed?

"I've thought about that. A lot. If they've changed, they've only gotten closer. Mostly, my relationship with my older brother and sister-in-law, which has always been good, deepened, because I asked them for help. It's not because they helped me that it changed, but *because I asked them for help.* That was the key factor. I've always thought of myself as self-reliant. It's hard for me to ask, to show I need them. My asking made them feel important to me. At first, we got very close. As time goes on, we can't keep up that intensity, but there's a residue of being closer than before. I discovered affection I didn't know existed."

Does being aware of your own mortality make you more alive to the sweetness of life or more angry at the universe?

"Good question. The answer is both. I feel bitter in many ways when I think, '*I really do have heart trouble. I'm not going to live to be the two-thousand-year-old woman.*'

"Yet there's something else. You don't know when they will come up with some miraculous panacea. When my father had his heart trouble, they never had this operation. So who's to say? Tomorrow morning, I can pick up the *Boston Globe*, and they'll have another operation, a permanent cure. I had three blocked arteries, but they could only Bypass two. That's why I have angina again. The worst one they couldn't do anything with because it was too small to Bypass. In other words, the diameter of the artery was smaller than the vein in my leg. They say I probably will have a heart attack some day. They say, 'Don't worry too much. The right side of your heart is not too important.'

"I guess it's true. Yet I feel the writing is on the wall. Again, it limits me. The first year after Bypass, I had no problems. I felt reborn. Suddenly, possibilities arose again. That's what I'm bitter about: the shutting down of possibilities. I'm acutely conscious of my limited time. That's pessimistic, but who's to say? Nobody in my family lived past fifty-six. If you believe heredity plays a role, then the cards are not so good. The other part is I'm not as afraid. In a way, I'm living more deliberately than I used to. I'm not denying myself things I was postponing until retirement age."

Now that you are fifty-two, have you ever been sorry for the things you haven't done with your life?

"That's one of life's great crises, coming to terms with the 'it's-too-late' business. Things you always thought you'd do that you're never going to do. That's part of the aging process, I guess. That's middle-age crisis. Whether I'd feel this way without the heart problem, who knows? How could I know I'd feel this sense of loss? Yet I feel it intensely."

You've had a successful career.

"If I hadn't had a career, who knows? I'm sure the extra stresses have contributed—but given my heredity and personality, it probably would have happened anyway, though perhaps not so early."

Do you ever think, "I wish I had married and had a family"?

"Yes. More so now. Because now, children are not a possibility. I always wanted both a career and marriage—*and* children—not either-or. The grass is always greener, but as you get older, if you have children, if the children are caring— People with children end up less lonely than people alone. Being alone as you get older is very hard. It's the worst. I have many friends who are better for me in many ways, much more supportive than my family ever was. They're better family than my family. Yet when the chips were down, it was my family that counted. But I do wish . . . Oh, I don't want to get old by myself."

Have you ever thought that heart disease and Bypass have closed off the option of marriage?

"Every once in a while I think, 'Who would want someone with a heart problem?' But it's not my heart, I think. It's my age. If the marriage option is closed, it's because middle-aged women in our society aren't very marketable."

You said that after Bypass you had psychic problems characteristic of the post-Bypass phase; yet you also said you felt reborn.

"Once I'd recuperated and was back in life again, once I could do all those things I couldn't do before, I felt reborn. While I was recuperating, I didn't feel reborn. No, I can't say that. Once I'd passed that stage, once I'd come back to work, when I could run up the street, go up and down three flights of stairs, do what I wanted when I wanted with no death threat hanging over my head, I felt life had opened like a flower. Like a Lawrentian flower, gorgeously, gaudily, vividly." Looking away, she stops. "I didn't mean to wax poetic. I hate people who carry on like that, but in the beginning, it's almost a sexual-spiritual feeling. Coming back to life, coming back to work, to the world, without being limited. Work, *my work*, mattered so much to me, yet after Bypass, it was the absence of pain, the absence of limitations, that made me feel so fully alive. Not the presence of work. You need the presence of work, of being involved in something important to you and to other people, but the operative factor is the absence of physical restrictions."

How long after Bypass did you return to work?

"Three months."

How long before you drove?

"Three months. They put a three-month ceiling on everything. They made me wait to drive because, if I were in an accident, my chest mightn't be sufficiently healed, and if I got hit by the steering wheel, my Bypass might cave in."

Driving also is stressful.

"Nobody mentioned that. I thought it was the physical danger to my fragile healing chest."

Do you think of your chest now as fragile?

"No, never."

Then?

"No, I just followed orders."

How long after Bypass did you resume sexual activity?

"I am not married, so my sexual activity is not as usual as I'd like. A few months, I guess."

Did you worry the first time, or the first couple of times? Did your doctor talk to you about intercourse?

"Nobody said a word. Maybe they thought sex didn't matter to me because I wasn't married. I did some reading. I spoke to a sex therapist. It's easier for women. We don't have to worry about getting an erection. We just have to worry about getting a man. I worried about being disfigured. I used to wear V-neck T-shirts, and they said, 'You won't be wearing those things any more.' That made me unhappy. I'm conscious of my scar, but I'm getting less self-conscious all the time. If I were younger, I'd mind lots more. If I were twenty-five or thirty-five, I'd mind a lot. At this stage, the scar doesn't make an appreciable difference. There was a young girl with me in the hospital, a girl in her thirties, who'd had Bypass. That's unusual for a woman. She said to her father, 'Who'd want me now, with this big scar down the front?' If you're young and female, when 'perfection' matters so much, it must be awfully difficult. Before Bypass, I was unhappy about the scar. As things turned out, I don't think about it—too much."

Like that girl, do you think, 'Who would want me?'

"If I get into a romantic situation, I think about it at first. Then you get over it."

I've only talked to one person who felt strongly about the scar, a man in his thirties from Las Vegas.

"Where they care about bodies, bodies, bodies."

Ironically, he's about one hundred pounds overweight. When I said, "Women who have mastectomies feel the same way," he cut me off with "This is much worse."

"It's not, I'm sure it's not. I've never had a mastectomy, thank God, but I'd feel much more mutilated than I do with a line between my breasts."

Do you sleep well at night?

"Most of the time. If I don't sleep well, it's because of menopause, not because of my heart problem. I have hot flashes, and I take Inderal, which keeps me awake. I don't take Inderal after five o'-clock any more. My doctor says, 'That's a paradoxical reaction, because most people get sleepy with Inderal.' When I first started it, Inderal gave me nightmares, especially if I took it at bedtime. I stopped the bedtime dose and the nightmares stopped."

Do they give you anything for hot flashes?

"Estrogen, but it makes me blow up like a balloon. I gained ten pounds in three days. There are no panaceas, no solutions to everything. Frankly, menopause can be worse than heart trouble, but it can't kill you."

What was the worst aspect of the operation?

"The worst part? Physically, the only bothersome part of Bypass was that respirator tube. It's torture. I'd do anything rather than have that tube again. And I was lucky. I only had it into the evening of the day of surgery. Some people have it for days. I don't know how they bear it. I got into ICU about noon, and they removed it about six or seven in the evening."

How did you feel when you awakened?

"Of course, I didn't know where I was. I thought I was in a trench somewhere. I could just see dim lights. I thought I'd fallen into a deep hole. But I came to quickly; my mind was clear. Then I knew exactly what was going on and what I was thinking. Of course, I couldn't talk. I started throwing up right then; they sent another tube down to aspirate. Not being able to talk was frustrating because that's when they came and told me they could only do two arteries. I was dying to ask questions. I wanted to know more. Afterwards, I never could get a satisfactory answer. They don't want to emphasize it, they don't want you to think about what didn't happen. They think that if they tell you fast and leave, you won't wonder, 'Was it the surgeon's fault or my fault? Was the surgeon too slow or inadequately dextrous? Are my arteries too diseased?'

"In the hospital (I'd forgotten all this, but talking now is bringing it back) I was angry because I couldn't get satisfactory answers to my questions. They said, 'That's it, back to square one.' They came in just as I was coming to and said, 'We could only do two, but everything's fine. We did everything we could. We even looked under the bottom of your heart and poked around, so don't worry.' I wanted to say, 'What does this mean?' but I couldn't talk with the tube in. I couldn't do anything. I couldn't lift my arm. The advice given me before the operation was, 'Never mind, you can write on a pad.' Can you imagine? I couldn't lift my arm and could hardly write a word on a pad, much less make a sentence. All that is a lot of hooey. A lot of what they tell you is a lot of hooey. My own doctor was in the clear on this because he told me before I went into the hospital that he'd be away, he wouldn't be able to come to the hospital the night before the operation. But the surgeon never came either.

"That night I was lonely and frightened. The worst part was the night before the operation. My brother and sister-in-law stayed with me way past the time allowed. Finally, like storm troopers, the nurses made them leave. Then all I had was interns puttering around. The surgeon should come to see you the night before the operation. It would have made such a difference if he had come by the night before and said, 'Now, in the morning this will happen. Don't worry, I'll be there. Everything will be fine.' I was so hurt, so angry, so lonely. I had these little nurses, who were very nice, and these obnoxious interns. My own doctor would have come by but he was out of town, so there I was, all by myself."

What did your surgeon charge you?

"He was cheap. He was the professor, but only charged $3,500."

Since Bypass, has your internist been a help to you?

"Yes. He's a dedicated man, I must say. As far as personality, well, I went to him because I was desperate. As I told you, I had to leave this other man, and I had to find somebody fast. His name was given to me. I just took him. Luckily, he took me on. As far as rapport and personality go, if there were twenty doctors in this room, I wouldn't choose him. But it's like one of those loveless marriages, where you fall in love with the person afterwards. I've come to like him enormously. He's this rare person, utterly and totally dedicated to his patients. He's always there for you. I feel enormously secure in his care. Perhaps a more personable, flashier doctor might be more fun, but who's to say? What matters is, *Are they there when you need them?"*

Does your doctor have an associate?

"Yes, but he didn't come by the night before either. The anesthesiologist sent her assistant, a little blonde, very pretty, who looked about nineteen years old. She said, 'I'm the anesthesiologist.' I said, 'You are?' I was terrified; I thought, 'Let me out of here.' She shouldn't have said that. She should have said, 'I'm the intern on the anesthesiologist's service, and she sent me.' I thought, 'This *kid* is going to anesthetize me.' I felt bereft—that's the word exactly. I wanted to put on my clothes and go home, where I belonged."

Do you think your bereftness contributed to your dependency and depression after Bypass?

"It took me awhile to get over the night before, and then those surgeons marching in with bad news while the tube was in so I couldn't quiz them. I was angry for a long time. I felt abandoned, a much different experience than I'd expected. Before the operation, before I went into the hospital, I guess I'd gotten spoiled because I'd had so much attention. Exhibit A: a fifty-year-old woman, still menstruating, needing Bypass or something like that. Suddenly, everything, about me was fascinating, and just as suddenly, on the big day, I felt, 'Nobody cares.' I went into it with a good attitude, but it was a much lonelier experience than I'd expected."

Would bibliotherapy—

"What's bibliotherapy?"

Books that talk about what people have been through, books that tell you what to expect physically and mentally, how to help yourself. Would such books have helped you?

"Definitely. I wanted to know a lot, and it was hard finding anybody who could tell me anything. First, there aren't many people who've had it. Sure, I know—a million Americans since '68, but it's tough to find them. Doctors aren't nuch help with networking. I found three people, but one was bitter, and all were self-centered. They wanted to talk about their own operations, not about me. I suppose that's what you're doing, isn't it? Getting together enough people so Bypassers can pick and choose who they want to listen to. One man, a CEO, said, 'What are you asking questions for? There's nothing you can do about it. You have to do what the doctor says, anyway.' For active, ambitious types, CEOs are astoundingly passive when it comes to doctors.

"Because I need to fend for myself, I wanted to know what I could do physically. Little things, womanish things, I guess: 'Do I need special clothes? Can I move my arms and button buttons? Can I put shirts on over my head? Can I wear panty hose?' Nobody ever told me. Of course, I didn't need special clothes, I could move my arms and button things, although clothing that buttoned in the front and didn't slip over the head was easier for the first few weeks so I didn't twist my scar out of kilter. Women who live alone ought to own those zipper-fasteners on a wire. Women pack suitcases ahead to go have babies; they know what to take. Not with Bypass. Bras with front closures are better, too. The night before the surgery my one visitor, the nurse, told me these things—a little late."

For you, the worst of Bypass was the not knowing?

"I knew what would happen and what procedures they'd do during the operation. For the doctor, Bypass is a pretty simple procedure. I'm beginning to sound like a surgeon. There's not much to know, and I did my own reading. I'm the kind who goes to the library, gets all the books, reads everything I can. I knew a lot on my own. But not enough. Nobody ever *didn't* answer questions, but they don't understand the simple things you need to know. Before you can frame the question, they're gone. The morning I left the hospital, the nurse came round and told me, 'Don't do this,' or, 'Do that.' I wanted to know long before. By telling you practical things, little things, they can make Bypass simple for the patient, too. Or at least, a little easier."

Physically, the tube bothered you most. Psychically, what was the worst part and how could it have been alleviated?

"The helplessness and the isolation afterwards. The loneliness. I wanted somebody with me all the time. I wanted to be pampered and taken care of. My sister-in-law, who is such a super person, understood so well. I'd sit on the couch, and she'd bring me my dinner. I didn't have to move. She'd talk to me, but not too much. She'd pick up the dishes and go out to the kitchen. That's what I wanted all the time. I wasn't physically incapable. I snuck out and did things I wasn't supposed to do. For instance, I love thrift shops. When they went out to get groceries, I put on my clothes and went to a thrift shop. Nobody knew.When they came back, I was in my nightgown and robe."

On the couch.

"On the couch. Right!" She laughs delightedly. "Like Camille. Stealing away to the thrift shop was fun. Responsibilities—forget it. That's the thing you can't do. You want somebody else to assume your responsibilities."

What did Bypass accomplish for you?

"Even though I now have some limitations, I'm about 85 percent restored. I feel younger, more hopeful."

Do you think Bypass prolonged your life?

"I can't say, because I could still have a heart attack at any time. Probably Bypass gave me some years. Statistically, if you had three occluded arteries, you are much more likely to have a heart attack than if you have one occluded artery or none."

Describe yourself psychically for me.

"I'm Type A all the way."

What's Type A to you?

"Competitive. Racing the clock. Never satisfied. Measuring everything in quantity rather than quality. No matter what you do, it's never enough. Pressure, pressure, pressure, much of it self-generated."

How are you at waiting in lines?

"I can't stand it. Waiting for a cab, getting the subway, I say, 'Come on, hurry up, hurry up.' I'm short-tempered, volatile, impatient, and, I suppose, passionate. About everything. I've always been that way."

Are you any better?

"I try."

Does Inderal change you?

"It's supposed to slow you down. It changes my personality."

Some people don't like the way it makes them feel.

"If it's too much, it makes you lethargic, but it turns me into a normal person. It even gives me confidence."

How?

"It's called the 'stage-fright' drug. It has that effect on me. I'm lucky, even in my side effects. When the doctor finished the operation, he was going to take me off it. I said, 'It gives me psychic benefits, which alleviate stress, not like a tranquilizer which could make me dopey. It makes me less competitive, but no less sharp.' Unfortunately, it also makes me awfully tired, which may slow down my brain when it shouldn't.'"

Philosophically, what are you like?

"I'm idealistic and spiritual without being religious, whatever that word means."

Do you think there is a God up there?

"Not a bit. I'm an atheist. An atheist and a socialist. I'm rebellious and skeptical. I'm very independent. I cannot stand restrictions. Stupidity drives me bananas. My adventurousness and curiosity got me through the operation. More than anything. It was a fascinating experience. I went into it all the way."

Before Bypass, what did you worry about?

"Not that I would die during the operation. No. I asked him, and he said, 'There's about a 2 percent chance.' I didn't think death was a possibility. I worried about two things: brain damage from anesthesia and that the shock of the operation would bring on diabetes, which runs through my family. Neither happened, to my knowledge."

Who or what makes your life worth living?

"No particular thing in my life. Friendships, love, human contacts, are the most important things anyway. Work is important. I like it, but I liked my other job better, before my heart acted up. It's satisfying. Since Bypass, work isn't as important to me as people."

You've gotten to the top in publishing. How did you get into this business?

"Close to the top," she edits. "It's the old story. I worked days, went to school nights. After my mother died, I went back home to Maine to take care of my father and my little brother, took courses at night, got my B.A. in English literature. After my father died and my brother grew up, I came to Boston and got into the publishing business. I thought Boston might be easier than New York. Boston's been good to me."

What would you tell somebody who's been advised to have Bypass?

"Even though the angina's returned, I'm delighted I did it. I'd go back to the same doctor, the same hospital; I'd do things the same way. I made the right decision. *If* I'd been better prepared for the aftermath, the afterevents, I'd have arranged for more support, although I don't know how I'd have gotten it. If you can arrange it, support is what people need."

Carefully, she straightens the piles of manuscripts on her desk, sets out her pens in neat rows, then looks sharply at me: "Tell me about you. Why are you writing this book?"

I've something to tell you about my family, just for you. My family history's like yours. For four generations. My father died at fifty-two. His middle brother died two years later. I remember my uncle Eddie saying at my uncle George's funeral, 'Everybody's here and thinking, "Okay, Eddie, your turn is in two years."' Uncle Eddie's first coronary was the night his daughter was graduated from high school. I don't like to tempt fate, but he's now eighty-four years old. So you just don't know. Sometimes, you avert the family curse.

"How very nice of you to tell me that! It makes me feel so good. I guess I'll have to save my money after all."

III

Transfer
Point

From the Admitting Office to the Cashier's Office

This section should be read before you ever walk in the hospital door, even before you have your office conference with the cardiovascular surgeon. As you read, keep your pad and pencil near, and jot down questions as they occur to you. When you go to the hospital, take this book with you.

While you are thinking over the Bypass choice, once you have opted for it, and after you get your hospital date, do some Bypass reading (see the Bibliography). Be sure to read Dr. Herbert Benson's *The Relaxation Response* and a good book on transcendental meditation. Even if you're not a believer in TM, try its techniques or the self-hypnosis techniques in the back of this book. It can't hurt. One second-time-around Bypasser, Vince Battaglio, maintains, "Using self-hypnosis on my second Bypass made all the difference. The first was a nightmare. The second was an interesting experience." Though Norman Cousins did not have Bypass, his *The Healing Heart* has worlds to open for the heart patient, his or her family, and the doctor.

Almost every hospitalization for Bypass begins in the admitting office and ends in the cashier's office. It begins in fear: "What did

I get myself into?" After even a successful Bypass, it ends in fear: "How will I get along outside the hospital?" Because the Bypassers here have talked about how they coped inside and outside the hospital, what follows is necessarily a brief overview. Should you wish to know more, the books in the Bibliography will help. One caution: every hospital does things a little differently.

Usually, patients are admitted to the hospital two days before Bypass.[1] Bring your medications, even vitamins, with you, as well as a list of them for the resident to see. Keep a copy of the list for yourself. Bring your Blue Cross/Blue Shield card or whatever insurance identification and requisite forms that you have. In a small kit, bring pajamas or nightgown, robe, slippers, comb, brush, toothpaste and toothbrush, two pencils and a notepad. Don't forget your glasses and other necessities such as hearing aid or dentures. Although you arrive at the requested time, you'll probably have to wait. Bring a good novel and this book, a deck of cards, or a small magnetic Scrabble game to while away the waiting. Practice the coughing, deep breathing, and self-hypnosis exercises.

Once admitted, you'll be taken to your room on a general surgical floor. There, a nurse will take the first of many checks—temperature, blood pressure, pulse, and respiration. After that, residents or "house officers," medical students, nurses and student nurses, lab technicians, x-ray technicians, pulmonary therapists, will keep you busy telling your history and that of your mother and father, giving blood, having a chest x-ray and an EKG. If you get bored recounting your own and your family's medical history, do what one Army general did: in between visitors, start working on a genealogical tree. At this writing, General Schaeffer's family tree has become a hundred-page "story of our family to hand down to succeeding generations."

Many hospitals will give you the Triflow gadget to practice your breathing exercises. If the hospital doesn't give you a Triflow, ask for it. Many hospitals have a social worker assigned solely to Bypass floors. If none comes to see you, ask for someone adept in Bypass counseling. Even if you don't think you need such help, you'll find it a comfort before and particularly after Bypass. Fre-

---

[1] To decrease hospital costs, some hospitals are doing preliminary tests on an ambulatory basis when possible and admitting patients the day before Bypass.

quently, hospitals have a Bypass coordinator, a cardiac nurse or social worker acting as patient-educator, patient-spokesperson, patient-doctor liaison. If such a person hasn't come calling on you on your first hospital day, ask if there is such a coordinator. No, you're not being a "difficult patient." If you and your family have a good understanding of Bypass and your care before and after surgery, you'll be better equipped to help yourself get better. *The Bypass patient's role is an active one.* You want to understand what will happen at each step of the way and how *you* can promote your recovery. Your doctors and nurses should be giving you additional information about your Bypass. If, after reading this book and any booklets the hospital may hand out, you have questions, ask the doctors and nurses caring for you. Jot down your questions in your notepad as they occur to you. Write down the answers. A pencil and notepad are required tools for every Bypasser.

Some hospitals have group meetings for you and your family with knowledgeable staff members. Some show video tapes of the operation and post-Bypass rehabilitation. Try to read this section again before such a meeting; bring your written questions with you. Arrange to meet your surgeon in the hospital as well as in his office. See him alone so you may ask questions you might not wish to ask in front of your family. But afterwards, those closest to you need a chance to ask their questions. Bypass is a family affair. Try to have one lengthy visit with the surgeon before being admitted to the hospital, first with you alone, then with your most intimate family member. If you travel to some faraway spot, this prehospitalization visit won't be possible. In that event, your referring cardiologist and internist at home should make themselves available for questions. Most Bypassers agree that a good internist, while not the person who does the surgery, is, nevertheless, the linchpin in helping them get through Bypass. Cultivate such a good understanding with your internist. He or she will stand you in good stead. But *you* must not be afraid to ask questions at any time; you should be prepared, if necessary, to insist on the opportunity. Because hospitals and doctors, like patients and their hearts, differ, take this book with you to the hospital for reference. The night before your Bypass, give it to a family member or friend to be returned to you when you leave the Intensive Care Unit for an intermediate care floor.

Somewhere along the line, you will have to sign a consent form giving permission for the doctors to perform your Bypass. Signing it means you have been informed of the arguments for and against the operation and that *you* assume *legal* responsibility for its outcome. Whether any of us ever is sufficiently informed to give "informed consent" may be a moot point, but without your signature the doctors won't operate. You do, however, have the right to ask questions, to read the form carefully, without being rushed, before signing. Refer to your notepad. Ask your questions. Jot down the answers on your pad. Much is happening to you, so it's hard to remember without notes. On the other hand, don't let all the dire possibilities listed on the consent form scare you—they *are* remote; the odds are decidedly in your favor.

At the Ochsner Medical Institutions in New Orleans, when the consent form is signed, smokers must sign a pledge never to smoke again. If Bypassers renege on the pledge, the Ochsner surgeons, of course, don't come after them and reclaim their grafts. They *do* make a telling point about the uselessness of having a Bypass if you're going back to smoking, fats, and high tension.

At some time during the day before Bypass, the anesthesiologist will come to see you. You should be sure to tell him or her of any allergies, any special dental work, any particular eye problems, you have had, even in the distant past. In some places, the anesthesiologist's fee is not covered by Blue Cross/Blue Shield. Avoid aggravation: check your coverage with both your surgeon and, if possible, the anesthesiologist before admission. If there's a problem, you should be able to negotiate terms. When you see the anesthesiologist in the hospital, you may want to know what kind of preoperative medication you'll get and when it will be given; what kind of anesthesia he or she is planning; how long after Bypass he or she waits to remove the endotracheal tube.

The anesthesiologist is an important person in your life. He or she not only is responsible for your sleeping through the operation but also, with the heart-lung technician, is the custodian of your heart-lung machine connection and of your endotracheal tube, your pipeline to the respirator. In some hospitals, the anesthesiologist is in charge of the Intensive Care Unit. During Bypass, the anesthesiologist usually stands at the head of the Bypass table.

Many hospitals will offer to take you on a tour of the ICU and even the operating room. Most prospective Bypassers are uneasy about taking this little trip. You don't have to go, but it's a good idea to talk to Bypassers themselves, not just "hear" the ones in this book. Again, the decision is yours. And you can change your mind.

The Evening Before Bypass

You'll receive your regular dinner tray. Nothing special. You won't be permitted to go out for dinner. You *can* ask if your family may bring in something special from the coffee shop.

You'll be shaved from chin to ankles, front and back, to reduce the chance of infection, to protect your incision from bacteria normally present on hair. After being shaved, you'll be instructed to scrub yourself clean with a special antibacterial soap. Some institutions require several such scrubbings; some settle for one. After these baths, you should practice the coughing and the deep breathing and self-hypnosis exercises.

Your family probably will be allowed to visit with you until about eight in the evening. You may want them to take your valuables and clothing home because you won't be able to have them in the Intensive Care Unit. If you'd prefer to keep your things with you, you can have your valuables placed in the hospital safe and your clothes hung up in the hospital clothes room. Do what makes you least edgy.

Some hospitals encourage families to come in briefly on the morning of your Bypass to wish you well. Other hospitals don't say anything about families. If you'd like your family there, the family can make arrangements with the nursing station. If you'd rather not have a family gathering in the morning, say so. This is your show.

After your family's visit, once you've showered and done the deep breathing and self-hypnosis exercises, you'll be given a sleeping pill. Take it. You've got a big day ahead. It's important to be rested. If your hospital waits for you to ask for sleeping medication, then ask. Just as much as you want your surgeon to have a good night's sleep, you also need one.

You're going to have nothing to eat or drink after midnight. Usually, the morning of Bypass, you'll be allowed to rinse your mouth with water and brush your teeth. Be sure *not* to swallow any water. No matter what may be placed by your bedside, eat or drink nothing after midnight. You need an empty stomach before general anesthesia.

Bypass

You'll be awakened at the crack of dawn to get ready for surgery. Some civilized institutions will let you call after nine the night before to ascertain the time that your operation is scheduled; they will awaken you accordingly. Others won't tell you specifically and will awaken everyone together. Most places will have you bathe or shower again with antibacterial soap. Now, you'll have to change into a hospital gown. Women must remove makeup and nail polish, because the color of lips and nail beds is important in assessing circulation during and after Bypass. If you choose to wear your wedding band, tell the nurse; she'll cover it with tape. If you wear dentures, you must remove them and give them to the nurse to place in a denture cup. Remove contact lenses, wigs, hairpieces. Hospitals differ as to who is the custodian of your glasses. If you're particularly dependent on glasses, be sure that they're in good hands. You'll want them sooner than you think. Arrange for a family member to bring an extra pair after you've resumed consciousness.

At some hospitals, for women Bypassers, the nurse inserts an indwelling catheter (a thin flexible tube) into the bladder while patients still are in their rooms. For male Bypassers, the bladder catheter is inserted in the operating room. The reason for the catheter? To drain urine from your bladder during surgery and for the first two days after the operation.

When the operating room has called for you, the nurse will give you an injection that will not sedate you but will help you relax and lessen your apprehension. Believe it or not, the injection works. It also makes your mouth feel dry. Once you've received this injection, stay in bed. Usually, the nurse puts the side rails up on the bed as a reminder that you must stay there. It's not an easy time, but the more you're able to go limp, the better the injection works. Here's another chance to practice the self-hypnosis or other relaxation techniques.

About twenty to forty-five minutes after you've had this injection, an attendant will take you to the operating room on a stretcher. As a patient, you'd probably prefer having that hospital-room injection put you out until the operation is over. That usually is not done. It's best for you to be unconscious for as little time as possible. Sometimes, the operating room may be behind schedule. What happens then? You lie on your gurney outside the operating room until all systems are go.

After someone helps you from the stretcher onto the operating table, you may be surprised by the number of people crowding into the operating room. All of the team will be there, at least nine of them: nurses, residents, research fellows, the anesthesiologist, the surgeon, the heart-lung technician. You'll even hear music piped into the operating room. The surgeon chooses the tapes. Some operate to rock, some to country-and-western, some to Bach and Beethoven. The operating room lights may make you blink from their brightness. Everybody will be wearing plastic caps, masks, gowns, and gloves; your surgeon probably will wear strange protruding glasses called loupes, similar to the small high-powered magnifying lenses used by jewelers.

There'll be an instrument table for hardware and small operating equipment, another for software such as sponges, dressings, and bandages; a physiological data monitor will display a continuous graph of your EKG, arterial blood pressure, venous pressure, blood gases, and temperature readings. To the side will be the heart-lung machine, constantly watched over by its caretaker, the heart-lung technician. The anesthesiologist will insert an intravenous tube into a vein in your arm so you can receive medications and fluids during Bypass. This I.V. needle is the only discomfort you'll feel, and it hurts only for a moment. Another technician will attach small adhesive patches wiring you to the heart-monitoring equipment. The I.V., the heart-monitor, and you will be linked together for several days after Bypass.

The anesthesiologist will give you anesthesia through the I.V. line and will keep you safely, painlessly, and deeply asleep until your operation is over. Just before you drop off to sleep, you may feel a catheter being inserted into the radial artery in your wrist so your arterial blood pressure can be directly monitored. You will not be aware of the anesthesiologist inserting a catheter into the jugular vein in your neck to monitor pressure and blood gases. You will not be aware of the endotracheal tube being put in to keep your airways open during Bypass and for twelve to twenty-four hours after the surgery.

For now you are well asleep. You, your heart, and your arteries are in the hands of experts. You've done your part; now it's their turn. And while for you Bypass is a big event, for an excellent cardiovascular surgeon Bypass is quite routine. In fact, some cardiac surgeons actually complain that Bypass is the dullest of operations, because aorta artery grafting consists mainly of doing the same things over and over. Ever mindful of the old Chinese curse "May you live in interesting times," we wish you the dullest—and the most successful—of Bypasses.

Just as you have slept through your Bypass, we fade out with you from the operating room to the Surgical Intensive Care (SICU), Cardiovascular Intensive Care Unit (CV-ICU), Coronary Care Unit (CCU), or whatever your hospital calls that place where highly skilled nurses and hi-tech equipment do what their name says: care for you intensively. The length of time you remain in ICU varies with the hospital, the doctor, and the patient. For the first twenty-four to forty-eight hours, you'll have continuous one-to-one nursing care. An ICU is a strangely noisy, sealed-off compartment, seemingly disconnected from the world. Many have no windows. You won't know whether it's day or night. Monitors whirr and beep, buzzers sound.

When you awaken, there'll be drainage tubes coming out of many orifices, an endotracheal tube passing through your mouth into your trachea (windpipe) and connected to a mechanical ventilator (respirator). By breathing for you, the mechanical ventilator lets you rest from the work of breathing on your own immediately following Bypass. As the oxygen is carried to your lungs, the ventilator whooshes loudly. To help it do its job, you must relax as much as possible, another good time to practice self-hypnosis. Because the tube—probably the most universally disliked part of Bypass—passes through your throat past your vocal cords, you won't be able to talk.

Before your Bypass, the nurse responsible for you in ICU may have been in to see you and practiced communicating signals with you. If not, you should have practiced two kinds of communication. First, while lying down, with your hand in one position (because the I.V. and catheter will be in your wrists when you awaken), practice writing on a pad with a fairly short pencil (it's easier). Second, practice tracing letters of words on the palm of your nurse's hand or in the palm of a family member's hand. Good nurses anticipate many of your needs. They know what Bypassers are feeling; they're sympathetic. In that first twenty-four hours, you will never be alone, so don't worry. Some hospitals do not permit your family in to see you for the first 48 to 72 hours. If this would upset you, change your Bypass plans, because these are hard-and-fast rules. Once every hour while you're awake, you must do the deep breathing and coughing exercises. Your nurse will help you with them.

While the endotracheal tube is in place, the nurse must clean the tube every hour by passing a suction catheter down the tube and suctioning the mucous secretions normally produced by your lungs. As the catheter is removed, it sucks up the mucous secretions from your airway and eases your breathing. Suctioning may make you feel as though you are gagging. Don't be afraid. Again, try self-hypnosis. As soon as the endotracheal vacuuming is over, you'll feel comfortable. Depending on hospital procedure, as well as on how much oxygen is present in your blood, the tube probably will be taken out by the next morning. After the tube is removed, your throat may be sore for several days.

You'll also have a nasogastric tube passing through your nose and into your stomach. Its purpose? Draining your secretions to prevent nausea and vomiting.

You'll have three electrocardiographic leads taped to your chest to transmit a continuous tracing of your EKG and heart rate onto the monitor screen. The monitor's alarms are exceedingly sensitive to movement. Don't be frightened by a false alarm.

You'll probably have two mediastinal tubes draining fluids from your chest cavity. The chest tubes make a gurgling that sounds as though it's raining outside. Usually, these tubes are removed by the afternoon of the day after Bypass; like everything else, this varies with the patient, the doctor, and the hospital.

There's more. The small catheter in your wrist will record your blood pressure continuously and transmit it to the monitor screen. The catheter enables blood samples to be drawn without your having to be stuck by a needle. Your nurse may ask you not to move your hand too much. Usually, this little catheter is taken out the day after surgery. You'll have a least two I.V.s through which you'll receive blood, fluid nourishment, and antibiotics. In case you've forgotten, you'll have a bladder catheter to drain urine. Usually, this is removed two days after Bypass. Besides all these drainage pipes and hookups, you'll be attached to lines recording the pressure in your heart. Generally, most of the seven tubes are removed the day after Bypass.

Will you be uncomfortable? In pain? How bad will it be? Everybody's pain threshold is different. No, this is not a cop-out. Read what Bypass veterans say about the pain. Many people mind the incision in the leg far more than the chest incision. Some people complain of shoulder and back pain from lying immobile so long during the operation. Others object to the sore throat following removal of the endotracheal tube. Sometimes, lying too long on an injection site makes someone's hip or side hurt. When you're recuperating from Bypass, don't suffer unnecessarily. Ask for pain medication. Many hospitals deliberately undermedicate. Many hospitals wait for the patient to *ask* for pain medication. The patient, unaware that he must ask, may think he shouldn't request painkiller. Some patients fret that pain medication might be addictive. In the dosages prescribed, medicine to relieve pain will *not* make you an addict. The moral of the story: if you're in pain, don't wait to ask for medication; postpone the heroics until you're well. One other word about pain: removing the chest tubes usually hurts. Ask your doctor, the resident, or the nurse to give you pain medication about half an hour before the chest tubes are taken out. It's like having Novocaine before having a tooth yanked out.

Once the endotracheal and nasogastric tubes have left, you can talk and eat. Julia Child doesn't prepare the clear liquid diet of gelatin and tea, but it'll be welcome fare, for thirst is a common complaint while the tubes are in place. Ask if you can have Fudgsicles or Popsicles. (If the hospital has none, a family member could stock the ICU refrigerator.) Your diet will progress to full liquids such as milk and juices, then to ice cream, and finally on to a low-salt diet. You may not be hungry, the hospital food may be unappetizing, but try to eat to build your strength. If there are specific foods you might like, some hospitals encourage you to let the nurse or the dietitian know. The family gofer[2] may be allowed to bring in food to tempt you. Check with the nurses.

After the drainage tubes are removed, you'll begin a serious walking regimen. Even before you walk (the doctors call it ambulate), on the night after Bypass, the nurse will help you sit up on the edge of the bed and dangle your legs over the side. Dangling helps you become accustomed to being in an upright position. Some places even stand you up and insist on weighing you. After that,

---

[2] A gofer is a Bypass essential. He or she works hard helping you. Remember to say thank you and to get your gofer a gift.

you'll sit up in a chair; soon you'll be walking, first assisted by your nurse, then on your own.

Like the coughing and breathing exercises, walking is crucial to a fast recovery. Walking improves your circulation and your ability to take deep breaths, so important for your lungs. You should increase the distance every day, but you shouldn't overdo. Pace yourself with frequent short walks rather than one overlong, exhausting walk. Learn to do nothing overmuch, balancing exercise and rest but walking at least three times a day.

A word about sitting: don't do too much. By resting your legs on the bed from the chair, you can keep your legs up to hip level. Do leg exercises. Don't cheat. Wear thigh-high surgical stockings. In the sitting position, unlike walking, the bend at your hips decreases the blood flow to and from your legs and may cause pooling of the blood in your legs. For the first week, you should sit only for meals and going to the bathroom. Which brings up another problem. Between the pain medication, the inactivity, and the not eating, you've got a good chance of being constipated. Once the tubes are out, ask your doctor to prescribe a stool softener.

The Bypassers here have talked about postoperative complications: lung complications especially for heavy smokers, phlebitis, arrhythmias (irregular heart beats), postcardiotomy syndrome or post pump syndrome (fever, chills, aching, chest pain), hallucinations, postoperative psychosis, postoperative bleeding, perioperative infarction, return of angina. But if you are a nonsmoker, reasonably trim, if you go to a good Bypass center and your surgeon himself has a good track record, probably you will recover fairly swiftly. Even the most common postoperative Bypass complications do not have a high statistical incidence and can be relieved by prompt therapy in a good Bypass center.

As you leaf through these Bypassers' accounts, you'll note one particular theme: almost everybody got depressed, had memory loss, even confusion. Some people felt blue on the fourth and fifth postoperative day; others didn't become depressed until they went home. Usually, depression lifted more quickly than memory returned. Severe depression occurs in about 30 percent of Bypassers. Certain physicians attribute memory loss to the length of time on the pump. Others blame depression on the insult to the body, on Bypass's physical stress and the body's responses to that stress.

While depression may not strike you, it's a good idea to plan an antidepression strategy. After you get home from the hospital, ask your spouse or friend to take a week off, even two, to walk with you, to take you for a drive, to cook your favorite foods, to keep you company. Schedule post-Bypass psychological counseling. It's money well spent.

As the Comfort Station Chapter advises, get dressed every morning, putter around the house, dust, set the table, clear the dishes, rinse, load the dishwasher. Not only will you be helping out, you'll be helping yourself fight post-Bypass blues. For the first two to three weeks, be sure to sequester two hours in the afternoon, and even an hour in the morning, for a rest, if not a nap. While you'll enjoy having company, visitors should know your calling hours and space their visits. Everybody should not arrive at once; nobody should stay longer than half an hour. *Festina lente*—make haste slowly—is the fastest route to recovery.

Conference Call

One of this book's major goals is to help future Bypassers obtain better medical care while they're having heart surgery. The *New England Journal of Medicine*, on October 19, 1982, reported that 55 percent of hospitals performing coronary artery bypass surgery are "suboptimal," a medical euphemism for inadequate at best, incompetent at worst. Such suboptimal hospitals do fewer CABS than necessary to keep their physicians, ancillary personnel, and even their equipment in top operating shape. In such places, Bypass costs no less, but patients get less: complication rates are higher; mortality rates are higher. Even within hospitals, individual surgeons' batting averages vary enormously.

The *New England Journal of Medicine* does not identify "optimal" and "suboptimal" hospitals. To avoid such places and to help themselves, patients and their families must learn to ask questions, to see the doctor with pencil and notebook in hand, both before and after Bypass. They must enlist their family physician's assistance in getting honest information about recommended surgeons and hospitals.

Unfortunately, the malpractice shadow tinges the relationship between doctors and patients. But if your physician knows that you are not asking antagonistically, that you're asking and writing down questions and answers to help you in your team effort to get you back to good health, he should be happy to talk to you. You're not going to ask your internist or cardiologist, "Is that surgeon any good?" He or she might reply, "Would I send you to a surgeon who wasn't the best?" But all the Bypassers I spoke with had questions they wish they had asked, information they recommended that prospective Bypassers obtain. Most agree that they didn't know enough to ask the right questions, that if they'd known what to expect, the unexpected would not have proven so worrisome.

Many Bypass veterans remark wonderingly on their reluctance to quiz their physicians and regret their silence. In this regard, one cardiologist-Bypasser, Dr. Eugene White, urged me to write, "Don't be intimidated. Ask everything on your mind. No question is silly or irrelevant. Be sure the doctor will give you all the time you want for your questions. While you're sitting around fretting and wondering, make notes. If the chances of success bother you, ask. If the length of time you'll be out of work worries you, ask. Don't keep things inside. If the cardiac surgeon does not have time to talk to you, tell your cardiologist and tell him you want someone else. Getting questions answered is of major importance to a Bypasser's peace of mind. Be sure to get them all answered. Satisfy yourself, because you'll do better in the hospital and afterwards."

Peter Stanwyck, president and CEO of a chemical engineering firm adds, "I'm unpopular with doctors because I insist on asking lots of questions, on their giving specific answers. When a physician looks past your shoulder or at his watch, ask him to make eye contact. You don't go to a doctor to be popular. You go to a doctor for advice, for experience, for technical skill in helping you—as best he can—to get better. Without having a chip on his shoulder, a patient has to say, 'We're talking about me and my life, my chances, how I will live my new life. I know you're busy, but you and I have to sit down and talk about my problems and solutions in meticulous detail.' "[1]

If your doctors object to spending time on something relatively routine for them, tell them Tom Fouretier's story about the phy-

---

[1] Dr. White and Mr. Stanwyck (both fictitious names) are among the many Bypassers whose accounts are regretfully omitted from this volume.

sician and the IRS man. One man's routine is another man's dark forest full of briers. From the twenty-one sets of questions here, make your own notes. Everybody's questions differ. Everybody looks at himself differently. These questions are for all the physicians responsible for your care and well-being; some are specifically aimed at your family practitioner or your internist (indicated by **I**), your cardiologist (indicated by a **C**), your cardiovascular surgeon (indicated by an **S**), or your anesthesiologist (indicated by an **A**). Depending upon your circumstances and community, the primary responsibility for "directing traffic" will reside with your family physician, internist, or cardiologist. Because so much depends on the nature and length of the doctor-patient relationship, it's important for you to have a physician who knows you, whom you can trust, who can be your traffic manager in Bypass and in the rest of your health care.

What follows is a distillation of Bypass veterans' questions. Some will pertain to you. Some will not. Whether you're having Bypass in your hometown or in a faraway place; whether you live in snowy Aroostook County, Maine, or in warm Beverly Hills, California, both geographical extremes where climate is a factor determining when you can go out and where the availability and density of physicians who specialize are markedly unequal; whether you're male or female, single or married, divorced or widowed—all will influence what you want to know and whom you ask. But ask you must.

Questions

1. (I, C) *Why do I need Bypass?* What will it do for me? Will I live longer? Will my life be better? Will I be free of pain? What benefits can I reasonably expect from Bypass? Could medicine help me just as well?

2. (I, C, S) *What are my odds?* Taking into account my age, sex, previous heart problems, family history, smoking history, pertinent medical history, how badly my arteries are blocked, how many arteries are involved, *what are* my *odds?* May I have a second opinion from a cardiologist in another hospital? (The American Heart Association recommends that, whenever possible, everyone get a second opinion.)

3. (C, S) *What vessels are involved in my heart disease?* How seriously blocked are they? May I see the angiographic films with you? Please draw me a sketch before and after Bypass and give it to me to keep. Do you think you'll be able to fix all the blocked vessels?

4. (I, C, S) *How many of your patients are better off since Bypass?* How many of these Bypassers now can do things better? How many of these Bypassers are worse off? What follow-up do you employ? One year? Two years?

5. (I, C) *What happens during the angiogram?* What percent of cardiac-catheterized patients go to Bypass? How many angiograms do you perform in a year? What's your complication rate?

6. (I) *How do doctors decide who is a good CABS candidate?* How much is the Bypass decision governed by how "aggressive" or how "conservative" are my internist, my cardiologist, my cardiac surgeon? How much is influenced by what facilities are available in my hometown or the doctor's hometown? How much is affected by how long I have to wait for surgery? How much of my surgeon's decision is shaped by his statistics? If I am refused as a candiate because I'm a poor risk, do you recommend I go for another evaluation? If so, where should I go?

7. (I) *What are the advantages and disadvantages of going away from home for Bypass?* What are the major Bypass centers in America? How do I find out about the hospital you're sending me to? How do I know about the surgeon? Please do not send me to a group and let me take potluck among the group. Where would you go if you needed Bypass? Who would operate on you?

8. (I, C, S) *How long must I wait for Bypass?* If I went to another hospital, in my town or out of it, would I wait less time? For me, with my disease, is waiting dangerous?

9. (S) *How many CABS does your hospital perform a year?* How many CABS do you personally perform a year? How many of your Bypassers have complications? In the hospital? In the first year? What are they? What is your average pump time? Will you, my surgeon, see me every day while I'm in the hospital? Will you sit down and talk to me with the door closed? How many times will you see me after I'm discharged? How often? What percent of your patients need second and third operations? After what period of time? How well do your second-time-arounders do? Will you be in town during the entire time I'm in the hospital? If not, who will? What doctor will see me every day? May I meet him or her before Bypass? Do you have well-trained resident physicians and cardiovascular fellows, not just physicians' assistants, good though they may be, *on twenty-four-hour duty in the hospital* during the week and on weekends? What do you charge? How much is covered by third-party medicine (Blue Cross and Blue Shield, other insurance plans)? How much will I have to pay? How does your fee and the hospital fee compare with the national average?

10. (I, C, S) *How long will I be in the hospital, before and after Bypass?*

11. (I, C, S) *Does the hospital make any special arrangements for my family?* If I go out of town, is there a place nearby for my family to stay? Is the neighborhood safe? Is there a special room in the hospital for my family to wait? How often does the staff keep my family posted? Will my family have Bypass and all the pre-Bypass and post-Bypass procedures explained to them? When I come to, will I be allowed to see my family? How often? If I am under sixty, should my children and siblings have complete physical exams, with EKG, stress test, cholesterol, triglycerides, and blood sugar, as recommended by the Johns Hopkins Preventive Cardiology Center and by the "Son of Framingham" study of sons and daughters of the original Framingham subjects?

12. (I, C, S) *Does the hospital have a formal postoperative rehabilitation program begun in the hospital and continued after I get home?* Does the hospital have nutritional counseling to help me modify my diet? Does the hospital have an occupational counselor, someone who will advise me about the impact of Bypass on my job and my career? Does the hospital have psychological counseling? Will a psychiatrist, psychologist, or psychiatric social worker see me regularly before and after Bypass and after I go home? What kind of cardiac rehabilitation is available in my town? Is there a behavior-modification program along the lines of Dr. Meyer Friedman's Recurrent Coronary Prevention Program? If not, how can I obtain such counseling? Will Blue Cross/Blue Shield pay for postoperative cardiac rehabilitation?

13. (S, C, A) *Tell me about the operation itself.* What do you do? How does it work? How long will I be unconscious? When do they put me out? How long will surgery take? How long do you leave the tube in? What about learning self-hypnosis to help tolerate the tube? If I'm embarrassed to ask for a painkiller, will someone realize I'm in pain and give it to me?

Before your Bypass, preferably before you go into the hospital, ask the anesthesiologist, "What kind of anesthesia will you give me? What are its side effects?" Be sure to ask the anesthesiologist, "What is your fee? How much is covered by Blue Cross?" Many anesthesiologists send bills in excess of the Blue Cross/Blue Shield allowance. If you're strapped for funds and he will not negotiate his fee, perhaps your cardiologist or your cardiac surgeon will speak to him for you. It's worth a try.

14. (I, C) *Will the Coronary Care Unit nurses be available when I need them?* When I'm transferred from the CCU to the general hospital floor, will I need special nurses? I hear that some hospitals don't have enough nurses. Is that true of the floors where I'll be? How many patients are assigned to each CCU nurse? How many patients are assigned to each general-floor nurse? Do you have a step-down, or transitional, floor with telemetry between the CCU and the general floor?

15. (I, C) *Before my Bypass, may I have a Triflow apparatus on which to practice my breathing exercises?* If I have to wait several weeks for Bypass, are there simple, nonrisky exercises I can do to get in better physical condition for Bypass and recovery?

16. (I, C) *When I get home, will I be able to take care of myself, or will someone need to take care of me for the first week or two?* What arrangements should I make? Some people I know were depressed by being home alone. Should my spouse take time off from work to stay home with me? Should I make arrangements with the Visiting Nurse Association or Meals-on-Wheels? After Bypass, how long will it take for my scars to heal? What can I do to help them heal more quickly? Should I wear surgical stockings on my legs? For how long? What kind do you recommend?

17. (I,C) *After Bypass, what are my chances of complications?* While I may not have any troubles, it's better knowing than not knowing. What should I do for:

   A. *Psychological problems:*

       Depression, weepiness, hopelessness for longer than three
          to five days
       Memory loss
       Loss of concentration
       Reduced attention span
       Confusion
       Disorientation

Trouble in thinking clearly

Weakness

Irritability

Speech defect or paralysis

B. *Physical symptoms:*

Chest pain—How do I distinguish between anginal chest pain and the pain of my scars knitting?

Shortness of breath on permitted activity or shortness of breath at rest

Severe fatigue unrelieved by rest[2]

Severe weakness unrelieved by rest[3]

Sudden unexplained weight gain (measured by weighing yourself every day at the same hour)

Any fever for more than three days

Fever, chills, headache, aches and pains

Any leg-swelling or calf-aching

Redness or heat around the incisional areas; persistent incisional pain, itching, aching; pus leaking from the incision

Persistent cough—particularly coughing that brings up green or yellow mucus—or pain on taking a deep breath.

Irregular heartbeats, either too fast or too slow

18. (I, C) *After Bypass, when can I resume my normal activities?* When can I return to work? Will there be any work limitations involving length of days, number of days, travel? How long will my recovery take? Will I have any restrictions on diet, on alcohol consumption, on exercise?

19. (I, C) *Will Bypass affect my sex life?* Will my desire be the same? As a male Bypasser, will I have any sexual dysfunction, any inability to have or maintain an erection, any inability to come to ejaculation? Do women Bypassers have any problems with desire or function? If I have any sexual problems from medication, will you change my medicine? Will you help me cope with any sexual dysfunction or groundless fears? Will you talk to my spouse so that she/he will not be afraid to have intercourse? How long after Bypass may I resume sexual activity? Must I take any precautions about

---

[2] Some fatigue is to be expected. Some Bypassers say that the bone-tiredness after Bypass may not lift for a year.

[3] Pace your walks and exercise. Always remember you must walk as far in returning as you did in going. It's like all of life.

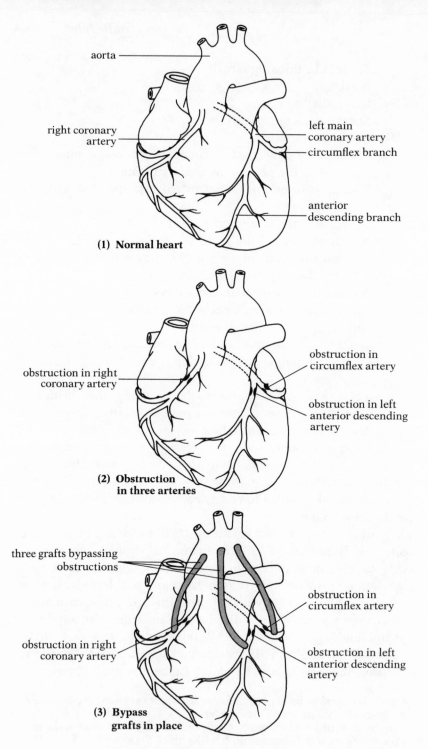

aorta

right coronary artery

left main coronary artery

circumflex branch

anterior descending branch

(1) Normal heart

obstruction in right coronary artery

obstruction in circumflex artery

obstruction in left anterior descending artery

(2) Obstruction in three arteries

three grafts bypassing obstructions

obstruction in circumflex artery

obstruction in right coronary artery

obstruction in left anterior descending artery

(3) Bypass grafts in place

Original drawing by Marvin Hoffman, M.D., adapted by Sandy McMahon my chest incision? I've heard that the new Bypasser should be the more passive partner, that the active-partner-astride and side-by-side positions are better for a new Bypasser. Do you agree? I've heard that, like swimming, sexual activity should be postponed for two hours after a heavy meal, after more than one drink, after exercise. Do you agree? Do I need to take a nitro before intercourse?

20. (I, C, S) *If you're a woman Bypasser, you may want to ask the following questions:* Should I arrange for part-time help at home after my discharge from the hospital? If so, for how long? Would it be a good idea for my husband or a friend to take a couple of weeks off from work after my hospital discharge? Can I wear panty hose to go home? should I take slacks to go home in? I've heard that women have a tendency to form keloids with the chest scar. Is there anything I can do to prevent this keloid- or hyper-trophic-scar formation? What kind of bra do you recommend I wear in the hospital to prevent keloids? What kind of makeup do you recommend to camouflage my scar? Do you have any post-Bypass exercises particularly geared to women? Do you have any post-Bypass counseling especially for women? Do you have any special counseling for their husbands or friends? Could you give me the names of some women Bypassers to call about their experiences?

21. (I, C) *Knowing that there aren't any guarantees, what kind of results, based on the statistics, do you expect I'll get?* How permanent are these results? I've heard of people needing second and third Bypasses; will that happen to me? What can I do to change my life, my attitude towards myself and my world, to enhance my Bypass results?

22. (I, C, S) Last but not least, do you have a hot line so I can talk to *you*, the doctor, not a nurse or a secretary? If not, how do I reach you if I need you?

Comfort Station: Easy Ways to Relieve Common Complaints

Coughing and Breathing Exercises

Before the operation, at most hospitals, the pulmonary therapist or the chief cardiac nurse will teach you breathing exercises and coughing techniques. Obviously, it is easier to learn before surgery than afterwards. Patients are taught how to blow into a small plastic tube, so that the exhaled breath pushes three little balls to the top of the breathing apparatus. Practicing these exercises at least once every three hours for two or three days before Bypass will help you remember in the foggy postoperative aftermath. If you practice occasionally with a nurse or an inhalation therapist watching, he or she can advise you whether you're "exercising" your breathing correctly.

Coughing hurts. However high or low your pain threshold, coughing will hurt. Before the operation, listen carefully to the therapist's instructions about how to cough; then *practice*. If by chance your doctor or hospital does not have someone to teach you breathing and coughing exercises, insist that you be shown at least twenty-four hours before surgery so you can practice on your own.

After Bypass, even before they let you sit up, they'll make you cough. You *must* cough because you *must* clear your lungs of secretions to prevent pneumonia or atelectasis (partially collapsed lung). Some hospitals tell you to hug a pillow or a turkish towel to support the incision and lessen the pain from coughing. The doctors at Walter Reed Hospital in Washington, D.C., recommend large stuffed animals. They are just soft enough and just firm enough. All over the cardiac surgery floor at Walter Reed, you can see thin-lipped generals and hard-nosed sergeants hugging giant pandas, Snoopy dogs, and teddy bears. Walter Reed provides its patients with stuffed animals. At most other places, you'll have to bring your own. Don't be embarrassed. It works. It's comforting, too.

Also take a small triangular wedge-shaped pillow with you. It will help you sleep.

How to Keep a Scar from Being Irritated

Some scars knit well and quickly, some scars knit painfully and scratchily, some scars are irritated by male chest hair growing back, some scars are irritated by a shirt or an undershirt rubbing against it, some scars form keloids. If your scar bothers you, try the ingenious contraption devised by the CEO of a corporation listed on the New York Stock Exchange. This chief executive officer, a "problem-solver by nature," bought polyurethane Styrofoam, about one inch thick, five to six inches wide, and about two to three inches longer than his chest scar. He cut a hole in the Styrofoam three inches wide and an inch longer than the scar. The Styrofoam lies on his chest. "It needs no adhesive," he reported, "because my undershirt, shirt, and tie hold it in place. It can't be seen by outsiders. It keeps the shirt and the undershirt from rubbing the healing scar or from irritating a keloid."

If you're female and big-breasted, take a bra to the hospital for wear once you've been moved from the Intensive Care Unit to the step-down floor or to the general nursing floor. One forty-three-year-old female Bypasser recommended a Bali Flower Bra, while a fifty-year-old nursing supervisor used a Mary Jane Sleeping Bra. The Bali fastens in the back; the Mary Jane fastens in the front and may irritate the scar.

Communicating

If you're female and decorous, talk over your feelings with your internist and your cardiologist before you book yourself into a Bypass. Most CCUs have only a sheet between beds. Frequently, you'll be uncovered. Often, the hospital will insist on your using a commode before you transfer from the CCU. In many places, you'll be the only woman in the unit. If this bothers you, discuss it with your doctor. There are a few institutions which have post-Bypass units for women only.

People complain about not being given a pencil and paper, about not being able to communicate during that period when they're awake but the endotracheal tube hasn't been removed. Until every hospital starts providing its CCUs with pad and pencil, bring your own. Further, be sure your wife, husband, friend, child, carry a spare pad and pencil. In the trip from the general floor to the operating room to the recovery room to the CCU, your pad and pencil may get lost. Have a prearranged signal set up with your special person, so he or she may give them to you in those first few minutes after you awaken.

A special person is not always with you, however. Some people like knitting their wounds alone. Others prefer the solace of someone they love standing by. Some hospitals don't permit families to see Bypassers until three days after surgery. If this separation would upset you and yours, you must arrange to go elsewhere. They won't bend their rules. Before you make your hospital arrangements, ask about rules for families.

Most Bypassers are beset by "hurry sickness," are too time-concious. Nevertheless, if you can see a clock in the CCU, it helps you to orient yourself. Like restaurant kitchens, CCUs often aren't designed by or for the people who use them. Frequently, there's no clock in sight. Once you're awake enough to care, which is sooner than you think, it helps to have a clock in view. Before your Bypass, ask your special person to bring a quartz clock, not one that ticks loudly and disturbs your fellow CCU-ers, and not one that's electric—you've got enough wires without adding more. Get a clock with large numbers, because your glasses won't be on your nose. Get a clock with the date, preferably one that tells whether it's day or night. Some CCUs have windows, but many do not. Patients need to see day become night, to see night fade and dawn herald a new day. Without windows, a clock will help you count the minutes towards getting better.

Some CCUs have small radios or TV sets attached to each bed. Others don't. If the CCU doesn't have a radio or a TV, a small portable radio slipped under your pillow may keep you company.

When Bypassers come to, sometimes they don't know the operation is over. Often, they worry that they've lost their place in the Bypass line. Some CCU nurses tell you right away: "The Bypass is done. You're doing fine." Some CCUs are better staffed than others. Before your Bypass, ask both your special family member and your doctor to give you the good news at the first flicker of your eyelids. Initially, you'll be slipping in and out of consciousness. It's best for them to repeat this news bulletin several times, to be sure you've registered the glad tidings.

Before you go home, ask someone to beg, borrow, or purchase an inflatable incliner, to be ready and waiting for you. These large, wedge-shaped vinyl pillows can be blown up like balloons, their size and firmness adjusted for comfort. Get two; they're small. At about $5.95, they're also cheap. Not only is such an incliner a comfort in the early postoperative weeks when sleep can be a problem, it's a good leg elevator to help your leg scars heal.

When you get home, be sure to get up in the morning and get dressed for the day. Do not hang around in a robe and slippers. When getting out of bed, don't let someone help you. They may pull too hard or pull the wrong way. Take it easy yourself. When you shower, be sure there's a rubber mat in the tub or shower. Keep a chair by the tub to grasp. If you feel a little weak in the knees, ask someone to sit in the bathroom while you're bathing. Don't use too hot or too cold water. When sitting or standing, be conscious of your posture. Sit or stand up straight. While sitting, always have your legs on a stool or chair. Don't let them dangle. It's bad for circulation. Don't cross your legs. Be sure to wear support hose every day.

When you go for a walk, wait an hour and a half after eating. Until you're able to drive yourself, you'll want to go for a drive as a passenger. Be sure to wear your safety belt, even to the corner. Don't let an auto accident injure your incision just because you've been careless about wearing a belt. If it's warm out and you sit outdoors, keep your incision out of the sunlight for six to eight weeks. Apply cocoa butter to the incision to help it heal.

At home, remember that you're not sick; you're recuperating. Help out with household chores. Do dishes, set the table. But don't iron, vacuum, lift trash heavier than ten pounds, or struggle opening tightly fixed bottle tops. Walter Reed Army Hospital gently reminds its patients: "Remember always to say 'please' and 'thank you' to family for the smallest favors. They deserve it."

Concentration and Relaxation Techniques

Almost everybody wishes for a willpower pill. Almost everybody recognizes the dangers of overeating, of overdrinking, of smoking, of quick-fired rages, of rushing to do more and more in less and less time. Usually, all we do is wish for the magic pill—without changing. Most of us don't recognize that fatigue, our most common symptom, frequently results from anxiety. Like a thief in the night, obsessive running around in circles "steals" energy. Feeling exhausted, we worry more, rush more, drain our resources even more.

One way of teaching ourselves not to yearn for food, drink, cigarettes, and revenge, one way to conquer anxiety, is through concentration and relaxation. While some doctors don't believe in behavior modification, in stress management, in domesticating the "relaxation response," most physicians are beginning to realize that frenzy-modulation is a necessity. Friedman and Rosenman's drills in *Type A Behavior and Your Heart* need to be memorized and used daily. They're lifesavers. Norman Cousins's humorous tapes and singing aloud works. Many Bypassers have commented on the helpfulness of self-hypnosis techniques, particularly in the hospital, and even after discharge. Here are some quick tricks:

1. *Concentration:* Focus your full attention on an object—your thumb, the corner of the room, the nightstand.

2. *Rhythmic breathing:* Take a deep breath, hold it for a second, and let it out. Then take a tauter breath, with a tighter hold and a fuller expiration. Now, move onto pendular breathing, easy in and hold, easy out. Focus your full attention on your breathing. See how many breaths you can count without losing track. Then start over.

3. *Relaxation:* Regular breathing relaxes the chest muscles. Better respiration helps muscle metabolism and enhances relaxation. Concentrate on relaxing toes (try to do it toe by toe), feet, calves. Gradually, and gently, let the relaxation ascend. When you bring relaxation to your neck and facial muscles, your eyes will want to close. They'll feel heavy. Don't force your eyes to remain open. Let them close. Yield to the relaxation.

4. *Disassociation:* In your mind, move to a secure and pleasant place—a park bench on a warm day, a boat on a lake, a lover's arms. Feel a warm breeze ruffling your hair, listen to the birds calling one another, smell the hyacinths, see a field of daffodils reflect the sunshine.

5. *Deepening:* Slowly get on a psychic elevator. As you descend each floor, registered on the elevator's light panel and visualized by your mind's eye, consciously will yourself to be more relaxed.

6. *Repetition:* To yourself, keep saying, "In every adverse, scratchy situation, I'll be *calm, confident, smiling, relaxed, self-aware, self-possessed.*"

7. *Instruction:* Focus on ways of changing *one* bad habit. Every time you lose your train of thought, go back to the train station and get back on the train again. Work on one thing at a time. If the list is too long, you'll be overwhelmed.

8. *Diet:* Keep repeating, "I will find green vegetables, fruit, fish and chicken fully satiating and fully satisfying. I'll cut them finely, chew them well. This food will fuel my energy. No part of it will be converted to plaque-building fat. I will shun fried foods, animal fats, cakes, candies, ice cream, and cookies." Try and make yourself believe it.

9. *Anxiety:* Tell yourself again and again, "Contentment will be mine. I'll master my worries rather than let them master me.

Checking and containing my annoyance level will energize my work and my play. Conscious delight in life's small joys will be my daily antidepressant."

Then one, two, three, awake.

Much of this may seem simple, even simplistic. It is. Nevertheless, it works.

Sex: The Three-Letter Word Doctors Are Reluctant to Use

Recently, you've experienced a major health crisis. Now, you're planning to go home. You've made it, yet often you may find yourself getting easily annoyed or depressed. Not being able to do certain things may frustrate or irritate you. Such emotional responses are normal. It takes time to return to your old routine. If you vent your anger on your family, they may be puzzled about how to react to you, how best to help you. Usually, the first few months after a Bypass are difficult for both the Bypasser and his or her family.

One question too infrequently asked or answered is: What about the resumption of sexual activity? Remember, sexuality and sensuality are intimately related. Good sex involves behavioral and emotional continuity. Even when some physical condition prohibits intercourse itself, individuals still can be satisfied by and satisfying to their partners, can express tenderness, affection, and passion, can give and receive sexual comfort and solace.

After cardiac surgery, Bypassers and their partners often worry, "How safe is it to resume sexual activity?" Obviously, sexual intercourse does call for some exertion, but most cardiologists agree that intercourse is no more demanding than climbing two flights of stairs. Unfortunately, intercourse is mistakenly considered highly strenuous. *This is not true.* Most Bypassers eventually resume their customary lovemaking without any restrictions at all.

Remind yourself of one rule: *keep communication channels open.* Frequently, sexual anxieties, an unaccustomed shyness, prevent a couple from talking about their sexual feelings for each other or from reaching out with affectionate gestures. Tenderness is a great healer. Such avoidance can cause unnecessary stress and frustration, can do both your hearts much more harm than sexual activity. Avoidance too quickly becomes habit. Anxiety becomes a self-actualizing prophecy. Don't wait too long.

Sexual intercourse between two partners in a long-term relationship only moderately increases the heart's work. Because of your Bypass and your hospitalization, you'll need "reconditioning" before your return to an active sex life and to other energetic physical activities. Reconditioning means slowly increasing your exertional capacity with regular exercise aimed at building your physical stamina. During the reconditioning period, your physician may provide you with an activity schedule to follow. If not, you can show him the schedule on p. 425 and ask him to fill in the prescribed exercise time limits. As you regain your strength and obtain clearance from your physician, you'll be able to engage in many activities which enrich your life, including sexual intercourse.

Although you may not be able to resume sexual intercourse immediately after Bypass, you can demonstrate loving signs of affection. Holding hands, kissing, caressing, all communicate closeness between partners, a feeling you both need. When the time comes, sooner rather than later—and don't wait too long—that you're ready to resume sexual activity, the following suggestions may help both of you:

1. Do not eat for at least three hours beforehand. A large amount of blood is redirected to the stomach when you are digesting food. This results in a decreased amount of blood circulating to other areas of the body. The heart muscle must exert a greater amount of effort to support added physical activity such as intercourse.

2. Keep the temperature in the room comfortably regulated, not too hot or too cold.

3. Do not consume any alcoholic beverages for at least three hours before sexual activity. Alcohol causes an increase in the heart-beat and makes the heart work harder.
4. Try to be comfortably rested. If you are too tired, sexual activity is more draining and more energy-consuming. The best time for exercise, such as intercourse or other forms of physical activity, is after a rest period or in the morning just after awakening.
5. Sex is easier when you are content and happy. When you are upset, worrying, or angry, your heart is under strain. These emotional reactions place an additional demand on the heart's work load.
6. Do not engage in sexual activity one hour before or after bathing or showering. Warm water causes the blood vessels in the skin to increase in size and thus to take up more blood. The heart must then pump faster and with greater force.
7. Engage in sexual intercourse when you have plenty of time and are in familiar surroundings; this also reduces the strain on your heart. Abruptly starting and stopping sexual intercourse can place added strain on your heart. Take your time and enjoy each other; do not rush!
8. Above all, don't worry. Let sex be fun, consolation, comfort, passion. Enjoy yourself and each other.

After Bypass, which positions for intercourse are best? Eventually, you may want to experiment with different positions. Most important, do what is comfortable. The male-on-top position is perhaps the most commonly used sexual technique, but it's physically taxing for the male Bypasser. For some individuals, it may be too strenuous and lead to some discomfort. Explore through trial and error what modifications are helpful. Some couples will continue with the male-on-top position because they don't experience any problems. Less stressful positions include partner on top, side by side, and sitting upright. Try to experiment with other comfortable positions, but remember that satisfaction depends on both of you feeling good about what you are doing. If a change causes too much discomfort or anxiety, the benefits of changing are decreased. In the long run, the decision remains with each individual couple.

If you experience chest pain (angina) with sexual exertion, your doctor may advise you to take your prescribed medication (such as nitroglycerin) fifteen to thirty minutes before engaging in sexual activity. Ask him. Probably, medication will reduce chest pain during intercourse. Consult your physician if continued chest pain occurs with sexual or any other form of physical activity.

Most Bypass information assumes you're male, over fifty, and married. Not every Bypasser fits this description. If you're female and married, in some ways, resuming sexual intercourse may be easier than for your male counterpart. Whatever are women's anxieties, women aren't dogged by concerns about "performance," that awful word often used to describe male erectile function during life's joyous moments. If you're female and single, widowed or divorced, you may worry about your partner's reactions to your scar. If your partner cares about you, usually, as Charlie Brown would say, "you've wasted a good worry." If you're exceedingly self-conscious about your scar, once it's begun healing you can apply a little facial foundation to camouflage it, even wear a frilly chemise. If you and your partner like each other, you'll soon find the foundation and the chemise unnecessary.

Males, no matter what their age, can have erectile or ejaculatory dysfunction, possibly caused by blood-pressure, cardiac, or ulcer drugs. For many years, doctors thought erectile dysfunction was psychological. Now they realize that most sexual problems are physiological. If you're having trouble, tell your doctor and ask him if he can change your medication. Talk to your partner. Don't be embarrassed. Don't *not* talk about it. Don't get tense. Don't practice avoidance. If you're living longer, live better; learn how to give your partner pleasure with your fingers, your tongue, even your toes. Giving pleasure will give you pleasure, even if you are not able to ejaculate.

After Bypass, sometimes the Bypasser's desire diminishes. Frequently, reduction in desire is attributable to those same drugs. Often, it's caused by plain old-fashioned fear of "breaking" the Bypass, hurting the heart by getting too excited. Remember this: *sex can't break your Bypass.* Extramarital sex, sex with someone much younger, or sex with someone new does exert your heart more. There's an old cardiologist's "joke": people with heart conditions should have intercourse only with someone to whom they've been married for over twenty years. While this advice reveals something about doctors' own attitudes towards matters sexual, nevertheless, it has an edge of truth.

Now for the silver lining: many Bypassers find Bypass has

renewed their sexual lives. With Bypass, their hearts pump more blood—everywhere. They've come to life. This may be true for you. Don't let fear or anxiety about erectile dysfunction harm your new sense of sexual possibility and fulfillment.

You are going to be the person primarily responsible for monitoring your health after discharge from the hospital. Be aware of how you feel and any changes in your tolerance of different physical activities, not just in relationship to sexual activity. Watch for the following:

1. A rapid heart rate that persists and is noticeably prolonged after intercourse
2. A "knocked-out" feeling of excessive fatigue on the day following intercourse
3. A new or greater degree of chest pain during or after intercourse, even when you use the chest-pain medication
4. Palpitations (a fluttering or pounding in the chest) continuing for fifteen minutes or more after intercourse
5. New or unusual sleeplessness following intercourse

Any persistent problems should be reported to your physician as soon as possible. In most cases, stopping the activity will stop the discomfort. Frequently, your doctor will tell you ways to help your heart pump better during sexual activity, ways to avoid cardiac interruptions of sexual pleasures.

Activity Sheet

Take this chart to your doctor and ask him to check off when you can begin each activity.

Activity	Weeks following discharge						
	2nd	3rd	4th	6th	8th	12th	26th
Shower, shave, shampoo							
Dress in street clothes							
Eat meals with family							
Walk around house and yard							
Walk—increase distance							
Climb stairs							
Sit up in chair as desired							
Ride in car							
Drive car alone							
Visitors (Brief = B) (Longer = L)							
Sexual activity							
Light housework, light home repair							
Prepare light meals							
Wash dishes							
Laundry							
Lift up to 10 pounds							
Lift more than 10 pounds							
Table and card games							
Clerical work: Balance checkbook (the pits) Typing							
Light gardening							
Travel by car for more than 1 hour							
Travel by plane							
Social life: Small groups							
Large groups							
Out to dinner in a restaurant							
Out to a movie, concert, or play							
Work: Half days							
Full days							
Full weeks							
Travel on business							
Sports: Golf							
Fishing							
Bicycling							
Swimming							
Tennis—doubles							

A Talk About Heart Disease
and its Prevention

This year, 1.5 million Americans will be struck by their first heart attack. This myocardial infarction (heart attack) will, for 50 percent of these victims, be the first symptom of coronary artery disease. Of this estimated 750,000, 20 percent will die immediately, felled by their first assault. Another 12 to 15 percent will die in the Coronary Care Unit, while 15 percent more will die during the first postinfarction year. Only half, then, of this million or more, once attacked, will be alive one year later. With fast action, many heart-attack deaths can be prevented. CPR is a lifesaver, as John Boggs's story demonstrates. Everyone should be trained and have a yearly refresher course in CPR. Everyone—not just heart patients—should post the doctor's, hospital's, and nearest ambulance service's phone numbers beside every telephone at home and at work.

In the United States, of the 25 million men between forty and sixty, approximately 4 percent (one million) have asymptomatic, silent but significant, heart disease. Because the CCU tends to be considered a man's world, because many more men have cardiovascular disease than do women of the same age, because pre-menopausal women's hormones tend to protect them against heart disease, there are few statistics for women, except that 21 percent of all Bypassers are female. In this country, coronary artery disease annually kills some 650,000 Americans, male and female. Coronary artery bypass surgery is one way doctors and patients fight heart disease.

Many Bypass prescriptions are written for people who never have had an outright heart attack—for people with angina, particularly angina uncontrolled by medication. Angina, that most common of heart ailments, is recurrent pain in the chest and left arm, caused by a sudden decrease of the blood supply to the heart muscle. But often angina is *not* pain and *not* in the chest. Like its near relative "anger," "angina" derives its name from the Greek *ankhone*, "a strangling," or *anchein*, "to squeeze," both common descriptions of anginal sensations. Tightness, burning, squeezing, numbness, pressure, fullness or heaviness, aching, tingling in the throat, chest, arms, or stomach, indigestion, shortness of breath, choking, pain in the jaw, gums, teeth, or earlobes, neck pain between the shoulders, all can be manifestations of angina. While angina's location varies with the individual, your angina usually strikes in the same place and is brief (from thirty seconds to five minutes). It may worsen and then slowly disappear; or it may be severe but fleeting. Heavy meals, walking uphill, walking in exceedingly cold or hot weather, striding against a strong wind, exercise or heavy lifting, fear, anger, or tension, sexual intercourse, and high altitudes, all make your heart work harder and may generate angina.

Stable angina can originate from a sudden excessive increase in the heart's demand for oxygen. Unstable, or variant, angina arises from a temporary decrease in the heart's limited oxygen reserves. *Neither stable nor unstable angina is a heart attack.* Nor are the aches and pains enumerated always symptoms of angina. While angina is a temporary warning, a heart attack is a sign of permanent damage. People with angina are twice as likely to have a heart attack than people without angina. If the course of your angina alters, if it occurs more frequently or more severely with milder stimuli, if it persists longer, if it's not relieved by your medicine, if it occurs at unusual times, then call your doctor right away. If you think you're having a heart attack, *don't wait. Get emergency medical help instantly.*

Wherever and whenever angina appears, it's caused by the heart muscle not getting enough oxygen-carrying blood to fuel its pumping. Angina is the heart's protest against overworking with inadequate fuel. For the heart is a double-force pump composed of four chambers—two auricles (the upper chambers) and two ventricles (the lower chambers)—and serviced by coronary arteries through which oxygenated (oxygen-carrying) blood flows to the body's vital organs. These arteries surround the heart like a crown (the Latin word *corona* means "crown"). Branching off the aorta are two main coronary arteries, the right and the left. Branching off the left coronary are two main limbs, the circumflex and the left anterior descending (LAD) artery.

When plaque builds up and hardens inside the artery wall, the artery gradually loses elasticity; blood flow through the narrowed artery slows to a trickle. Just as sludge reduces flow in a drainpipe, so, too, do fatty cholesterol deposits decrease blood flow in an artery until it becomes severely narrowed or completely blocked. With insufficient blood and oxygen delivered to the heart's muscle cells, the heart muscle fed by this blood vessel begins to wither; it may even die. If tissue dies from not receiving enough oxygen-nourishing blood, the heart is attacked by a myocardial infarction.

Bypass surgery, today the most common major operation performed in the United States, permits blood to bypass a clogged artery, much as a highway detour permits cars to go around roads clogged by traffic. The obstructed area is bypassed by constructing a detour for blood flow through a healthy blood vessel, usually a section of saphenous vein taken from the leg, or from the internal mammary artery (two vessels in the chest wall), or both. The original obstructions remain. The new roadways are subject to the same traffic jam. Like highway repairs, Bypass is *not* a cure. The tragedy of Bypass is that its veterans often look upon it as a "fix" and go back to the same old ways that first brought them to the Bypass table. No matter how complete the revascularization (restoration of blood flow), no matter how many arteries are repaired, Bypass only reduces symptoms. For a variety of reasons, many as yet little understood, grafted veins and mammary arteries may close down in a few years. Depending on the location and the extent of blockage, the blood flow, even initially, may not be fully restored.

Recent studies have shown that the internal mammary artery graft remains patent (open and working) longer than the saphenous vein, that Persantine and aspirin help keep the grafts open, that not smoking (smoking is the *number-one* cardiac risk factor), restricting dietary fats, exercising moderately and sensibly, modifying AIAI—anger, irritation, aggravation, and impatience, the components of the hostile, competitive Type-A personality—all help protect the heart's muscles, valves, and pipes. In the fifteenth century, Leonardo da Vinci, artist, sculptor, engineer, inventor, and anatomist, called the heart "an admirable instrument." The great Leonardo was, as usual, right. Pumping four quarts of blood a minute, 1,400 gallons, or eleven tons, of fresh blood a day, beating an average of seventy beats a minute, more than 100,000 beats a day, 37 million beats a year, this pump, no bigger than a fist, needs all the help it can get from its owner. And every owner has a vested interest in helping his heart: heart disease kills more Americans than any other ailment.

What causes coronary artery disease? Atherosclerosis, commonly known as coronary artery disease, is a particular kind of hardening of the arteries in which the arterial channels gradually become blocked with fatty deposits. Atherosclerosis is a disease *process*, caused by many factors. To repeat: Bypass does *not* stop this process. It does not remove existing obstructions. Creating new byways, Bypass goes around blockages so that life-nourishing blood again can flow. To keep the old circulation open and the new grafts from closing, the owner of a newly Bypassed heart has his work cut out for him. He must *not* look upon Bypass as a cure; he must see CABS as a new chance for a new and better way of life, an atherosclerosis-retarding life.

In Point of Departure, we talked about risk factors: maleness, age, family history, smoking, elevated blood pressure, obesity, elevated cholesterol and triglycerides, sedentary way of life, and chronically hostile Type-A behavior. Obviously, you can't change your sex, your age, your relatives. For the rest, you can alter or postpone the evil decree. If you smoke, *stop!* Smoking is three times more likely to kill you with a heart attack than with lung cancer. If you give up smoking, your 50 to 200 percent greater chance of a heart attack will diminish slowly until it's almost equal to non-smokers' chances of heart trouble. Of the one thousand individuals in this admittedly nonstatistical study, only fifty have ever not smoked! Female smokers are at as great a risk as male smokers, more so if they use oral contraceptives. Cigars, pipes, and low-tar cigarettes are just ways to kid yourself.

As for hypertension (high blood pressure), the NHLBI says 10 to

15 percent of all Americans have hypertension and need medication. Millions more have borderline high blood pressure. Yet only five million are on regular medication and have their hypertension under control. Like heart trouble, high blood pressure is not an old people's disease. Everyone, even children, should have a blood-pressure check yearly. Current blood-pressure treatment utilizes stepped care. Step one is simple: avoid table and cooking salt and foods high in sodium content; if necessary, take diuretics, which hasten salt loss through urinary excretion. If your blood pressure doesn't respond, further steps add incrementally stronger medications, alone or in combination. High blood pressure, known as the silent killer, is easy to ignore. Blood-pressure pills are easy to forget. If your antihypertensive pills trouble you with their side effects (headaches, weakness, fatigue, inability to concentrate, upset stomach, thirst, rash, muscle cramps, aching joints, nervousness, depression, decreased libido, impotence), don't suffer in silence. Tell your doctor. Ask him to try other antihypertensive drugs which may be easier for you to tolerate. You may have to try several medications or combinations to arrive at the least side-effective, most blood-pressure-effective, therapy for you.

The American diet is a major coronary risk factor. Every day, many of us commit slow suicide with a knife and fork. For its cholesterol cover story "And Now the Bad News . . . ," *Time* magazine's cover showed a platter of bacon and eggs, the egg-eyes weeping, the bacon-mouth curling dolefully downwards. Ironically, the story was preceded by a report on Wendy's successful ad, "Where's the beef?" its high-cholesterol fast food, and by an ad for Bright cigarettes, even more lethal to the heart than the standard American diet.

Since 1961, the American Heart Association has been crying in the wilderness to get Americans to change their eating habits. The U.S. Senate's Select Committee on Nutrition and Human Needs established national dietary goals: (1) reducing dietary fat intake from 42 percent to 30 percent; (2) reducing saturated fats from 16 percent to 10 percent; and (3) reducing daily cholesterol intake from six hundred milligrams to three hundred milligrams. Just as the American tobacco industry fights smoking-can-kill-you statistics, so, too, does the American dairy industry fight these indictments of saturated fatty foods. The operative word is "saturated." There are two types of fat, saturated and unsaturated, bad and good. Foods of animal origin, fat on red meat, bacon, lard, butter, cheese, cream, ice cream, all have saturated fats. With the exception of cream, most saturated fat solidifies at refrigerator temperature. Unsaturated fats, such as corn, sunflower, safflower, cottonseed, peanut, and soybean oils, may act to lower cholesterol levels. Unsaturated fat is healthy. Saturated fat is unhealthy. Unfortunately, the American diet is loaded with saturated fats, from bacon and eggs and buttered toast for breakfast, to a hamburger, french fries, and ice cream for lunch, to a big steak, lamb, or pork-chop dinner with a baked potato smothered in sour cream, a salad soaked with blue-cheese dressing, and topped off with pie à la mode. Sounds good, doesn't it? But it's a plaque-building heart-destroyer.

Fast foods, be they hamburgers, pizza, fried chicken, luncheon meats, hot dogs or sausage, deliver cholesterol faster. Dairy products such as milk, butter, cheese, and margarine are solid saturated fats. Dessert orgies, offering fare such as ice cream, pies, cookies, doughnuts, and cakes, are loaded with saturated fats, as are convenience foods and so-called gourmet meals of shellfish drenched in rich French sauces. Cholesterol lurks among such ethnic delights as ravioli or matzoh balls. To live longer, we must learn to eat better, for recent studies show that some atherosclerosis is reversible.

None of this is new. The famous Framingham Study, begun in 1948 by the Public Health Service, studied five thousand adults and concluded that the blood cholesterol level is a major factor in determining heart-attack risk. Nor is diet something to be watched just by old folks. Autopsies performed on American and Asiatic soldiers revealed startling differences: twenty-two-year-old American servicemen showed consistent evidence of coronary artery blockages, significant thickening of their arterial walls. Their Asiatic counterparts had relatively clean arteries. Why? Americans eat a high-fat diet; Asiatics eat a low-fat diet rich in saltwater fish, now shown to reduce the risk of heart attack.

Now a Federally-sponsored ten-year study has shown conclusively that lower blood-cholesterol levels lessen the chances of heart attacks. This NGLBI-funded study of 3,800 men from thirty-five to fifty-nine with cholesterols above 265 milligrams percent demonstrated that every 1 percent lowering of cholesterol produced a 2 percent cut in coronary heart disease. The cholesterol researchers stated unequivocally that these findings should be applied to younger men and women with moderately elevated cholesterols. Dr. Basil Rifkind, director of the research project, stated that at least 100,000 of the annual heart-attack deaths could be saved by an anticholesterol regimen. Many researchers believe such findings should influence the diets of children, who may need calcium-rich milk but don't need whole milk or ice cream. They also need to be pushed to exercise vigorously. "Eat, drink, and be merry, for tomorrow we may die" may be a *carpe diem* rallying cry, but eating the "ordinary" American diet, so rich in saturated fats, could be a self-fulfilling prophecy. Because coronary artery disease runs in families, people with bad family histories sometimes shrug off heart-protecting measures as useless. These findings demonstrate that nurture can defeat nature, that heart care can vanquish a hereditary predisposition to heart disease.

A panel convened by the National Institutes of Health in December 1984, called for an all-out, aggressive national campaign to urge all of us who think we're eating well to start eating better. For the first time, elevated blood cholesterol was indicted as a *direct cause* of heart disease, not merely listed as a "risk factor." Dr. David Steinberg, chairman of the panel, said this study clearly indicated the cause-and-effect linkage between cholesterol and heart trouble.

What's an "elevated cholesterol level"? Above 180 milligrams percent for persons under thirty, above 200 milligrams percent for people over thirty. Average American cholesterol levels range between 220 and 260. *But "average" is dangerous*: half the American population dies of heart disease.

Physicians talk, and you should learn, about HDL and LDL, or high-density lipoproteins and low-density lipoproteins. The higher the HDL, the better. HDL helps the body excrete LDL, the fatty deposits lining arterial walls. HDL even prevents LDL clogging of the arteries. The HDL:LDL ratio is important. Exercise reduces LDL, elevates HDL. While two ounces of alcohol also cuts down the LDL, pushes up the HDL, more than two ounces is harmful.

Every day, physicians are learning how crucial are those lipoproteins. In a study of eighty-two Bypassers ten years after surgery, Montreal's Dr. Lucien Campeau and colleagues concluded that "atherosclerosis in these patients was a progressive disease, frequently affecting both the grafts and the native vessels, and that

*the course of such disease may be related to the plasma lipoprotein
levels"* (italics mine). Translated into language laymen use, these
findings mean that you should do everything you can to reduce
your LDL and elevate your HDL. It's as simple as that.

The Numbers Game (see p. 437) section and the cookbooks listed
in the Bibliography are good places to begin your self-instruction
in plasma lipoprotein levels. Ask your doctor for help in fighting
the cholesterol battle. But your doctor doesn't live with you. You
live with you. Learn what's bad for you, what foods to avoid. Keep
those American Heart Association lists posted in your car, your
kitchen, your office, and in your wallet. Look at them. Read labels
on products. Be an informed consumer. Get your favorite restaurant to serve low-fat meals.

All those diet books at the top of the best-seller lists suggest the
most pervasive of American myths: you can get thin and stay thin
without really trying. It's a lie. Being careful about what you eat
is a lifetime proposition. Habits, not dietary crashes, lose weight
and keep weight off. Such dietary habits *do* help prevent coronary
atherosclerosis and heart disease.[1]

Heartaches and stress are causally connected. More than 350
years ago, one of the fathers of modern medicine, Dr. William
Harvey, wrote: "Every affection of the mind that is attended with
either pain or pleasure, hope or fear, is the cause of an agitation
whose influence extends to the heart." Yet, as Dr. Thomas Graboys
notes in the *New England Journal of Medicine* (August 30, 1984), not
until Drs. Meyer Friedman and Ray Rosenman first described and
indicted Type-A behavior[2] as "coronary prone" in the late 1950s
did physicians address "systematic direct scientific inquiry" towards the "intimate association between neural factors and the
heart." Even so, a quarter-century later, physicians still back off
from implicating psychological or emotional stress as a risk factor.

In August 1984, Dr. Friedman published the results of an NHLBI-
funded study on modifying Type A, that AIAI pattern of anger,
irritation, aggravation, and impatience, of "free-floating" hostility,
time-urgency, joyless striving after pie in the sky. Friedman et al.
found that behavioral counseling to alter A-ness in coronary victims can halve the chances of a repeat myocardial infarction. Among

---

[1] See Your Heart Is What You Eat, p. 435.
[2] See the list of Type-A characteristics on p. 436.

594 behavioral-counselees, 44 percent reduced their A-ness, versus 25 percent in the control group. Further, of 328 heart-attack veterans going the full three-year route in Friedman's Recurrent Coronary Prevention Program, 79 percent cut down their A qualities, as opposed to 49 percent with only cardiological counseling. Most important, said Dr. Friedman, of the A counselees, "the risk of a new heart attack by the third year of the study was only 2.5 percent annually compared to 5 percent for the control group."

In this country, we believe the myth of Type A as characteristic of ambitious CEOs and venture capitalists. But myth it is. In England, Drs. Rose and Marmot found an *inverse* relation between coronary artery disease and social class. Dr. R. A. Karasek and colleagues noted significantly higher cardiac death rates among middle managers, "workers frustrated by the occupational paradox of considerable demands but little or no latitude in decision-making." Dr. Graboys calls it an "Orwellian recipe in which the estranged worker, besieged from above and below, mixes internal rage and incessant frustration into a fatal brew." Other factors hurting the heart are depression, chronic anxiety, role-uncertainty, lack of adaptability and personal resources, situational stress, and marital discord. Noting Dr. William Ruberman's data substantiating Dr. Harvey's and Dr. Friedman's contentions of "a causal role for biobehavioral stress in cardiac death," Dr. Graboys urges physicians to "explore the psychosocial causes of stress . . . impairing a patient's ability to resist the adversity of heart disease [which] may ultimately lead to a chronic and debilitating sense of despair and futility."

In the meantime, Bypass veterans and everybody else would do well to try Dr. Friedman's A-changing techniques. Smiling at others, laughing at yourself, surely will improve your life, which is good enough for starters. As for diet, Dr. Friedman says fatty meals are the "fuse exploding a Type-A bomb into a heart attack."

Thus, after Bypass and *before*, much of the responsibility for keeping your arteries open belongs to you, the artery-owner. Bypass can help your heart, and this book and these Bypassers can help you get through coronary artery bypass surgery. But not needing a heart operation or a repeat revascularization is best of all.

Your Heart Is What You Eat: Some Guidelines

1. Eat almost no red meat. If you indulge, eat lean cuts cooked without added fat. Eat poultry, without the skin, and fish, that lovely "brain" food. Eat no sausage meats or bacon, no hot dogs, salami, hot pastrami, or organ meats.
2. Use 1 percent fat or skim milk. Eat yogurt and cottage cheese made from skim milk.
3. Eat almost no ice cream. Substitute water ice or tofu-based frozen dessert, *not* ice milk or frozen yogurt, unless made from skim milk.
4. Eat very little hard cheese. Eat no cream cheese or creamy semisoft cheeses. Use low-fat cottage cheese, low-fat ricotta, low-fat mozzarella.
5. Eat no butter. Eat less margarine and oil. Use margarines with a high polyunsaturated:saturated-fat ratio, such as Fleischmann's, Mazola, Old Stone Mill, Promise (2:1), Hain (2.5:1), Diet Fleischmann's, Diet Mazola, Mrs. Filbert's Family Spread, Parkay Light Spread (2:1). Best of all is Weight-Watchers Reduced Calorie Margarine, with a 3:1 ratio.
6. Limit egg-yolk consumption to two to four yolks weekly, including yolks used in cooking and baking. One egg yolk equals the day's recommended cholesterol allotment.
7. Avoid processed foods made with saturated fats, especially with coconut and palm oils. Avoid nondairy "creams" made with coconut oil. Eat more dietary fiber, especially beans.
8. Don't eat fatty salad dressings, sauces, gravies or shellfish.
9. Eat saltwater fish twice weekly.

Type-A Characteristics

- setting impossible goals and being AIAI—angry, impatient, aggravated, irritated—when falling short of the mark
- possessed by belief in the formula that *self-esteem* $= \dfrac{Achievement}{Expectations}$
- almost always competing with self and others, believing you should have achieved more
- blaming people closest to you, constantly feeling thwarted
- constantly warring with self, with others, with time
- thinking or doing two things at once
- walking fast, eating fast, leaving the table right after eating
- moving fast, often bumping into or tripping on objects
- compulsive about own punctuality; irritated if kept waiting
- sitting on the edge of chair as if braced to go into orbit
- frequent knee-jiggling, finger-tapping, thumb-twiddling, lip-clicking, head-nodding
- talking incessantly or not responding at all except in outbursts; staccato speech pattern
- hurrying others' speech, interrupting them
- not listening to others
- gesticulating vehemently while talking, particularly clenching and pounding fists
- speaking in absolutes: "Always!" "Never!"
- substituting numbers for ideas, measuring success in numbers
- mistrusting ideas, words, people's motives
- playing almost every game to win, even with children
- sighing deeply when speaking of past or present difficulties
- reactivating rage when describing anger-producing past events
- frequent grimacing, rare smiling, uneasy hostile laughing
- frequent inappropriate use of obscenity
- believing that if you want something done, you must do it yourself
- becoming unduly aggravated if forced to wait in line or drive behind a slow-moving vehicle
- periorbial pigmentation (dark shadowing around the eyes)

The Numbers Game

There's nothing like a Bypass to inspire an instant crash course in lay cardiology. While "patients oughtn't to practice medicine without a license," as one young resident insisted, the educated Bypasser helps himself more than does the ignorant one. Many Bypass veterans have asked about the normal ranges of cholesterols and triglycerides. The American Heart Association suggests cholesterol levels be held at 180 to 200 milligrams percent. Nathan Pritikin, not a physician but a passionate adversary against our fatty diet, argued, "People with cholesterol levels of 260 mgm. or more have a 500% greater chance of dying from heart disease." For people interested in Pritikin, but without the $7,500 for a four-week session at his Longevity Center, Pritikin has published a worthwhile diet book. The problem with Pritikin, with Joe Piscatella's recipe book, with the American Heart Association recipe book, is motivation.

Like birth-control pills, cholesterol control doesn't work unless you use it. Some physicians maintain that sodium is more lethal than cholesterol: "Eat your ice cream, but throw away the salt shaker," they'll say, licking the carton of chocolate Häagen-Dazs. With cholesterol and sodium, it's not either-or. "If it weren't for our fatty diet," Meyer Friedman believes, "Type A wouldn't be so harmful." Friedman states unequivocally: "Although some epidemiologists and physicians consider a serum cholesterol elevated only if it exceeds 270 mg/100 ml, it seems far more likely that any serum cholesterol level consistently above 200 may be considered hypercholesterolemic." Ironically, it's not merely five-star French restaurants or the standard American diet of bacon and eggs for breakfast, hamburger, coke and ice cream for lunch, steak and french fries for dinner, that's hypercholesterolemic. Often, hospital food is salty and fatty. Unlike French restaurants and "he-man" American fare, hospital food doesn't even taste good.

Lowering your cholesterol today is easier than it was ten years ago. McDonald's and Burger King now have salad bars. The punchline "Where's the beef?" will have to be taken over by politicians and little old ladies with an inborn resistance to cholesterol. Besides diet, two easy ways to raise your HDL, that much-needed protection, are exercise and two ounces of alcohol daily. Exercise must be checked out with your doctor. More than two ounces of alcohol upsets the delicate HDL/LDL balance. One cardiologist suggests jogging two miles every day to the liquor store. It's worth a try. The operative words are, of course, "every day."

The famous Framingham Heart Study, now thirty-five years old, has found the ratio of total cholesterol to HDL cholesterol to be the single best indicator of future heart attack. To learn your ratio, divide your cholesterol level by your HDL level, or divide the amount of bad fat by the amount of good fat. Half the average risk of heart disease would be less than 3.4, as opposed to the average risk of heart disease in Americans, which is 4.4 for men, 5.0 for women. The average heart attack victim's ratio is from 4.5 to 6.4 in women, from 5.4 to 6.1 in men. Twice the average risk is 7.1 for women, 9.6 for men. Triple the risk would be 11.0 for women and 23.4 for men. These values are weighted cardiologically rather than arithmetically. Triglycerides, another kind of blood fat, also influence coronary risk, particularly in women. Blood triglycerides can be lowered by weight loss and by a diet low in fats and high in fiber.

IV

Envoi:
Looking
Back,
Looking
Ahead

Now that you have shared a part of the lives of these cardiac-surgery pilgrims, you will have discovered that their human voices not only speak to us, but also are our own voices, in the strictest sense the voices of America. Vicarious experience is no substitute for living. However vicarious, the experience embodied in these human beings' travail and triumph teaches us how to change the shape of our lives, to keep ourselves from needing heart surgery, but in the event of need, how to cope with it and its aftermath. Thus, do not ask to whom and for whom this book speaks: it speaks for you, for me, and for our mutual friends—to all of us.

Prospective Bypassers for whom the details of these intimate experiences are illuminating can take this light with them wherever they go. So, too, can their families and friends. All should be more able to meet the crises of cardiac surgery intelligently and successfully, more able by far to seek out the information their doctors might have given them if the doctors only had taken the time, if the patients, so deafened by the noises in their heads and the fears in their hearts, only could hear and remember.

Why does it matter so for patients to know? Because, as ever, knowledge is power. First, knowledge helps to determine what advice to follow in making individual decisions. And second, having opted for surgery, Bypassers suffering from excessive anxieties have a six-fold higher mortality rate than do heart patients with "normal" pre- and postoperative anxiety. What you don't know *will* hurt you. Reading this book, learning about what other people did to come through, should help Bypassers and their family conquer their fears.

Bypass is controversial both medically and economically. Dr. Thomas Preston, long a foe of heart surgery, claims it's "scandalously overused." The National Institute of Health study under Dr. Eugene Passamani argues that 12 to 15 percent of Bypasses might be unnecessary or postponed until some later date. Yet the NIH study itself contained a 23 percent "crossover" of medically managed patients eventually requiring Bypass because of intractable heart problems. Of the Bypassers in these pages and outside their covers, nobody knows, obviously, how long or how well they would have lived had they not had surgery. Most of the Bypassers here have done remarkably well, perhaps better than the national average. All the Bypassers in the book are alive, most feel well, although their successes had nothing to do with their selection for this volume. Since Bypass, Dr. Ben Rand has had a heart transplant. While seeking a new heart, Dr. Rand reported, "My Bypass grafts were all that kept me alive." Sister Cecilia has had angioplasty for a closed Bypass vessel: "The nuns say, 'Why couldn't they have operated on your mouth as well?' " Carole Cosby flew for the first time, went to Europe, has gone for biofeedback, and is feeling "miraculously better." Of the one thousand Bypassers either interviewed on tape or written to, the longest record for the original Bypass is fifteen years. Three of the one thousand Bypassers have died, one leaving his Bypassed brother with an identical angiogram.

The difference between completed questionnaires and interviews was extraordinary, between what's on paper and what's said face-to-face, between handwriting and the human voice, between people's public and private faces. Most Bypassers spoke not just about their operations with amazing candor, but about their lives. Their revelations were a slow, incremental unfolding of personality. In our talks, medical matters served as the key to larger psychological and philosophical issues. Reflecting on their lives, the roads taken and not taken, they were acutely conscious and self-conscious of details. Their aim, above all, was, as Joseph Conrad said, to make us *see*. And in seeing, to make us feel, understand.

One Bypasser even called his wife at the funeral home where she was making arrangements for her mother's funeral to ascertain the surgeon's name. In fact, many people had forgotten their surgeon's name. And if they complained that a physician was hurried, uninformative, unsympathetic, inattentive, overcharging, unwilling to discuss sexual or rehabilitative questions, uninterested in a drug's or the operation's side effects on mood, libido, erectility, they would then be gingerly about telling the doctor's name or hospital. While some Bypassers were offended by their physicians' manner and manners, others thought their physicians had done well by them, the best they could, had been considerate and kind.

Women particularly remarked that physicians were unsympathetic, puritanical, censorious, and passed off legitimate symptoms as nothing. Three women whose interviews are not printed here bitterly recalled being restrained by straitjackets after Bypass. Carole Cosby speaks for many women Bypassers when she protests against the CCU's male orientation, when she objects to the violation of her privacy. While much has been written about support systems for men Bypassers after they come home from the hospital, almost nothing is said about the problems facing women Bypassers, particularly those like Moira Kitt and Carole Cosby, who lived alone. Even women who did not live alone felt abandoned during the first two weeks at home. Several women wished their husbands had taken a week or two off from work, yet were ashamed to ask them.

Physicians, Bypassers, and non-Bypassers alike repeated the myth that female heart disease and need for Bypass were the result of women's careers, of stress in the work place. As one man mistakenly but succinctly put it, "If women are going to go after men's jobs, then they have to be prepared to get men's diseases."

Yet most of the forty women interviewed did not have careers. If they had jobs, they were traditionally "female" jobs—secretaries, teachers, dental hygienists, bookkeepers, housewives. Conventional women, they found their stresses right at home. Demanding, impatient husbands, divorces, disappointments with children, the deaths of children, took grievous tolls. Few women Bypassers interviewed were educated past high school; remarkably few had job skills. Only one woman, a black teacher, had her doctorate; none had any disposable income, extra money to spend on themselves. Most were immaculate housekeepers. Most felt the house, the care and feeding of husband and children, were their responsibilities alone. One woman had baked six cakes and put them in the freezer before she went to the hospital: "That way, my husband could bring in a cake for everybody on each of the shifts." Several had cooked and frozen meals for their husbands before they went off to the hospital. Most felt guilty for being sick; many felt somehow defective for having "caught" a "male" disease.

Yet some men, like Dr. Jordan Bredely, felt strangely guilty, too. Outraged by their heart disease, young men in their twenties and thirties burned with resentment at what they erroneously thought of as "an old man's disease." For all the medical community's arguments pro and con about Type-A characteristics and modifying them, almost everyone at every age I surveyed fit Dr. Friedman's description of the flaming A-plus. Most of these men and women had smoked more than the national average: of one thousand Bypassers, *only fifty had never smoked at all.* Although they recognized smoking's role in bringing them to Bypass, although some blamed themselves for having imposed a family history of heart disease upon their children, few enjoined their children not to smoke.

Heredity is, of course, an important factor, particularly among young people with heart trouble. But there's so much we don't know. We don't know whom cardiac genes will choose, whom they will exempt. Like his uncle Stowe, Stowe Phillips has familial hypercholesterolemia, yet his mother and father are healthy. Of the physicians, Jason Master, Ben Rand, and Abraham Stearin have heart disease, as did their parents, but their siblings do not. In many instances, heart trouble struck these people at a younger age than it did their parents, which surely is a commentary on the way we live now. Stresses, our response to stresses at home and at work, smoking, and diet seem to tip the scales against the newer generation.

How careful heart-surgery veterans are about fatty meals depends, for the most part, upon the strictness of their doctors. Hence, the importance of self-education in eliminating or reducing risk factors. As the five doctors' accounts here make clear, doctors are as subject to the weaknesses of flesh and spirit as the rest of us.

The twenty-five physician-Bypassers interviewed for this book present more than the medical profession's statistical share of Bypass. More knowledgeable than lay people, at the same time they share and express the average Bypasser's helplessness in the hands of medical personnel.

George Bernard Shaw said, "Money is the root of all good." Money not only governs many surgeons' attitudes toward their patients and their craft; it influences patients' views of their Bypasses. Total costs for surgeon, anesthesiologist, cardiologist, internist, and hospital ranged from $13,000 to $46,000. Even the most satisfied CABS veterans' answers varied in response to the question "If you yourself had had to pay all the costs, would you have had your coronary artery bypass surgery?" Dr. Pierre Borget worries how younger people will finance older people's medical needs. Nathaniel White, another Bypasser whose history is omitted here, recalled what happened when his thirty-seven-year-old brother was advised to have Bypass: "He came home, told no one, got his affairs in order. Within a year, he was dead. Who's to say if he was right or wrong? Increasingly we'll see people evaluating what their lives are worth in dollars and cents to themselves and to their families. I can't blame him, even though I miss him. If I hadn't had insurance, who knows what I'd have done?"

In the best of all possible worlds, none of us would need Bypass surgery. If we did, not only could we afford to pay for it, but we would live healthier lives to prevent coronary artery disease. We would eat less and eat fewer saturated fats; we would exercise regularly; we would not smoke; we'd be temperate in our use of alcohol and drugs. We would avoid stress and reduce the flames of our fiery responses; our culture would try to minimize the tensions to which we are so vulnerable. We'd learn to deal with anxiety, anger, depression, haste, and obsessive perfectionism; we would not feel chained to the hands of the clock, not be propelled by external forces and impelled by internal forces beyond our control. We would not be fighting with ourselves and others for a control always just beyond our grasp. None of us, in short, would be sick at heart.

Someday, too, new medical means might help us keep well. Lasers, streptokinase, and angioplasty might dissolve or crush our clots and plaque; genetic manipulation might alter our hereditary weaknesses; new forms of psychotherapy might make us better able to deal with thwarting, impatience, and despair, might help us change our hearts without the aid of a surgeon's knife.

In the future, perhaps such healthier ways of life, new technology, new medications, and a more nourishing society will render coronary artery bypass surgery and books like this obsolete. In the meantime, however, we must use what we have. Coronary artery bypass surgery offers many patients stricken with heart disease a second chance, new hope, new vigor, and probably added years. To them, this book speaks; and the courage and persistence of the people here embodied should serve as a beacon to us all.

Glossary of Medical Terms

Ambulate: To walk.

Anastomosis: The union, or connection, of branches, as of rivers or blood vessels. The surgical connection of separate or severed hollow organs or vessels to form a continuous channel. Also called grafting.

Aneurysm: A bulging or ballooning out of a blood vessel wall or a part of the heart muscle.

Angina pectoris: A temporary discomfort, pain, or tightness in the chest, throat, arm, shoulder, back, neck, or jaw, the symptom of insufficient blood supply to the heart muscle.

Angiogram: An x-ray study of a blood vessel showing the course of a radiopaque substance injected into the bloodstream. A cardiac angiogram reveals the extent and location of blockages in the coronary arteries. Also called arteriogram.

Angiography: A method of visualizing the coronary arteries and pinpointing the locations and extent of blockages. Dye is injected into the coronary arteries through a catheter; its path is traced to indicate location, extent, and pattern of any blockages. Also called angiocardiography.

Angioplasty: Percutaneous transluminal coronary angioplasty (PTCA). A method of compressing blockages against the vessel walls by inserting and inflating a tiny balloon into the narrowed blood vessel, thereby widening a path for increased blood flow.

Anticoagulant: A drug to delay blood clotting, such as heparin or Coumadin, which tends to prevent new clots from forming or existing clots from enlarging, but does not dissolve existing clots.

Aorta: The main artery leading from the heart and carrying oxygen-rich blood from the heart to all body organs.

Arrhythmia: An alteration in the rate and/or regularity of the heartbeat.

Arteriogram: See *Angiogram*.

Artery: A blood vessel transporting oxygen-rich blood away from the heart to the body's organs. The exception is the *pulmonary artery*.

Aspirate: To remove liquids or gases from a space by suction.

Atelectasis: An inability of the lungs to expand fully.

Atheroma: A deposit of fatty (and other) substances in the inner lining of the artery wall, characteristic of atherosclerosis.

Atherosclerosis: The build-up of fatty substances, calcium, and fibrous tissues on the inner walls of an artery, causing a narrowing of the blood vessel and reduction in available blood supply. The arterial walls become thick, hardened, and inelastic, like an old rubber band. Sometimes referred to as hardening of the arteries or arteriosclerosis.

Atrium: One of the two upper chambers of the heart. The right atrium receives unoxygenated blood from the body. The left atrium receives oxygenated blood from the lungs. Adult capacity is about 57 cc. Also called auricle, although this term is now generally used to describe only the tip of the atrium.

Auricle: See *Atrium*.

Autoimmune response: Production by the body of antibodies against constituents of its own tissues, which can result in a number of serious illnesses.

Beta blocker: Certain drugs blocking beta receptor sites found on the body's cells; these sites are sensitive to adrenalin, which speeds up the heartbeat. Sometimes called adrenergic blocking agents.

Blood pressure: The force of blood against the walls of the arteries. Systolic blood pressure is the pressure against the wall of an artery at the time the heart contracts. Diastolic blood pressure is the pressure against the wall of the arteries between contractions, when the heart is relaxed. Readings are shown as follows:

$$\frac{\text{Systolic}}{\text{Diastolic}} = \frac{120}{80}$$

Bradycardia: Abnormally slow heart rate.

Bypass graft: A new pathway created during heart surgery to allow blood to flow around a narrowed section in a coronary artery.

CABS: Coronary Artery Bypass Surgery.

CCU: Abbreviation for Coronary Care Unit.

Calcium antagonist: Any of a new category of drugs that block the uptake of calcium by the myocardial cells, dilate the coronary arteries, and may relieve the symptoms of angina pectoris.

Cardiac: Pertaining to the heart. Sometimes used to refer to a person who has heart disease.

Cardiac arrest: The cessation of cardiac output and effective circulation when the heart stops beating.

Cardiac catheterization: Examination of the heart by introducing a catheter into a vein or artery and passing it through the heart. See *Angiography*.

Cardiac cripple: An old-fashioned phrase used to denote someone whose activities have been severely diminished by heart disease.

Cardiac imaging: Any one of a variety of new computerized techniques to visualize the heart and its coronary arteries without using invasive methods such as cardiac catheterization (angiography).

Cardiac output: The amount of blood pumped by the heart per minute.

Cardiac rehab: Any rehabilitation program for people who have had a heart attack or Bypass surgery. Some programs stress diet and exercise. Others, such as Dr. Meyer Friedman's San Francisco prototype, also work on Type-A behavior modification. Frequently, participants learn as much from one another as from their instructors.

Cardiopulmonary resuscitation: A combination of chest compression and mouth-to-mouth breathing used to keep oxygenated blood flowing to the brain until advanced cardiac life support can be initiated in a person whose heart is beating ineffectively or has arrested. Usually referred to by the abbreviation CPR.

Cardiovascular: Pertaining to the heart and blood vessels.

Cathecholamine: The term for both norepinephrine and epinephrine, produced by the adrenal glands. Norepinephrine increases the heartbeat rate and constricts muscle cells in the blood vessel walls. Epinephrine causes blood vessels in the skeletal muscles to relax, which in turn increases the flow of blood to the muscles during exercise.

Catheter: In cardiology, a thin plastic flexible tube which can be guided through blood vessels into the heart to take measurements, ascertain blockage, inject x-ray dye or drugs. The catheter is usually inserted into a vein or artery in the arm or leg. A physician, monitoring its progress on a screen, gently threads it into the heart. During catheterization, the patient also can watch the catheter's movement on the fluoroscopy screen. Catheters can be used for other purposes in relation to other organs of the body.

Cerebrovascular accident: An impeded blood supply to some part of the brain. Also called cerebral vascular accident, apoplexy, or stroke.

Chelation therapy: A technique approved in the United States to treat heavy metal poisoning. Some practitioners say it can be used to treat coronary artery disease.

Cholesterol: A fatty substance, produced by the body; its levels can be increased by intake of cholesterol-containing foods. Most experts believe there is a causal relationship between cholesterol levels and coronary artery disease.

Chronic stable angina: Angina pain persisting for six months or more, unchanged in intensity and controlled by medication.

Claudication: Pain in the legs after walking certain distances, caused by defective blood circulation.

Coagulation: The change from a liquid to a thickened or solid state.

Collateral circulation: Circulation of blood through nearby smaller blood vessels when a main blood vessel is blocked. The heart's own lifesaving method.

Congestive heart failure: A backing up of blood in the veins leading to the heart, often accompanied by accumulation of fluid in various parts of the body. It results from the heart's inability to pump all the blood returning to it.

Coronary artery: Either of two arteries arising from the aorta, arching down over the top of the heart, and conducting blood to the heart muscle.

Coronary Artery Bypass Surgery, or Coronary Artery Bypass Graft: Surgery to improve the blood supply to the heart muscle when narrowed or blocked coronary arteries reduce the flow of oxygen-containing blood, vital to the heart's pumping. During Bypass, one or more narrowed or blocked segments of coronary artery are tied off; nondiseased vessels taken from elsewhere in the body, usually the saphenous leg veins and/or the internal mammary artery, are grafted above and below the blockage to ensure that the heart muscle is supplied with its necessary blood and nutrients.

Coronary occlusion: An obstruction or narrowing of one of the coronary arteries that shuts off blood flow to some part of the heart muscle, which then dies because of lack of oxygen.

Coronary thrombosis: Formation of a clot in one of the arteries conducting blood to the heart muscle. A form of coronary occlusion.

Crepitation: A creaking or rattling sound.

Crescendo angina: A condition characterized by persistent pain unrelieved by medication, lasting more than half an hour, and usually accompanied by electrocardiographic changes revealing a diminished blood supply to the heart muscle. Sometimes called preinfarction angina.

Cupping: Vigorous pats on the back to encourage lung-cleansing coughing. An old-fashioned phrase for what is sometimes described as a pulmonary toilet.

Cyanosis: Blueness of skin caused by insufficient oxygen in the blood.

Defibrillator: An electronic device that stops an incoordinate contraction of the heart muscle fibers and may help to reestablish normal rhythm.

Digitalis: A tried-and-true drug made from foxglove leaves. Discovered by William Witherspoon in the eighteenth century, digitalis strengthens the contraction of the heart muscle, slows the rate of contraction of the heart, and promotes the elimination of fluid from body tissues.

Distal runoff: The area of the coronary artery beyond an obstruction.

Diuretic: A substance, such as thiazines, diazines, xanthines, and mercurials, that promotes the excretion of urine.

Dressler's syndrome: See *Postcardiotomy syndrome.*

Dyspnea: Difficult or labored breathing.

Echocardiogram: A method of diagnosing certain heart problems (for instance, valve disease). Ultrasound is transmitted into the body, and the echoes returning from the surface of the heart are electronically plotted and recorded.

Edema: Swelling due to abnormally large amounts of fluid in the body tissues.

Ejection fraction: A measurement of the pumping capacity of the heart muscle that can be obtained through a ventriculogram or during catheterization. Expelling 50 to 70 percent of the left ventricle's contents with each beat is normal.

Electrocardiogram: Called ECG or EKG, it is a graphic record of electric impulses produced by the heart as it contracts and relaxes.

Embolus: A blood clot that forms in a blood vessel in one part of the body and travels to another part to obstruct circulation.

End diastolic pressure: Measurement of the pressure at the end of the diastolic phase of heart pumping, when the heart is most relaxed. Taken during catheterization, it is another means of determining the heart muscle's vigor.

Endocarditis: Inflammation of the heart's lining and valves.

Endotracheal tube: A breathing tube.

Enzymes: Tests for myocardial damage. Blood enzyme levels are usually elevated after a myocardial infarction. See also *Streptokinase* and *Thrombolysis.*

Familial hypercholesterolemia: High levels of blood cholesterol that run in families.

Fibrillation: Uncoordinated contractions of the heart muscle occurring when individual muscle fibers take up independent irregular contractions.

HDL: High-density lipoprotein, which removes blood cholesterol and lowers the atherosclerotic risk. The higher the HDL, the better.

Heart attack: A nonspecific term usually referring to a myocardial infarction.

Heart block: Interference, either partial or complete, with the conduction of the heart's electrical impulses.

Heart-lung machine: A machine used during heart surgery to supply oxygen and blood to the body as a substitute for the work of the heart and lungs. Also called the Bypass machine.

Hemorrhage: Loss of blood from a blood vessel. In external hemorrhage, blood escapes from the body. In internal hemorrhage, blood passes into tissues surrounding the ruptured blood vessel.

Hypercholesterolemia: Excess cholesterol and animal-fat substances—above 200 milligrams percent—in the blood. Sometimes called hypercholesteremia.

Hypertension: A persistent elevation of blood pressure above the normal range, commonly called high blood pressure.

Hypotension: Blood pressure below the normal range, commonly called low blood pressure.

Hypothermia: In heart surgery, a means to induce lower body temperature and slow metabolism by cooling the blood going from the heart-lung machine to the patient. Cooled body tissues require less oxygen and are less likely to be injured by diminished oxygen supply.

Hypoxia: Less-than-normal content of oxygen in the organs and tissues of the body.

ICU: The abbreviation for Intensive Care Unit.

Infarct: Injury to or death of tissue resulting from inadequate blood supply. Myocardial infarct refers to impairment or death of an area of heart muscle because of insufficient blood flow through its sources of supply, the coronary arteries.

Infarction: The formation of an infarct.

Intra-aortic balloon pump: A temporary device to help a weakened heart pump fresh blood: a balloon inflates at the tip of a catheter snaked up into the aorta from its point of insertion in a leg artery. It helps reduce the load on the heart, enabling it to work less.

Intravenous: Going into or by way of the veins, as in intravenous feeding or intravenous solutions. Often abbreviated as I.V.

Ischemia: A local deficiency of oxygen (usually brief), usually caused by an obstruction in or constriction of one or more blood vessels.

Keloid: A thick scar resulting from excessive growth of fibrous tissue.

Labile hypertension: Blood pressure that varies frequently, often because of excessive response to stress.

LDL: Low-density lipoprotein, which carries blood cholesterol, increases plaque, and increases atherosclerotic risk. The lower the LDL, the better. The HDL:LDL ratio is an important marker.

Left ventricular hypertrophy: Thickening of the left ventricle muscle because of an increased pressure load, possibly caused by high blood pressure.

Lipid: Any fat or fatty substance.

Lipoprotein: A combination of fat (lipid) and protein molecules bound together.

Mammary artery: One of two blood vessels located in the upper chest wall. These are sometimes used for Bypass grafts. Also called internal mammary.

Mediastinum: The center of the chest behind the breastbone and between the lungs. The heart's home.

Mended Hearts: A national volunteer organization of veterans of heart surgery who visit and support one another before and after the operation. Other such groups are Bridgeport's Heart Beats Club and the various Zipper clubs around the country.

Myocardial infarction: Damage to or death of a part of the heart muscle due to lack of oxygen. Also called heart attack, coronary occlusion, or coronary thrombosis.

Myocardial revascularization: Heart surgery that creates new pathways for blood to flow to the heart muscle. Also called Bypass surgery.

Myocardium: Heart muscle.

N-G tube: Nasogastric tube.

Nitrate: Any of a group of chemical compounds that dilate small vessels.

Nitroglycerin: A nitrate that relaxes the muscles of the blood vessels. One of the vasodilators, it is often used to relieve attacks of angina pectoris and spasm of the coronary arteries.

Normotensive: Characterized by normal blood pressure.

Nuclear ventriculogram: A diagnostic procedure that reveals the wall motion of the heart's left ventricle and tells the patient's ejection fraction.

Pacemaker: The heart has an inborn, "natural" pacemaker called the SA, or sinoatrial, node, located in the right upper chamber. "Pacemaker" refers to an artificial device that can provide small electrical signals to stimulate the heart rate and thus control the heart's beat by a series of rhythmic electrical discharges.

Palpitation: A fluttering sensation of the heart, due to alteration in the heart rate or rhythm, which is felt by the person.

Paroxysmal auricular fibrillation: See *Fibrillation, Palpitation.*

Percutaneous transluminal coronary angioplasty: PTCA. See *Angioplasty.*

Pericarditis: A painful inflammation of the membrane surrounding the heart.

Pericardium: A closed sac surrounding the heart and roots of the great vessels. The sac is formed by two walls.

Peripheral bruit: Arterial sound usually caused by plaque in a vessel.

Phlebitis: Inflammation of a vein, often in the leg. Sometimes a blood clot is formed in the inflamed vein.

Polyunsaturated fat: A fat, such as liquid vegetable oil, corn oil, or safflower oil, capable of absorbing additional hydrogen. A diet high in polyunsaturated fat tends to lower the amount of cholesterol in the blood.

Postcardiotomy syndrome: Fever or aching, usually within the first few weeks after Bypass. Sometimes it is first manifested as chest pain, which can be confused with angina. All chest pain should be promptly reported to your physician. Postcardiotomy syndrome and postpump syndrome, which also consists of fever, chills, achiness, headache, resemble each other. Both mandate the attention of your physician, who can usually prescribe medications for relief.

Prinzmetal's variant angina: A phenomenon whereby spasms temporarily constrict coronary arteries and cause pain.

Pulmonary artery: The large artery conveying unoxygenated (venous) blood from the lower right chamber of the heart to the lungs, it is the only artery in the body carrying unoxygenated blood—all others carry oxygenated blood to the body.

Pulmonary toilet: Regular forced coughing and breathing to clear lungs of secretions and to prevent pneumonia.

Pulse: The expansion and contraction of an artery with each heartbeat, which may be felt over several parts of the body, such as the wrist and throat.

Radioisotopic scanning: A diagnostic technique involving labeling of tissues and organs by injecting radioisotopes into the bloodstream. The emitted radioactivity is detected by a scanner and a record of the scan is made. Such techniques include Multiple Gated Acquisition (MUGA), radioisotope ventriculogram, and thallium scan (also called myocardial imaging).

Rales: A crackling sound heard during stethoscopic examination of the chest that indicates fluid or secretions in the air sacs of the lungs.

Respirator: A breathing machine connected to the breathing tube in the patient's throat. Until the anesthesia wears off completely and the patient is able to breathe on his or her own, the patient usually remains on a respirator.

Resting electrocardiogram: A record of the electrical activity on the surface of the heart while the patient is resting.

Risk factor: A characteristic or habit that tends to increase the likelihood of heart disease and stroke: male sex, age, family history of heart disease, smoking, blood pressure, obesity, elevated cholesterols, Type-A behavior, glucose intolerance, all are risk factors.

Saphenous vein: Either of two large superficial veins of the foot, leg, and thigh, one on the inner side and the other on the outer and posterior side.

Saturated fat: Usually solid animal fat, occurring in milk, butter, meat, eggs. The American diet, high in saturated fats, tends to increase the amount of cholesterol in the blood.

Septum: The muscular wall dividing the two chambers on the left side of the heart from the two on the right.

Stable angina: Angina pain that has persisted for a long time—six months or more—unchanged in intensity and controlled by medication.

Stepped care: The term used to describe stages of therapy.

Sternum: A long, flat bone located in the middle of the chest. Also called the breastbone.

Streptokinase: An enzyme sometimes used to dissolve blood clots. See *Thrombolysis*.

Stress test: A record of the heart's electrical activity, pulse, and blood pressure while the patient exercises on a bicycle or a treadmill. This tests how well the heart works at delivering oxygenated blood during physical exertion.

Tachycardia: Abnormally fast heart rate.

Thallium scan: A common form of radioisotopic scanning. Thallium has an affinity for heart muscle. If the injected thallium does not migrate to a certain area, that part of the heart muscle is assumed to be injured or dead.

Thallium stress test: A stress test performed after injection of thallium.

Thrombolysis: Use of streptokinase or a tissue plasminogen activator to dissolve blood clots of an acute myocardial infarction, effective only if performed within three hours of an MI. Also known as thrombolytic therapy.

Triglyceride: A fat in the blood indicated as a causal factor in coronary artery disease.

Type A: A behavior pattern, first identified as a coronary risk factor in 1958 by Friedman and Rosenman, characterized by free-floating hostility, time-urgency, and AIAI—anger, irritation, aggravation, impatience. Although some cardiologists disagree, Friedman's latest studies show behavior modification can cut coronary recurrence in half.

Unstable angina: Intense and prolonged angina while resting, with little or no response to medication; angina that has increased in frequency and intensity in the past three months; angina experienced within thirty days after a heart attack; new angina.

Vasodilator: A drug to relax the arterial walls, often used in treating high blood pressure and heart disease.

Vein: Any vessel that carries blood from various parts of the body back to the heart.

Ventricle: One of the two lower chambers of the heart.

Ventricular gallop: A heart sound, often the first sign of congestive heart failure.

Pharmaceutical Addenda

The interviewees have mentioned several pharmaceutical agents, some by their trade names, others by their generic names. Inasmuch as they may have multiple medical indications and uses, only their chemical names and in some cases their general familial action (such as beta blocker or calcium channel antagonist) are defined below. Some major pharmaceutical agents in the medical management of heart disease are grouped by families (for instance, nitrates or beta blockers) and defined as such in the *Glossary*. That some pharmaceutical agents are listed here and others are not in no way comments on their efficacy. Only drugs specifically mentioned by Bypassers are here.

Adapin: Doxepin hydrochloride, an antidepressant, anti-anxietant. See *Sinaquan*.

Corgard: Nadalol, a nonspecific beta-adrenergic receptor blocking agent (commonly known as a beta blocker). See *Inderal*.

Desyrel: Trazodone hydrochloride, an antidepressant.

Digoxin: One of the digitalis family. See *Lanoxin*.

Hydrodiuril: Hydrochlorothiazide, a diuretic and antihypertensive, the number-one prescription drug in the United States, with 78 million prescriptions written annually.

Inderal: Propanol hydrochloride, the first beta-adrenergic receptor blocking agent (commonly known as a beta blocker) in the United States. Now one of many such drugs of this family. See *Corgard*.

Indocin: Indomethacin, a nonsteroidal, anti-inflammatory agent.

Isordil: Inosorbide dinitrate, a smooth-muscle relaxant used in treating angina pectoris.

Lanoxin: Trade name for digoxin.

Lasix: Furosemide, a potent diuretic.

Nifedipine: Generic name for *Procardia*, a calcium channel antagonist.

Nitrobid capsule: Controlled-release capsule of nitroglycerin. Sometimes prescribed as an ointment.

Nitro-Dur Transdermal Infusion System: A patch applied to the skin through which nitroglycerin is absorbed continuously into the systemic circulation.

Persantine: Dipyramidole, a coronary vasodilator, sometimes used with aspirin after Bypass to try to prevent graft closure.

Pronestyl: Procainamide hydrochloride, an anti-arrhythmic agent.

Quinidine: An anti-arrhythmic agent with many trade names.

Sinaquan: Doxepin hydrochloride. See *Adapin*.

Tagamet: Cimetidine hydrochloride. A histamine H^2 receptor antagonist, it inhibits gastric-acid secretion.

Tenormin: Atenolol, yet another beta-selective, adrenoreceptor blocking agent (commonly known as a beta blocker). See *Inderal*, *Corgard*, and *Timolide*.

Timolide: Timolol, another beta blocker.

Valium: Diazepam, an anti-anxietant and another of the most frequently prescribed drugs in the United States.

Bibliography

While the history of Bypass is a fascinating chapter in medical pioneering, only recent books which might interest the concerned reader have been included here. Particularly significant works are marked with an asterisk.

Books

*American Heart Association. *Heart Facts*. New York: E. P. Dutton, 1985.
*———. *Heartbook*. New York: E. P. Dutton, 1981.
*American Medical Association. *Guide to Heart Care*. New York: Random House, 1984.
*Benson, Herbert. *The Relaxation Response*. New York: William Morrow, 1975.
*Bierman, E. K. *Diet and Coronary Heart Disease*. Dallas: American Heart Association, 1978.
*Brecher, Edward. *Love, Sex and Aging*. Boston: Little, Brown, 1984.
 Carrera, Michael. *Sex: The Facts, the Acts and Your Feelings*. New York: Crown Publishers, 1981.
 Comfort, Alex. *The Joy of Sex*. New York: Crown Publishers, 1972.
*Cousins, Norman. *Anatomy of an Illness*. New York: W. W. Norton, 1980.

*———. *The Healing Heart: Antidotes to Panic and Helplessness*. New York: W. W. Norton, 1983.

*———. *Human Options*. New York: W. W. Norton, 1983.

DeBakey, M., and Gotto, A. *The Living Heart*. New York: Grosset and Dunlap, Charter Books, 1977.

Epstein, Joseph. *Ambition: The Secret Passion*. New York: E. P. Dutton, 1980.

Freeman, A. M. *Anxiety and Anxiety with Depressive Symptoms in the Patient with Cardiac Disorders*. Chicago: Pragmaton Publications, 1983.

*Friedman, Meyer, and Rosenman, Ray. *Type A Behavior and Your Heart*. New York: Alfred A. Knopf, 1974.

*Friedman, Meyer, and Ulmer, Diane. *Treating Type A Behavior and Your Heart*. New York: Alfred A. Knopf, 1984.

Hackett, T. P., and Cassem, N. H. *Coronary Care: Patient Psychology*. Dallas: American Heart Association, 1975.

*Halperin, Jonathan, and Levine, Richard. *Bypass*. New York: Times Books, 1985.

*Hochman, Gloria. *Heart Bypass*. New York: St. Martin's Press, 1982.

Kaplitt, Martin J., and Borman, Joseph. *Concepts and Controversies in Cardiovascular Surgery*. New York: Appleton-Century-Crofts, 1983.

Kra, Siegfried. *Coronary Bypass Surgery: Who Needs It?* New York: W. W. Norton, 1985.

Lear, Martha. *Heartsounds*. New York: Simon and Schuster, 1981.

Lesher, Steven, and Halberstam, Michael. *A Coronary Event*. New York: Popular Library, 1978.

*Lynch, J. J. *The Broken Heart: The Medical Consequences of Loneliness*. New York: Basic Books, 1979.

*McGill, Michael. *Keeping It All Inside: Why Men Can't Open Up to Those Who Love Them*. New York: Holt, Rinehart and Winston, 1984.

Melzak, Z. A. *Bypass: A Simple Approach to Complexity*. New York: John Wiley, 1983.

Nash, David. *Coronary! Prediction and Prevention*. New York: New American Library, 1980.

Nierenberg, Judith, and Janovic, F. *The Hospital Experience: A Complete Guide to Understanding and Participating in Your Own Care*. New York: Bobbs-Merrill, 1978.

Nolen, William. *Surgeon under the Knife*. New York: Coward, McCann, and Geoghegan, 1976.

Ochsner, J., and Mills, N. *Coronary Artery Surgery*. Philadelphia: Lea and Febiger, 1978.

Preston, Thomas. *Clay Pedestal*. New York: Raven Press, 1981.

———. *Coronary Artery Surgery: A Critical Review*. New York: Raven Press, 1977.

Prinzmetal, Myron, and Winter, William. *Heart Attack: New Hope, New Knowledge, New Life*. New York: Simon and Schuster, 1958. This book is out of print but is well worth hunting up in the library or in used-book shops.

Ramsey, Paul. *The Patient as Person*. New Haven: Yale University Press, 1970.

Reinfeld, Nyles V. *Open Heart Surgery: A Second Chance*. Englewood Cliffs, N.J.: Prentice-Hall, 1983.

*Scheingold, L. D., and Wagner, N. *Sound Sex and the Aging Heart*. New York: Human Sciences Press, 1974.

*Schover, Leslie. *Prime Time: Sexual Health for Men over Fifty*. New York: Holt, Rinehart and Winston, 1984.

Selzer, Richard. *Confessions of a Knife*. New York: Simon and Schuster, 1979.

———. *Mortal Lessons*. New York: Simon and Schuster, 1976.

Sontag, Susan. *Illness as Metaphor*. New York: Farrar, Straus and Giroux, 1978.

Thomas, Lewis. *Lives of a Cell*. New York: Bantam Books, 1974.

———. *The Youngest Science*. New York: Viking Press, 1983.

Troup, Stanley, and Greene, William, eds. *The Patient, Death, and the Family*. New York: Charles Scribner's Sons, 1974.

*Waxberg, Joseph. *Bypass*. New York: Appleton-Century-Crofts, 1981.

Wertenbaker, L. *To Mend the Heart*. New York: Viking Press, 1980.

*Yalof, Ina. *Open Heart Surgery*. New York: Random House, 1984.

Cookbooks

American Heart Association. *Cooking without Your Salt Shaker*. Dallas: American Heart Association, 1980.

Anderson, Jean. *Unforbidden Sweets*. New York: Arbor House, 1982.

Bagg, Elma W. *Cooking without a Grain of Salt*. New York: Bantam Books, 1981.

Brenner, Eleanor. *Gourmet Cooking without Salt*. Garden City, N.Y.: Doubleday, 1981.

Cavaiani, Mabel. *Low Cholesterol Cookbook*. Chicago: Contemporary Books, 1980.

———. *Low Cholesterol Cuisine*. Chicago: Contemporary Books, 1981.

Claiborne, Craig. *Craig Claiborne's Gourmet Diet*. New York: Times Books, 1980.

Darak, Arthur. *Great Eating, Great Dieting Cookbook*. New York: Thomas Y. Crowell, 1978.

Eselman, Ruth, and Winston, Mary. *American Heart Association Cookbook*. New York: Ballantine Books, 1980.

Field, Florence. *Gourmet Cooking for Cardiac Diets*. New York: Crowell-Collier, 1962.

Goodman, Harriet W., and Morse, Barbara. *Just What the Doctor Ordered*. New York: Holt, Rinehart and Winston, 1982.

Jones, Suzanne. *Low Cholesterol Food Processor Cookbook*. Garden City, N.Y.: Doubleday, 1980.

Leviton, Roberta. *Jewish Low Cholesterol Cookbook.* Middlebury, Vt.: Eriksson, 1978.

Ornish, Dean. *Stress, Diet and Your Heart.* New York: Holt, Rinehart and Winston, 1982.

Piscatella, Joseph. *Don't Eat Your Heart Out.* New York: Workman, 1984.

Pritikin, Nathan. *The Pritikin Permanent Weight-Loss Manual.* New York: Grosset and Dunlap, 1981.

Pritikin, Nathan, and Pritikin, Ilene. *The Official Pritikin Guide to Restaurant Eating.* New York: Berkeley Books, 1984.

Roth, June. *Salt Free Cooking with Herbs and Spices.* Chicago: Contemporary Books, 1975.

Stern, Ellen, and Michaels, Jonathan. *The Good Heart Diet Cookbook.* New Haven: Ticknor and Fields, 1982.

Walsh, Jean. *Low Cholesterol Cookbook.* Secaucus, N.J.: Chartwell, 1977.

Whittlesey, Marietta. *Killer Salt.* New York: Avon Books, 1977.